METHODS IN MOLECULAR BIOLOGY

Series Editor
John M. Walker
School of Life and Medical Sciences
University of Hertfordshire
Hatfield, Hertfordshire, AL10 9AB, UK

For further volumes:
http://www.springer.com/series/7651

Light Microscopy

Methods and Protocols

Edited by

Yolanda Markaki

UCLA School of Medicine, Department of Biological Chemistry, Los Angeles, CA, USA

Hartmann Harz

Biozentrum der LMU Munchen, Planegg-Martinsried, Germany

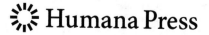 Humana Press

Editors
Yolanda Markaki
UCLA School of Medicine
Department of Biological Chemistry
Los Angeles, CA, USA

Hartmann Harz
Biozentrum der LMU Munchen
Planegg-Martinsried, Germany

ISSN 1064-3745   ISSN 1940-6029   (electronic)
Methods in Molecular Biology
ISBN 978-1-4939-8305-6   ISBN 978-1-4939-6810-7   (eBook)
DOI 10.1007/978-1-4939-6810-7

Cover image: Photoactivated localization microscopy (PALM) detecting a bacterial membrane protein. Shown is a *Bacillus subtilis* cell expressing FloA-mNeonGreen. FloA is a bacterial flotillin-like protein, involved in membrane compartmentalization. PALM images were acquired in TIRF. Detected signals were filtered for PSF width (100–200 nm) and photon count (200–1000 photons). The average localization precision of detected FloA-mNeonGreen molecules is 25 nm.

Printed on acid-free paper

This Humana Press imprint is published by Springer Nature
The registered company is Springer Science+Business Media LLC
The registered company address is: 233 Spring Street, New York, NY 10013, U.S.A.

Preface

Recent achievements, such as the development of a new generation of nanoscopes surpassing the Abbe's diffraction limit or high-resolution approaches for deep imaging, such as light-sheet or two-photon excitation microscopy, have revolutionized light microscopy. In addition to the progress made in optical systems, novel genetically encoded fluorescent reporters and labeling methods allow investigation of biological processes as never previously achieved. Equally important, the information collected from imaging experiments has been dramatically augmented by the development and optimization of a plethora of image analysis tools and computational solutions that provide unbiased and systematic quantitative imaging. Today, therefore, light microscopy encompasses an extraordinary range of applications that can meet the needs of any biological system under investigation.

In this regard, we aimed at creating a book, which functions as a roundup user manual, addressing up-to-date light microscopy approaches and toolsets offered for live or fixed cell observations. Imaging strategies outlined in this book include confocal laser scanning and spinning disk confocal microscopy, FRET (fluorescence resonance energy transfer), FRAP (fluorescence recovery after photobleaching) and laser microsurgery experiments, light-sheet and two-photon excitation microscopy, PALM (photoactivated localization microscopy), STED (stimulated emission depletion), TIRF (total internal reflection fluorescence), and optical coherence microscopy. Here we describe the use of these imaging methodologies to study properties of a multitude of biomolecular targets in a broad range of model systems, ranging from bacteria over tissue to whole animal imaging.

These advanced fluorescence light microscopy methods are exploited to pinpoint and track single molecules, visualize and follow individual cells in living animals or plants, monitor biomolecular spatiotemporal dynamics, or obtain super-resolved images at nanometer resolution. Focus is placed on system instrumentation parameters providing step-by-step guidelines for microscope and experimental setup, as well as sample preparation protocols. Moreover, sophisticated labeling and detection methods are introduced, including tissues clearing, genetically encoded voltage indicators, reciprocal probes, or biosensors. Finally, detailed workflows on data analysis and data quantification are presented dependent on the imaging setup, target, or biological process of interest, including automated and high-content analyses.

This book can offer to the inexperienced user the possibility of a straightforward strategy to address biological questions by selecting the appropriate imaging system, preparation protocol, and data evaluation method based on the experimental model available. In parallel we are wishing to reinforce the experienced user with a variety of additional cutting-edge applications that can be complementary to routine practices and can increase the array of acquired observations and datasets. Finally, we anticipate that the book will additionally prove to be a robust teaching guide for light microscopy practical courses.

Editing this book has been a lengthy but most enjoyable quest. Firstly, we would like to thank our authors who accepted our invitation and generously introduced their expertise and protocols to the scientific community, while patiently went over revisions. We have been overwhelmed with the information and detailed methodologies, as well as image quality included in the manuscripts, which have indeed exceeded our original expectations. We are familiar with the pains and joys of image acquisition and analysis and we are grateful for their efforts and dedication in bringing this work forward. Further, we would like to thank our series editor Prof. John M. Walker for his critical advice and help on the book preparation, as well as the staff at Humana Press for inviting us and greatly assisting us to edit this book and for giving us the opportunity to produce what we feel is today's Light Microscopy. Happy imaging!

Los Angeles, CA, USA   *Yolanda Markaki*
Martinsried, Germany   *Hartmann Harz*

Contents

Preface. . . . . *v*

Contributors. . . . . *ix*

1   Introduction to Modern Methods in Light Microscopy. 1
    Joel Ryan, Abby R. Gerhold, Vincent Boudreau, Lydia Smith,
    and Paul S. Maddox

PART I   ADVANCED FLUORESCENCE MICROSCOPY: SAMPLE PREPARATION,
          FLUOROPHORES AND MODEL SYSTEMS

2   Three-Dimensional Live Imaging of Filamentous Fungi
    with Light Sheet-Based Fluorescence Microscopy (LSFM) 19
    Francesco Pampaloni, Laura Knuppertz, Andrea Hamann,
    Heinz D. Osiewacz, and Ernst H.K. Stelzer

3   Light-Sheet Fluorescence Microscopy: Chemical Clearing
    and Labeling Protocols for Ultramicroscopy 33
    Nina Jährling, Klaus Becker, Saiedeh Saghafi, and Hans-Ulrich Dodt

4   Two-Photon Intravital Microscopy Animal Preparation Protocol
    to Study Cellular Dynamics in Pathogenesis 51
    Erinke van Grinsven, Chloé Prunier, Nienke Vrisekoop,
    and Laila Ritsma

5   Imaging of Brain Slices with a Genetically Encoded Voltage Indicator 73
    Peter Quicke, Samuel J. Barnes, and Thomas Knöpfel

6   FRET Microscopy for Real-Time Visualization of Second Messengers
    in Living Cells. 85
    Axel E. Kraft and Viacheslav O. Nikolaev

7   Imaging the Dynamics of Cell Wall Polymer Deposition
    in the Unicellular Model Plant, *Penium margaritaceum* 91
    David Domozych, Anna Lietz, Molly Patten, Emily Singer, Berke Tinaz,
    and Sandra C. Raimundo

8   Targeted Ablation Using Laser Nanosurgery. 107
    Naga Venkata Gayathri Vegesna, Paolo Ronchi, Sevi Durdu,
    Stefan Terjung, and Rainer Pepperkok

PART II   SUPER AND HIGH-RESOLUTION OPTICAL IMAGING

9   Sample Preparation and Choice of Fluorophores for Single
    and Dual Color Photo-Activated Localization Microscopy (PALM)
    with Bacterial Cells 129
    Juri N. Bach, Giacomo Giacomelli, and Marc Bramkamp

10   STED Imaging in *Drosophila* Brain Slices   143
     Sandra Fendl, Jesús Pujol-Martí, Joel Ryan, Alexander Borst,
     and Robert Kasper

11   Two-Color Total Internal Reflection Fluorescence Microscopy
     of Exocytosis in Endocrine Cells   151
     Adam J. Trexler and Justin W. Taraska

12   Optical Coherence Microscopy   167
     Rainer A. Leitgeb

PART III   QUANTITATIVE AND COMPUTATIONAL IMAGE ANALYSIS

13   Designing Image Analysis Pipelines in Light Microscopy:
     A Rational Approach.   185
     Ignacio Arganda-Carreras and Philippe Andrey

14   Automated Analysis of Intracellular Dynamic Processes   209
     Yao Yao, Ihor Smal, Ilya Grigoriev, Maud Martin, Anna Akhmanova,
     and Erik Meijering

15   Quantitative Image Analysis of Single-Molecule mRNA Dynamics
     in Living Cells.   229
     José Rino, Ana C. de Jesus, and Maria Carmo-Fonseca

16   Analysis of Protein Kinetics Using Fluorescence Recovery
     After Photobleaching (FRAP)   243
     Nickolaos Nikiforos Giakoumakis, Maria Anna Rapsomaniki,
     and Zoi Lygerou

17   Fluorescence-Based High-Throughput and Targeted Image Acquisition
     and Analysis for Phenotypic Screening.   269
     Manuel Gunkel, Jan Philipp Eberle, and Holger Erfle

Index *281*

Contributors

ANNA AKHMANOVA • *Department of Cell Biology, Faculty of Science, Utrecht University, Utrecht, The Netherlands*

PHILIPPE ANDREY • *Institut Jean-Pierre Bourgin, INRA, AgroParisTech, CNRS, Universite Paris-Saclay, Versailles, France; Sorbonne Universites, UPMC Univ Paris 06, Paris, France*

IGNACIO ARGANDA-CARRERAS • *Ikerbasque, Basque Foundation for Science, Bilbao, Spain; Computer Science and Artificial Intelligence Department, Basque Country University (UPV/EHU), Donostia-San Sebastian, Spain; Donostia International Physics Center (DIPC), Donostia-San Sebastian, Spain*

JURI N. BACH • *Faculty of Biology, Ludwig-Maximilians-University, Munich, Germany*

SAMUEL J. BARNES • *Division of Brain Sciences, Imperial College London, London, UK*

KLAUS BECKER • *Department of Bioelectronics, FKE, Vienna University of Technology, Vienna, Austria; Center of Brain Research, Medical University of Vienna, Vienna, Austria*

ALEXANDER BORST • *Max Planck Institute of Neurobiology, Munich, Germany*

VINCENT BOUDREAU • *University of North Carolina at Chapel Hill, Chapel Hill, NC, USA*

MARC BRAMKAMP • *Faculty of Biology, Ludwig-Maximilians-University, Munich, Germany*

MARIA CARMO-FONSECA • *Instituto de Medicina Molecular, Faculdade de Medicina, Universidade de Lisboa, Lisboa, Portugal*

HANS-ULRICH DODT • *Department of Bioelectronics, FKE, Vienna University of Technology, Vienna, Austria; Center of Brain Research, Medical University of Vienna, Vienna, Austria*

DAVID DOMOZYCH • *Department of Biology, Skidmore College, Saratoga Springs, NY, USA*

SEVI DURDU • *Cell Biology Cell Biophysics Unit, EMBL Heidelberg, Heidelberg, Germany*

JAN PHILIPP EBERLE • *BioQuant Center, ViroQuant-CellNetworks RNAi Screening Facility, University of Heidelberg, Heidelberg, Germany*

HOLGER ERFLE • *BioQuant Center, ViroQuant-CellNetworks RNAi Screening Facility, University of Heidelberg, Heidelberg, Germany*

SANDRA FENDL • *Max Planck Institute of Neurobiology, Munich, Germany*

ABBY R. GERHOLD • *Institute for Research in Immunology and Cancer, Université de Montréal, Montreal, QC, Canada*

GIACOMO GIACOMELLI • *Faculty of Biology, Ludwig-Maximilians-University, Munich, Germany*

NICKOLAOS NIKIFOROS GIAKOUMAKIS • *Laboratory of Biology, School of Medicine, University of Patras, Rio, Patras, Greece*

ILYA GRIGORIEV • *Department of Cell Biology, Faculty of Science, Utrecht University, Utrecht, The Netherlands*

ERINKE VAN GRINSVEN • *Department of Respiratory Medicine, Laboratory of Translational Immunology, University Medical Center Utrecht, Utrecht, The Netherlands*

MANUEL GUNKEL • *BioQuant Center, ViroQuant-CellNetworks RNAi Screening Facility, University of Heidelberg, Heidelberg, Germany*

ANDREA HAMANN • *Institute of Molecular Biosciences and Cluster of Excellence Frankfurt Macromolecular Complexes, Department of Biosciences, Goethe Universität Frankfurt am Main, Frankfurt am Main, Germany*

NINA JÄHRLING • *Department of Bioelectronics, FKE, Vienna University of Technology, Vienna, Austria; Center of Brain Research, Medical University of Vienna, Vienna, Austria*

ANA C. DE JESUS • *Instituto de Medicina Molecular, Faculdade de Medicina, Universidade de Lisboa, Lisboa, Portugal*

ROBERT KASPER • *Max Planck Institute of Neurobiology, Munich, Germany*

THOMAS KNÖPFEL • *Centre for Neurotechnology, Imperial College London, London, UK; Division of Brain Sciences, Imperial College London, London, UK*

LAURA KNUPPERTZ • *Institute of Molecular Biosciences and Cluster of Excellence Frankfurt Macromolecular Complexes, Department of Biosciences, Goethe Universität Frankfurt am Main, Frankfurt am Main, Germany*

AXEL E. KRAFT • *Institute of Experimental Cardiovascular Research, University Medical Center Hamburg-Eppendorf, Hamburg, Germany*

RAINER A. LEITGEB • *Christian Doppler Laboratory OPTRAMED, Center for Medical Physics and Biomedical Engineering, Medical University of Vienna, Vienna, Austria*

ANNA LIETZ • *Department of Biology, Skidmore College, Saratoga Springs, NY, USA*

ZOI LYGEROU • *Laboratory of Biology, School of Medicine, University of Patras, Rio, Patras, Greece*

PAUL S. MADDOX • *Department of Biology, University of North Carolina at Chapel Hill, Chapel Hill, NC, USA*

MAUD MARTIN • *Department of Cell Biology, Faculty of Science, Utrecht University, Utrecht, The Netherlands*

ERIK MEIJERING • *Departments of Medical Informatics and Radiology, Biomedical Imaging Group Rotterdam, Erasmus University Medical Center, Rotterdam, The Netherlands*

VIACHESLAV O. NIKOLAEV • *Institute of Experimental Cardiovascular Research, University Medical Center Hamburg-Eppendorf, Hamburg, Germany*

HEINZ D. OSIEWACZ • *Institute of Molecular Biosciences and Cluster of Excellence Frankfurt Macromolecular Complexes, Department of Biosciences, Goethe Universität Frankfurt am Main, Frankfurt am Main, Germany*

FRANCESCO PAMPALONI • *Physical Biology Group, Buchmann Institute for Molecular Life Sciences (BMLS), Goethe Universität Frankfurt am Main, Frankfurt am Main, Germany*

MOLLY PATTEN • *Department of Biology, Skidmore College, Saratoga Springs, NY, USA*

RAINER PEPPERKOK • *Cell Biology and Cell Biophysics Unit, EMBL Heidelberg, Heidelberg, Germany; Advanced Light Microscopy Facility, EMBL Heidelberg, Heidelberg, Germany*

CHLOÉ PRUNIER • *Department of Molecular Cell Biology, Leiden University Medical Center, Leiden, The Netherlands*

JESÚS PUJOL-MARTÍ • *Max Planck Institute of Neurobiology, Munich, Germany*

PETER QUICKE • *Department of Bioengineering, Imperial College London, London, UK; Centre for Neurotechnology, Imperial College London, London, UK; Division of Brain Sciences, Imperial College London, London, UK*

SANDRA C. RAIMUNDO • *Department of Biology, Skidmore College, Saratoga Springs, NY, USA*

MARIA ANNA RAPSOMANIKI • *Laboratory of Biology, School of Medicine, University of Patras, Rio, Patras, Greece; IBM Research Zurich, Rüschlikon, Switzerland*

JOSÉ RINO • *Instituto de Medicina Molecular, Faculdade de Medicina, Universidade de Lisboa, Lisboa, Portugal*

LAILA RITSMA • *Department of Molecular Cell Biology, Leiden University Medical Center, Leiden, The Netherlands*

PAOLO RONCHI • *Cell Biology Cell Biophysics Unit, EMBL Heidelberg, Heidelberg, Germany; Electron Microscopy Core Facility, EMBL Heidelberg, Heidelberg, Germany*

JOEL RYAN • *LMU Munich, Biocenter Martinsried, Munich, Germany*

SAIEDEH SAGHAFI • *Department of Bioelectronics, FKE, Vienna University of Technology, Vienna, Austria; Center of Brain Research, Medical University of Vienna, Vienna, Austria*

EMILY SINGER • *Department of Biology, Skidmore College, Saratoga Springs, NY, USA*

IHOR SMAL • *Departments of Medical Informatics and Radiology, Biomedical Imaging Group Rotterdam, Erasmus University Medical Center, Rotterdam, The Netherlands*

LYDIA SMITH • *University of North Carolina at Chapel Hill, Chapel Hill, NC, USA*

ERNST H.K. STELZER • *Physical Biology Group, Buchmann Institute for Molecular Life Sciences (BMLS), Goethe Universität Frankfurt am Main, Frankfurt am Main, Germany*

JUSTIN W. TARASKA • *Laboratory of Molecular Biophysics, National Heart, Lung, and Blood Institute, National Institutes of Health, Bethesda, MD, USA*

STEFAN TERJUNG • *Advanced Light Microscopy Facility, EMBL Heidelberg, Heidelberg, Germany*

BERKE TINAZ • *Department of Biology, Skidmore College, Saratoga Springs, NY, USA*

ADAM J. TREXLER • *Laboratory of Molecular Biophysics, National Heart, Lung, and Blood Institute, National Institutes of Health, Bethesda, MD, USA*

NAGA VENKATA GAYATHRI VEGESNA • *Cell Biology and Cell Biophysics Unit, EMBL Heidelberg, Heidelberg, Germany*

NIENKE VRISEKOOP • *Department of Respiratory Medicine, Laboratory of Translational Immunology, University Medical Center Utrecht, Utrecht, The Netherlands*

YAO YAO • *Departments of Medical Informatics and Radiology, Biomedical Imaging Group Rotterdam, Erasmus University Medical Center, Rotterdam, The Netherlands*

Chapter 1

Introduction to Modern Methods in Light Microscopy

Joel Ryan, Abby R. Gerhold, Vincent Boudreau, Lydia Smith, and Paul S. Maddox

Abstract

For centuries, light microscopy has been a key method in biological research, from the early work of Robert Hooke describing biological organisms as cells, to the latest in live-cell and single-molecule systems. Here, we introduce some of the key concepts related to the development and implementation of modern microscopy techniques. We briefly discuss the basics of optics **in the microscope**, super-resolution imaging, quantitative image analysis, live-cell imaging, and provide an outlook on active research areas pertaining to light microscopy.

Key words Microscopy, Technology, Super-resolution, Image analysis, Live-cell

1 Introduction to Light Microscopy

Since the late 1800s, scientists have pushed the boundaries of optical resolution in search of biological understanding. Accordingly, innovation in light microscopy has paralleled major steps forward in understanding cellular mechanisms. Here we outline how variations on basic physical principles have generated diversity in light microscopy technologies and ultimately, mechanistic insights into biology.

Optical microscopy, no matter the technology, follows laws of physics that define how light interacts with matter. Light traveling from one medium to another with a higher refractive index (e.g., from air to glass) will (1) slow down and (2) change direction following Snell's law of refraction. In parallel, diffraction describes how light bends around the edges of an object. Huygens's principle states that objects diffract light in a manner directly proportional to their size and spatial distribution. These basic principles can be harnessed in an optical system using lenses to form an image via the controlled convergence and divergence of light. The combination of refraction and diffraction determine what form this image will take. The ability of an imaging system to generate the

Yolanda Markaki and Hartmann Harz (eds.), *Light Microscopy: Methods and Protocols,* Methods in Molecular Biology, vol. 1563, DOI 10.1007/978-1-4939-6810-7_1, © Springer Science+Business Media LLC 2017

image of a point source of light is given by the point spread function (PSF, [1]). Effectively, the PSF describes the degree of blurring imposed by a given imaging system, after the light refracts and diffracts its way through the optical path (including the sample). The size of the PSF is set by the numerical aperture, which defines the widest angle of light that can be collected by the lens. The wider the numerical aperture, the smaller the PSF, the better the resolution (i.e., the ability to differentiate between two small, closely spaced objects). For conventional light microscopy, the highest achievable resolution is around 200 nm. Since biological phenomena are studied at all scales, it has been a great challenge in the field to go beyond this resolution limit.

Light interacts with matter in very predictable ways allowing for optical system design. Depending on the refractive index, transmittance, and dispersive properties of a material, light can be made to perform optical "tricks" to generate contrast in otherwise clear samples. Technological advances in transmitted light microscopy have allowed biologists to visualize previously inaccessible cellular features. For instance, Frits Zernike was awarded the Nobel Prize in Physics (1953) for his invention of the phase contrast microscope, which transforms optical path and refractive differences into contrast [2]. As the nucleus has a higher refractive index than the cytoplasm, light travelling through each can be modulated independently to create either constructive (bright) or destructive interference (dark). The resulting contrast-enhanced image permits improved visualization of both cellular compartments, as compared to standard brightfield images. Further, as the amount of interference is linearly related to the refractive index of a material, phase contrast microscopy can also be used to quantify features such as bulk protein concentration [3]. Later, Shinya Inoue used polarized light microscopy to exploit the birefringence generated by sub-resolution microtubules in the mitotic spindle, leading to the first description of microtubules as protein based fibers connected to chromosomes [4]. An additional triumph of transmitted light microscopy was the invention of video enhanced Differential interference contrast (DIC) imaging at the Marine Biological Laboratory in the 1980s. Using this technology, Vale and colleagues discovered the kinesin motor protein that transports vesicles along microtubules in neurons [5].

In the early 1990s two innovations irreversibly shaped the way we use microscopy in biology: digital detectors and green fluorescent protein (GFP). GFP opened the door for biologists to express fluorescent chimeric versions of their proteins of interest in living organisms [6]. Clearly access to this technology opened experimental space that was previously closed; however, in order to utilize that space, new tools were required. Charge coupled devices (CCDs) are very sensitive photon detectors easily coupled to a personal computer for image recording [7, 8]. At about the time

GFP burst on to the scene, CCDs were becoming increasingly affordable and available to biologists. The fortunate coincidental arrival of these two technologies pushed fluorescence-based light microscopy to the fore and created a revolution in cell biology.

Throughout this volume, methods to optimize light collection as well as clever tricks to generate super-resolved images are described. In addition, techniques to adapt light microscopy for live imaging studies and analysis methods to extract quantitative data from imaging experiments are covered. These technologies, among others, represent the seemingly never ending quest of scientists to extract more and more information from cellular images.

2   Super-Resolution Imaging

A key advantage of fluorescence microscopy is the ability to observe cellular processes as they happen, in vivo, providing not just spatial–temporal information, but also insight into how these events unfold within the native cellular, tissue or organismal environment. Spatial resolution in fluorescence microscopy is constrained by diffraction. The Abbe resolution law relates the finest periodic structure that can be discerned in its image to the wavelength of light and numerical aperture of the lens used. In theory, this limits resolution to approximately 200 nm (e.g., half of the wavelength of blue light) in the lateral plane and 900 nm in the axial plane. As individual proteins, macromolecular complexes (e.g., ribosomes) and certain subcellular structures (e.g., synaptic vesicles) are themselves significantly smaller than 200 nm, a major challenge in fluorescence microscopy has been to extend its in vivo observational power to macromolecular and molecular scales.

While in a perfect optical system, resolution is determined by Abbe's law; in practice, achieved resolution rarely reaches the theoretical limit. Achievable resolution is intimately linked to image contrast, which depends upon the signal-to-noise ratio [1]. Optical aberrations in the specimen itself, as well factors such as microscope alignment and immersion incompatibilities can introduce background or noise, which compromise contrast and reduce effective resolution. A significant source of noise, particularly when imaging relatively thick biological samples, comes from fluorescence originating outside the targeted focal plane. Consequently a common strategy to improve resolution is to reduce this out-of-focus fluorescence. This can be done computationally, as in deconvolution of an image, by blocking detection of out of focus light, as in a confocal pinhole, or by restricting the excitation of fluorophores to a smaller volume.

A widely used, successful implementation of the latter is total internally reflected fluorescence (TIRF) microscopy. In TIRF microscopy, the excitation beam is angled such that it is entirely reflected at the coverslip–sample/solution interface, generating an evanescent wave that propagates into the sample, exciting only those fluorescent molecules within roughly 100 nm of the coverslip [9]. TIRF microscopy enhances axial resolution to roughly 100 nm, and, by largely eliminating background, increases the signal-to-noise ratio, thereby also improving lateral resolution to that predicated by physics. While TIRF microscopy has become a prevalent tool in the study of events occurring at the cell surface (e.g., exocytosis and endocytosis and cytoskeletal dynamics), the cell interior cannot be accessed.

Alternative methods have been developed that enable better axial resolution throughout the depth of a cell. By sandwiching a specimen between two opposing objectives, 4Pi and I^5M microscopy have achieved axial resolutions approaching 100 nm in complex biological samples [10, 11]). 4Pi microscopy may perform better in live cell imaging applications [12] and has been used to investigate how mitochondrial morphology changes in response to dietary conditions in live yeast cells [13]. However, both methods are inherently constrained to relatively thin biological samples (80–200 μm) that fit within the narrow working distance of the two opposing high numerical aperture objectives.

Structured illumination microscopy (SIM) provides a roughly twofold improvement in both lateral and axial resolution [14, 15]. Finer periodic structures in a sample will diffract light at a higher angle, hitting the objective lens close to the edge of its aperture or missing it altogether; hence the dependency of resolution on lens numerical aperture in Abbe's law. SIM makes use of the phenomenon of moiré fringes, whereby a new, coarser pattern is generated when two finer, unaligned patterns are superimposed. In SIM, the excitation light is finely patterned. The interference pattern created when this structured illumination interacts with fine sample features is broad enough (i.e., the diffracted light angle is low enough) to be collected by the lens. The illumination pattern is rotated to defined angles and the underlying sample features are computationally extracted from this set of images. SIM has the benefit of working with standard fluorophores and biologically compatible imaging conditions and permitting multi-color, 3D imaging of whole cells. However, as the final image is a composite of multiple image acquisitions, overall acquisition time and sample stability must be considered, as well as the possible introduction of artifacts during image reconstruction. Nevertheless, multi-color, 3D SIM has revealed previously undetected aspects of nuclear organization [16] and time-lapse 3D SIM has been used to probe the dynamics of long-range homology searching during DNA double-strand break repair by homologous recombination [17].

Imaging methods, such as SIM, that use patterned excitation light are still inherently diffraction limited. The finest achievable illumination pattern, whether a point or a periodic structure, when projected through an objective lens, is also subject to Abbe's law. When the emitted light is proportional to the excitation light (i.e., linear fluorescence), the Abbe limits for detection and illumination sum and a maximum twofold increase in resolution is possible [18, 19].

To truly break the diffraction limit, nonlinear properties of fluorescent molecules (i.e., switching behaviors or saturable on/off states) have been exploited. These super-resolution or nanoscopy techniques have demonstrated 10–50 nm resolution and fall into two classes—the targeted approach and the stochastic or localization-based approach [20, 21]. The stochastic or localization-based approach relies on the principle that the position of a single emitter can be precisely calculated as the centroid of its blurred diffraction spot, provided that it is isolated in space from its neighbors and emits a sufficient number of photons to overcome error in the statistical fitting process [22]. Spatial separation is achieved through use of photoactivatable or switchable molecules and illumination conditions that ensure that, at any given moment, only a few, sparsely distributed molecules are emitting. A super-resolution image is then assembled from a series of acquisitions (thousands), in which the position of individual molecules is calculated. This approach was first realized in biological imaging as photoactivated localization microscopy (PALM) [23], fluorescence photoactivation localization microscopy (FPALM) [24] and stochastic optical reconstruction microscopy (STORM) [25]. Notably, an extension of PALM has been used to dissect the molecular structure of the focal adhesion complex [26]. While a huge number of variations on the stochastic/localization-based approach have emerged (see ref. [20] and references therein), major limitations, such as high labeling density, long acquisition times, and poor overall suitability to live cell imaging, remain [27].

In the targeted approach, an illumination pattern is applied such that a particular state of the fluorophore (e.g., the "ON" state) is reversibly inhibited everywhere except at certain sub-diffraction sized points, which are scanned across the sample to generate the super-resolution image [20]. Examples of the targeted approach include stimulated emission depletion (STED) [28], reversible saturable/switchable optical linear fluorescence transition (RESOLFT) [29] and nonlinear SIM (NL-SIM) [30] microscopy.

STED is, so far, the most broadly developed targeted technique [20]. STED uses the on/off state of a fluorophore, with a focused excitation laser driving molecules into their excited/emitting state and a second overlaid doughnut-shaped laser, with a zero intensity center, deexciting molecules by stimulated emission. The combination of the two beams effectively shrinks the size of the excitation spot well below the diffraction limit [28]. The STED technique has been adapted to accommodate multi-color and 3D imaging and implementations that decrease acquisition time and laser intensities, have made STED a viable option for live imaging [20]. Impressively, STED has been used in intravital live imaging of the mouse brain to monitor changes in dendritic spine morphology at ~70 nm resolution [31].

The primary limitations of STED are its relatively slow scanning speed and high laser intensities. Parallelized implementation of the RESOLFT approach has started to address these issues. Using structured illumination to generate ~100,000 doughnuts with zero intensity centers and relatively fast, lower laser intensity-driven, fluorescent protein photoswitching, larger fields of view can be more rapidly recorded, with reduced phototoxicity and bleaching, while maintaining theoretically diffraction-unlimited resolution [32]. NL-SIM, with its potential for rapid acquisition, larger fields of view and significantly lower laser intensities, may provide a promising solution for super-resolution live cell imaging, particularly the capacity for 3D whole cell live imaging offered by combining NL-SIM with lattice light sheet microscopy [33].

The technological advancements described above mark major advancements in the quest for improved, molecular-scale resolution in fluorescence microscopy. So far the speed of optical innovation has generally outpaced its application in the biological sciences. However, as these technologies become more broadly accessible, they will undoubtedly yield numerous biological insights. The large-scale adoption and utility of many of these techniques requires parallel developments in the field of image analysis, as well as further adaptation to accommodate the specific challenges in live imaging applications.

3   Image Analysis

The interaction of light with a sample, no matter what the imaging technique, can be recorded on a digital detector and translated into a digital image that is composed of pixels. The sample area represented by each pixel is dictated by the magnification of the objective, and the specifications of the camera or the acquisition settings of the scanning device. Each pixel carries a single intensity value, which is proportional to the amount of light collected by the detector at that specific position in the sample. Approaching an image as a two dimensional array of pixels with discrete intensity values allows for quantification of the associated intensity values and the spatial distribution of an object of interest. Adding a third dimension in depth allows for further quantification of the object's spatial distribution, while adding a time dimension can yield a wealth of mechanical properties including directionality of movement, velocity and acceleration. Clearly, viewing an image as a multidimensional array of pixel intensity values opens numerous doors for extracting quantitative data; however, we note that the validity of any image analysis is rooted in the quality of the image being analyzed. Image-based observations of biological features or behaviors represent data sets rich with readily extractable information. Quantitatively measuring image properties not only provides the opportunity for statistically testing hypotheses but also provides quantitative parameters for modeling biological processes and generating new hypotheses.

In designing image analysis protocols, identifying the biological process and the quantitative parameter to be measured is central. Being able to focus an analysis protocol on a particular parameter makes initial image-processing and analysis steps faster and subsequent data analyses more straightforward. Broadly, analysis pipelines can be divided into image processing, feature segmentation and quantification, and data analysis. At each of these steps opportunities arise to hone in the analysis pipeline on a given feature of interest or to automate repetitive tasks to improve efficiency.

Image-processing is a fixed sequence of operations on the raw imaging output that generates a new set of images that are more amenable to segmentation and further analysis. On the one hand, processing may include simple operations such as background subtraction, filtering, and projections. These operations produce new images with enhanced features or reduced size. On the other hand, more complex image processing operations, such as the reconstruction algorithms for PALM [23] and STORM [25], can generate a single super-resolution image from thousands of raw images, in each of which only a fraction of the object of interest is detected.

A frequent goal in image-processing is to enhance feature contrast to permit image segmentation, i.e., partitioning an image into sets of pixels that reflect a feature of interest. For example, small cellular features such as centromeres, centrosomes, or other protein complexes can be readily labeled with fluorescent probes and identified computationally. Isolating these features can be accomplished based on fluorescence intensity, shape, and contrast relative to the surrounding media. A simple segmentation could be a binary operation to group all pixels that fall within the feature of interest as signal (white) and everything else as background (black).

Being able to segment an object of interest from an image often represents a limiting step in image analysis, as it can be difficult to define parameters that reproducibly distinguish the object from its surroundings. However, a decent segmentation facilitates subsequent analysis and may generate new quantifiable parameters. For example, measuring the area occupied by a feature in two dimensions [34] or quantifying morphological parameters such as aspect ratios and roundness can be achieved through segmentation. Alternatively, computational identification of confounding features provides an opportunity to remove them to improve the analysis of others. For example, the plasma membrane is a protein-rich structure whose resident proteins also have a cytoplasmic component. Being able to quantify the cytoplasmic component versus the plasma membrane component depends on the ability to identify the plasma membrane, remove it computationally and quantify the resulting cytoplasmic signal. Such feature removal strategies are particularly powerful for analyzing complex samples such as embryos with many confounding features, including layers of plasma membranes, rows of cells and nuclei, or overlapping developmentally distinct tissues.

Applying both image processing and segmentation approaches to time-lapse data sets generates additional challenges in following features between frames, but also unlocks the potential for extracting new information. In studying microtubule dynamics, for example, several groups have used the analysis of time-lapse data sets to extract dynamic biological parameters such as catastrophe, rescue, shrinkage, and growth rates [35]. In other complex samples, tracking individual particles, cells, or nuclei can provide a wealth of dynamic descriptors, including directionality, velocity, and acceleration of movements. For example, tracking the multitude of nuclei in the developing Drosophila embryo through several rounds of mitotic division is proving to be essential in the study of transcription activation and pattern formation [36]. However, it is important to note that as the microscopy technique being used increases in dimensionality and image-processing and segmentation operations become applied to an increasing number of images, the computational workload increases exponentially highlighting the need for implementing automation in image analysis pipelines.

Additionally, it is important to understand sources of bias in any computational analysis method. For example, manual analysis is prone to user bias, where the user unintentionally biases the data extraction in one direction, often favoring a hypothesis, or manually picking the "best" samples to analyze. On the other hand, computational analysis can lead to artifacts due to subtle differences between samples. For example, feature segmentation based solely on pixel intensity can be problematic when even subtle differences in expression levels exist, with the number of thresholded pixels biased in favor of the sample with the highest expression. In this regard, it is important to carefully consider each step of the analysis pipeline, to catch sources of bias before drawing conclusions.

In recent years, computational image analysis has also contributed to the development of high-throughput microscopy systems. Briefly, computational analysis pipelines are applied to extract biologically meaningful information from large datasets acquired on systems designed to capture images automatically and in large quantities. High-throughput screens have been carried out using diverse light microscopy approaches, including a genome-wide screen using RNA interference in cultured cells to identify genes that contribute to mitotic spindle assembly [37], and a screen for interactions between nuclear proteins by applying fluorescence correlation spectroscopy in a high-throughput manner [38]. In both cases, robust analysis pipelines enabled the analysis of multiple parameters in order to extract meaningful biological information, highlighting the value of employing automated image analysis in large data sets.

Covered in this book are several techniques that require image analysis approaches to reconstruct images, quantitatively analyze biological parameters, or reveal and quantify new parameters in complex data sets. Although the past decade has seen tremendous momentum in the development of new microscopy techniques that allow biologists to go deeper into and faster though samples, the development of image analysis tools has not followed suit [39]. With the development of microscopy techniques capable of generating terabytes of data within minutes, the need for new analysis tools has become well established and will likely be sustained for years to come.

4 Live-Cell Imaging

While single time-point observations have yielded fundamental biological insights, most biological processes are highly dynamic, necessitating live, real-time observation. Live-cell imaging requires concessions to minimize the detrimental effects of fluorescence imaging (e.g., phototoxicity). Furthermore, the ability to investigate cellular behaviors within complex tissues or even entire organisms requires imaging solutions that permit observation at much greater distances from the objective lens.

For many biological questions, chemical fixation and staining is an adequate approach. However, there are many limitations to only imaging and quantifying fixed samples. This technique results in a lack of information about the temporal dynamics or life span of the structures of interest. The lack of temporal information from only observing fixed samples was noted by French biologist and cinematographer Jean Comando at the beginning of the twentieth century. He commented in his work that fixed samples marked "arbitrary steps in what was actually a continuous process" [40]. It is also generally accepted that the fixation process can alter the structure or organization of cellular components. Julius Ries, who published the first time-lapse films of cell division during sea urchin embryogenesis, noted that fixed samples were inadequate for understanding living cells not only because of the artifacts of fixation, but their inherent stillness [41]. By imaging live biological samples, one can remove the known limitations of fixation and observe a wealth of temporal and dynamic information.

The first and foremost consideration in an experimental design for live-cell imaging is the necessity to maintain the viability of the sample being imaged. Each type of sample, be it cultured cell, tissue explant, or entire organism will vary in its requirements for buffers, temperature, CO_2, and susceptibility to contamination. These requirements must be fulfilled throughout any imaging experiment, in a way that is amenable to imaging. In other words, vital conditions must be maintained while keeping the sample accessible to the microscope objective. Many solutions to these challenges are commercially available for cultured cells and thin tissues, from glass-bottom tissue culture dishes, to environmental chambers that control temperature, humidity, and CO_2 levels.

Another unique feature of live imaging is the propensity of living organisms to move. As a result, many organism-specific methods have been designed in order to maintain the sample at the focal plane and in the field of view [42]. The ideal solution would be to immobilize the sample while minimizing negative physiological effects. The most common methods of immobilization are pharmacological paralyzation and mechanical restraint. Pharmacological paralyzation often involves inhibitors of neuronal activity, thereby blocking animal locomotion. Mechanical restraint can employ microfluidic capillaries or gels, such as low melting point agarose, to restrain small animals. Each of these techniques has the potential to induce negative effects on sample viability, and must be carefully considered during experimental design. An alternative computational approach to the sample motility problem is real-time sample tracking. For example, during time-lapse acquisition of cultured cells, the fluorescence center of mass is determined at each timepoint. The distance traveled by the cell is then calculated, and fed back into the system to reposition the cell at the center of the field of view [43].

A crucial consideration in live-cell imaging is the optimization of the imaging settings that will be used to acquire the data. This includes laser power and the frequency and duration of illumination. For fixed samples, the primary consideration for optimizing imaging settings is the risk of irreversibly photobleaching the fluorophores available in the sample. In live samples, not only is there a risk of photobleaching, but also phototoxic effects on the viability of the cells being imaged. Phototoxicity resulting from sustained or frequent illumination can perturb biological processes and lead to cell death. Importantly, the effects of phototoxicity can be variable (e.g., healthy, control cells may be largely unaffected, while mutant or otherwise treated cells may be sensitized) and also heterogeneous even within the same sample population [44]. As a result, it is important to consider how the cell responds to excitation illumination and adjust the imaging conditions appropriately in order to observe the biological process of interest without compromising the physiology of the cell. This consideration is especially important with super-resolution imaging systems, which often require higher levels of laser illumination than diffraction-limited imaging methods.

There exist many probes appropriate for live-cell imaging. The most commonly used probes are genetically encoded fluorescent proteins, such as GFP. Besides GFP, there exist a myriad of different fluorescent proteins and sensors, with varying spectral properties, brightness, and responsiveness. Methods to deliver a plasmid, DNA, or RNA construct encoding a fluorescently labeled protein of interest into a sample include transfection, electroporation, and micro-injection. Recently, many research groups have established CRISPR/Cas9-mediated genome engineering techniques to generate stable lines in which the endogenous protein is tagged. In some cases, however, expression of a fluorescent protein can lead to cellular toxicity, or dysfunction of the fusion protein generated. Regardless of the labeling method, care must be taken to ensure that the labeled sample is viable and the fusion protein is functional.

While live imaging of cultured cells and embryonic development has become standard practice in the field, there is a limit to how well cells in culture and, for some biological questions, embryos can recapitulate the full range of behaviors exhibited by cells within their native environment. To understand how, for example, adult stem cell division is orchestrated relative to the niche poses an additional set of imaging challenges, given how deep these cells can be within the tissue. In this regard intra-vital imaging has seen huge development in recent years. Intra-vital imaging uses long-wavelength illumination (usually above 700 nm) to excite fluorophores, both with one- and multi-photon excitation. Light of longer wavelength is less absorbed by biological material than light of shorter wavelengths, and allows excitation of fluorophores deeper within a tissue. This, in combination with organism-specific methods for maintaining live, healthy samples, has dramatically increased the range of organisms in which researchers can observe biological phenomena as they unfold.

5 Outlook

In the past few years, much attention has been given to the development of super-resolution microscopy, highlighted by the 2014 Nobel Prize in chemistry awarded to key developers of the technique. In parallel, the development of light-sheet microscopy has also generated excitement, opening up new avenues of developmental biology by imaging entire live organisms at the cellular level [45]. From a technical point of view, these methods seem to be in stark contrast: super-resolution looks to image smaller structures, more often in fixed cells, while light-sheet implementations look to image larger structures at lower resolution in live organisms.

Nonetheless, from a conceptual point of view, each sub-field of microscopy has similar aims: to clearly see a relevant biological structure or process, while avoiding detection of other structures that may blur the image.

In this regard, limiting illumination or detection of fluorescence to only that from a structure of biological interest has largely driven innovation in microscopy. In many cases, rethinking the use of different physical properties of the optical system and fluorophores has propelled the development of novel imaging strategies. There exist many examples of this; some of which are illustrated in the methods described in this book. As discussed earlier, the optical configuration of total internal reflection microscopy (TIRF) takes advantage of the refractive properties of light to generate an evanescent wave at the surface of a coverslip, thereby exciting only fluorophores in close proximity to the surface of the coverslip. This has proven to be ideal for imaging the cell membrane and the cytoskeletal cortex, as well as isolated protein complexes, thereby allowing the observation of reconstituted biological processes [46].

In addition, the photophysics of fluorophores can also be harnessed to determine a range of molecular states and interactions. A widely utilized example of this is Förster (or fluorescence) resonance energy transfer (FRET). In FRET an excited fluorophore, the donor, transfers its energy to an acceptor fluorophore, which then emits and is detected. This energy transfer occurs only if the two molecules are in close proximity, in the 1–10 nm range, thus permitting detection of molecular events such as conformational changes, protease cleavages, and receptor–ligand interactions [47].

Lastly, to image deep within biological tissues, multi-photon microscopy relies on an intrinsic photophysical property of fluorophores and how light interacts with matter. In this optical system, fluorophores are excited if two (or more) photons are absorbed in close succession from long wavelength (infrared) excitatory light. The implementation of multi-photon excitation in an imaging system leads to a confined excitation volume, and the use of infrared excitatory light allows imaging deep within biological tissues. With these characteristics, multi-photon microscopy has contributed enormously to understanding neuronal networks [48] and has opened up the field of intravital imaging [49].

In sum, TIRF, FRET, and multi-photon microscopy are examples among many which highlight how very different physical properties of light and fluorophores can be harnessed within an optical system to accomplish different imaging goals.

Interestingly, there are many instances of reengineering limitations or "caveats" of microscopy to reveal novel information. For example, fluorophores undergo irreversible photobleaching after sustained illumination, which can lead to signal deterioration. However, careful calibration and analysis of these bleaching events enables single-molecule counting [50], as well as localization-based super-resolution microscopy. In addition, spatially targeted photo-bleaching of fluorophores lead to the development of fluorescence recovery after photobleaching (FRAP), which enables monitoring and measurement of the ensemble binding dynamics of fluorescently labelled proteins in living cells [47]. These examples are among many which demonstrate how the perceived limits of microscopy can be repurposed into revealing biologically relevant information.

Closely following the development novel microscopy systems, much effort has gone into developing specialized fluorophores that are better suited for particular imaging modalities [51]. These include photoactivatable and photoconvertible fluorophores for localization microscopy, dyes that are better suited to the emission characteristics of STED [52], and fluorophore pairs that have higher FRET efficiency [53]. In parallel, the development and refinement of biosensors, wherein fluorescent reporters are used to indirectly monitor "untaggable" processes, such as changes in voltage during neuronal activity, is constantly progressing, and being adapted to more specialized imaging systems [54].

The techniques described in this book showcase a series of innovative microscopy experimental setups. Each method targets a particular range of biological questions, thereby allowing imaging of samples at distinct scales of biology, from the nanoscale to the development of whole organisms. In this methods book, cultured cells, plants, bacteria, and model organisms are featured, and highlight the diverse usage of microscopy in biological research. These methods offer a detailed description of sample preparation, system setup and calibration, image acquisition, and data analysis to extract biologically meaningful information. Any imaging modality makes compromises between resolution, speed, SNR, and sample viability, and in all cases, the authors stress the importance of careful sample preparation and careful analysis of the resulting datasets. It is hoped that sharing these methods and making them more accessible will lead to a better understanding of a diverse range of biological structures and processes.

References

1. Stelzer (1998) Contrast, resolution, pixelation, dynamic range and signal-to-noise ratio: fundamental limits to resolution in fluorescence light microscopy. J Microsc 189 (1):15-24. doi:10.1046/j.1365-2818.1998.00290.x

2. Zernike F (1955) How I discovered phase contrast. Science 121(3141):345–349

3. Barer R, Ross KA (1952) Refractometry of living cells. J Physiol 118(2):38P–39P

4. Inoue S (1953) Polarization optical studies of the mitotic spindle. I. The demonstration of spindle fibers in living cells. Chromosoma 5(5):487–500

5. Vale RD, Reese TS, Sheetz MP (1985) Identification of a novel force-generating protein, kinesin, involved in microtubule-based motility. Cell 42(1):39–50

6. Chalfie M, Tu Y, Euskirchen G, Ward WW, Prasher DC (1994) Green fluorescent protein as a marker for gene expression. Science 263(5148):802–805

7. Inoué S, Spring K (1997) Video microscopy, 2nd edn. Plenum Press, New York

8. Inoue S, Spring K (1997) Video microscopy: the fundamentals. Plenum Press, New York

9. Axelrod D (1989) Total internal reflection fluorescence microscopy. Methods Cell Biol 30:245–270

10. Schrader M, Bahlmann K, Giese G, Hell SW (1998) 4Pi-confocal imaging in fixed biological specimens. Biophys J 75(4):1659–1668. doi:10.1016/S0006-3495(98)77608-8

11. Gustafsson MG, Agard DA, Sedat JW (1999) I5M: 3D widefield light microscopy with better than 100 nm axial resolution. J Microsc 195(Pt 1):10–16

12. Bewersdorf J, Schmidt R, Hell SW (2006) Comparison of I5M and 4Pi-microscopy. J Microsc 222(Pt 2):105–117. doi:10.1111/j.1365-2818.2006.01578.x

13. Egner A, Jakobs S, Hell SW (2002) Fast 100-nm resolution three-dimensional microscope reveals structural plasticity of mitochondria in live yeast. Proc Natl Acad Sci U S A 99(6):3370–3375. doi:10.1073/pnas.052545099

14. Gustafsson MG (2000) Surpassing the lateral resolution limit by a factor of two using structured illumination microscopy. J Microsc 198(Pt 2):82–87

15. Gustafsson MG, Shao L, Carlton PM, Wang CJ, Golubovskaya IN, Cande WZ, Agard DA, Sedat JW (2008) Three-dimensional resolution doubling in wide-field fluorescence microscopy by structured illumination. Biophys J 94(12):4957–4970. doi:10.1529/biophysj.107.120345

16. Schermelleh L, Carlton PM, Haase S, Shao L, Winoto L, Kner P, Burke B, Cardoso MC, Agard DA, Gustafsson MG, Leonhardt H, Sedat JW (2008) Subdiffraction multicolor imaging of the nuclear periphery with 3D structured illumination microscopy. Science 320(5881):1332–1336. doi:10.1126/science.1156947

17. Lesterlin C, Ball G, Schermelleh L, Sherratt DJ (2014) RecA bundles mediate homology pairing between distant sisters during DNA break repair. Nature 506(7487):249–253. doi:10.1038/nature12868

18. Schermelleh L, Heintzmann R, Leonhardt H (2010) A guide to super-resolution fluorescence microscopy. J Cell Biol 190(2):165–175. doi:10.1083/jcb.201002018

19. Heintzmann R, Ficz G (2006) Breaking the resolution limit in light microscopy. Brief Funct Genomic Proteomic 5(4):289–301. doi:10.1093/bfgp/ell036

20. Eggeling C, Willig KI, Sahl SJ, Hell SW (2015) Lens-based fluorescence nanoscopy. Q Rev Biophys 48(2):178–243. doi:10.1017/S0033583514000146

21. Nienhaus K, Nienhaus GU (2016) Where Do We Stand with Super-Resolution Optical Microscopy? J Mol Biol 428(2 Pt A):308–322. doi:10.1016/j.jmb.2015.12.020

22. Betzig E (1995) Proposed method for molecular optical imaging. Opt Lett 20(3):237–239

23. Betzig E, Patterson GH, Sougrat R, Lindwasser OW, Olenych S, Bonifacino JS, Davidson MW, Lippincott-Schwartz J, Hess HF (2006) Imaging intracellular fluorescent proteins at nanometer resolution. Science 313(5793):1642–1645. doi:10.1126/science.1127344

24. Hess ST, Girirajan TP, Mason MD (2006) Ultra-high resolution imaging by fluorescence photoactivation localization microscopy. Biophys J 91(11):4258–4272. doi:10.1529/biophysj.106.091116

25. Rust MJ, Bates M, Zhuang X (2006) Sub-diffraction-limit imaging by stochastic optical reconstruction microscopy (STORM). Nat Methods 3(10):793–795. doi:10.1038/nmeth929

26. Kanchanawong P, Shtengel G, Pasapera AM, Ramko EB, Davidson MW, Hess HF, Waterman CM (2010) Nanoscale architecture of integrin-based cell adhesions. Nature 468(7323):580–584. doi:10.1038/nature09621

27. Betzig E (2015) Single molecules, cells, and super-resolution optics (Nobel Lecture). Angew Chem Int Ed Engl 54(28):8034–8053. doi:10.1002/anie.201501003

28. Hell SW, Wichmann J (1994) Breaking the diffraction resolution limit by stimulated emission: stimulated-emission-depletion fluorescence microscopy. Opt Lett 19(11):780–782

29. Hofmann M, Eggeling C, Jakobs S, Hell SW (2005) Breaking the diffraction barrier in fluorescence microscopy at low light intensities by using reversibly photoswitchable proteins. Proc Natl Acad Sci U S A 102(49):17565–17569. doi:10.1073/pnas.0506010102

30. Gustafsson MG (2005) Nonlinear structured-illumination microscopy: wide-field fluorescence imaging with theoretically unlimited resolution. Proc Natl Acad Sci U S A 102(37):13081–13086. doi:10.1073/pnas.0406877102

31. Berning S, Willig KI, Steffens H, Dibaj P, Hell SW (2012) Nanoscopy in a living mouse brain. Science 335(6068):551. doi:10.1126/science.1215369

32. Chmyrov A, Keller J, Grotjohann T, Ratz M, d'Este E, Jakobs S, Eggeling C, Hell SW (2013) Nanoscopy with more than 100,000 'doughnuts'. Nat Methods 10(8):737–740. doi:10.1038/nmeth.2556

33. Li D, Shao L, Chen BC, Zhang X, Zhang M, Moses B, Milkie DE, Beach JR, Hammer JA

3rd, Pasham M, Kirchhausen T, Baird MA, Davidson MW, Xu P, Betzig E (2015) ADVANCED IMAGING. Extended-resolution structured illumination imaging of endocytic and cytoskeletal dynamics. Science 349(6251):aab3500. doi:10.1126/science.aab3500

34. Maddox PS, Portier N, Desai A, Oegema K (2006) Molecular analysis of mitotic chromosome condensation using a quantitative time-resolved fluorescence microscopy assay. Proc Natl Acad Sci U S A 103(41):15097–15102. doi:10.1073/pnas.0606993103

35. Lacroix B, Bourdages KG, Dorn JF, Ihara S, Sherwood DR, Maddox PS, Maddox AS (2014) In situ imaging in C. elegans reveals developmental regulation of microtubule dynamics. Dev Cell 29(2):203–216. doi:10.1016/j.devcel.2014.03.007

36. Bothma JP, Garcia HG, Ng S, Perry MW, Gregor T, Levine M (2015) Enhancer additivity and non-additivity are determined by enhancer strength in the Drosophila embryo. Elife:4. doi:10.7554/eLife.07956

37. Goshima G, Wollman R, Goodwin SS, Zhang N, Scholey JM, Vale RD, Stuurman N (2007) Genes required for mitotic spindle assembly in Drosophila S2 cells. Science 316(5823):417–421. doi:10.1126/science.1141314

38. Wachsmuth M, Conrad C, Bulkescher J, Koch B, Mahen R, Isokane M, Pepperkok R, Ellenberg J (2015) High-throughput fluorescence correlation spectroscopy enables analysis of proteome dynamics in living cells. Nat Biotechnol 33(4):384–389. doi:10.1038/nbt.3146

39. Danuser G (2011) Computer vision in cell biology. Cell 147(5):973–978. doi:10.1016/j.cell.2011.11.001

40. Landecker H (2009) Seeing things: from microcinematography to live cell imaging. Nat Methods 6(10):707–709

41. Ries J (1909) Kinematographie der Befruchtung und Zellteilung. Arch für mikroskopische Anat 74(1):1–31

42. Aufderheide KJJC (2012) Immobilization of living specimens for microscopic observation. Curr Microsc Contrib Adv Sci Technol 2:833–839

43. Rabut G, Ellenberg J (2004) Automatic real-time three-dimensional cell tracking by fluorescence microscopy. J Microsc 216(Pt 2):131–137. doi:10.1111/j.0022-2720.2004.01404.x

44. Magidson V, Khodjakov A (2013) Circumventing photodamage in live-cell microscopy. Methods Cell Biol 114:545–560. doi:10.1016/B978-0-12-407761-4.00023-3

45. Weber M, Huisken J (2011) Light sheet microscopy for real-time developmental biology. Curr Opin Genet Dev 21(5):566–572. doi:10.1016/j.gde.2011.09.009

46. Martin-Fernandez ML, Tynan CJ, Webb SE (2013) A 'pocket guide' to total internal reflection fluorescence. J Microsc 252(1):16–22. doi:10.1111/jmi.12070

47. De Los SC, Chang CW, Mycek MA, Cardullo RA (2015) FRAP, FLIM, and FRET: Detection and analysis of cellular dynamics on a molecular scale using fluorescence microscopy. Mol Reprod Dev 82(7-8):587–604. doi:10.1002/mrd.22501

48. Helmchen F, Denk W (2005) Deep tissue two-photon microscopy. Nat Methods 2(12):932–940. doi:10.1038/nmeth818

49. Weigert R, Porat-Shliom N, Amornphimoltham P (2013) Imaging cell biology in live animals: ready for prime time. J Cell Biol 201(7):969–979. doi:10.1083/jcb.201212130

50. Zhang H, Guo P (2014) Single molecule photobleaching (SMPB) technology for counting of RNA, DNA, protein and other molecules in nanoparticles and biological complexes by TIRF instrumentation. Methods 67(2):169–176. doi:10.1016/j.ymeth.2014.01.010

51. Fernandez-Suarez M, Ting AY (2008) Fluorescent probes for super-resolution imaging in living cells. Nat Rev Mol Cell Biol 9(12):929–943. doi:10.1038/nrm2531

52. Butkevich AN, Mitronova GY, Sidenstein SC, Klocke JL, Kamin D, Meineke DN, D'Este E, Kraemer PT, Danzl JG, Belov VN, Hell SW (2016) Fluorescent rhodamines and fluorogenic carbopyronines for super-resolution STED microscopy in living cells. Angew Chem Int Ed Engl 55(10):3290–3294. doi:10.1002/anie.201511018

53. Bajar BT, Wang ES, Lam AJ, Kim BB, Jacobs CL, Howe ES, Davidson MW, Lin MZ, Chu J (2016) Improving brightness and photostability of green and red fluorescent proteins for live cell imaging and FRET reporting. Sci Rep 6:20889. doi:10.1038/srep20889

54. Miyawaki A, Niino Y (2015) Molecular spies for bioimaging—fluorescent protein-based probes. Mol Cell 58(4):632–643. doi:10.1016/j.molcel.2015.03.002

Part I

Advanced Fluorescence Microscopy: Sample Preparation, Fluorophores and Model Systems

Chapter 2

Three-Dimensional Live Imaging of Filamentous Fungi with Light Sheet-Based Fluorescence Microscopy (LSFM)

Francesco Pampaloni, Laura Knuppertz, Andrea Hamann, Heinz D. Osiewacz, and Ernst H.K. Stelzer

Abstract

We describe a method for the three-dimensional live imaging of filamentous fungi with light sheet-based fluorescence microscopy (LSFM). LSFM provides completely new opportunities to investigate the biology of fungal cells and other microorganisms with high spatial and temporal resolution. As an example, we study the established aging model *Podospora anserina*. The protocol explains the mounting of the live fungi for the light sheet imaging, the imaging procedure and illustrates basic image processing of data.

Key words Advanced light microscopy, Light sheet-based fluorescence microscopy, Live cell imaging, LSFM, SPIM, DSLM, *Podospora anserina*, Ascomycetes, Mycology, Microbiology, Aging model, Autophagy

1 Introduction

Advanced fluorescence microscopy, including confocal microscopy [1, 2], is a standard tool to study filamentous fungi at cellular and subcellular levels [1–3]. Fluorescence microscopy is essential for in vivo studies of dynamic processes and provides spatially and temporally resolved information of organelles such as the endoplasmic reticulum, mitochondria, and the Golgi apparatus [2].

We describe a detailed step-by-step user guide for the live imaging of fungal mycelia and hyphae with the cutting-edge technology Light Sheet-based Fluorescence Microscopy (LSFM) [4]. As an example, we apply the protocol to the filamentous fungus *Podospora anserina*.

1.1 Podospora anserina

Podospora anserina is a filamentous fungus that is characterized by a limited, short lifespan [5, 6]. After germination of ascospores, the progeny of a sexual reproduction, the developing colony (mycelium) grows by extension at the tips of filamentous cells. After a strain-specific period of linear growth, growth slows down

Yolanda Markaki and Hartmann Harz (eds.), *Light Microscopy: Methods and Protocols*, Methods in Molecular Biology, vol. 1563, DOI 10.1007/978-1-4939-6810-7_2, © Springer Science+Business Media LLC 2017

until it completely ceases and the mycelium dies at the periphery. This easily identifiable phenotype, the availability of mutant strains and the plethora of potential experiments make *P. anserina* an ideal model for the investigation of the basic mechanisms of aging [7–12]. Over the years, several specific *P. anserina* strains have been generated and molecular pathways have been identified, which are involved in the control of aging and life span [10], e.g., autophagy. For microscopic analyses of pathways related to autophagy, transgenic strains expressing fluorescent fusion proteins are available [8, 11, 13]. In our protocol, we employ the *P. anserina* GFP::PaATG8 strain. PaATG8 is the fungal homologue of the LC3 protein in mammalian cells. The GFP-tagged PaATG8 allows to monitor autophagosomal dynamics in live fungus [13].

1.2 Light Sheet-based Fluorescence Microscopy (LSFM)

Imaging dynamic processes in living organisms with fluorescence microscopy has developed into an essential tool in biology [14–16]. Time-lapse fluorescence microscopy provides information on cellular and subcellular processes over time in whole organisms and single cells. Three-dimensional imaging is essential to analyze the interplay of cells in multicellular organisms. The main challenges of fluorescence microscopy are minimizing phototoxic effects in live specimens, minimizing photobleaching and achieving a high three-dimensional recording speed. These challenges are addressed by spinning-disk confocal fluorescence microscopy [17], heavily optimized wide-field fluorescence microscopy (OMX) [18], and light sheet-based fluorescence microscopy (LSFM) [19, 20]. The youngest and most promising of these three techniques is LSFM. The principles of LSFM are described in Fig. 1. In LSFM, a laser light sheet illuminates the sample with an extremely low energy of about 2 µJ at 488 nm in the illumination plane [20, 21]. LSFM takes advantage of modern CCD and CMOS cameras, which provide a high recording speed. While in second-generation LSFMs such as the Digital Scanned Light Sheet-based Fluorescence Microscope (DSLM), a speed of six planes/second was achieved (one plane consisting of 2048 × 2048 pixels) [20], third-generation microscopes record >100 images per second [22]. A key advantage of LSFM over confocal microscopes is the high dynamic range of the images, which is essential for subsequent high-performance image processing. With LSFM, the long-term fluorescence imaging of zebrafish (*Danio rerio*) and fruit fly (*Drosophila melanogaster*) embryos for up to 72 h have been achieved without impairing embryonic development [20, 23]. The high speed of the light sheet microscope has allowed to follow the mitosis and migration in toto of more than 16,000 cells in the zebrafish embryo. LSFM has also been applied to study developing lateral roots in *Arabidopsis thaliana* [24], to investigate the development of *Tribolium castaneum* [25, 26], and, not the least, to study the behavior of three-dimensional cell cultures and multicellular spheroids [27–31].

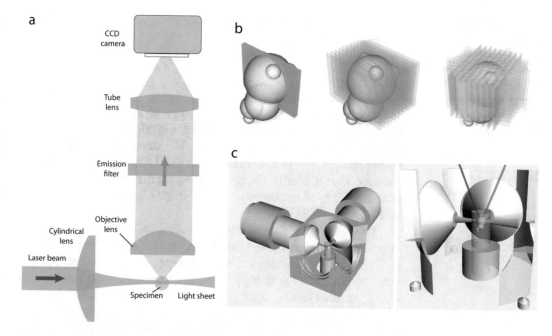

Fig. 1 Principles of Light Sheet-based Fluorescence Microscopy (LSFM). (**a**) Setup of a single plane illumination microscope (aka SPIM [19]). (**b**) Principles of LSFM imaging. *Left*: a single plane in the specimen is illuminated by a light sheet and overlaps with the focal plane of the detection lens. Hence, only the plane that is observed is also illuminated, resulting in lower photobleaching and lower phototoxicity. *Center*: by moving the specimen through the stationary light sheet, a three-dimensional stack of images is recorded. *Right*: by rotating the specimen multiple-views image stacks are obtained. Combining multiple different views of the specimen increases the resolution along the *z*-axis. (**c**) Close-up of a specimen chamber, showing both the illumination and detection objective lenses oriented at a 90° angle with respect to each other

2   Materials

2.1   Chemicals and Small Laboratory Equipment

1. *Low-melting point agarose aliquots*: prepare a 1 % solution of low-melting point agarose (gel point 26–30 °C, e.g., Sigma A9414) in PBS. Aliquot the agarose solution in 2 ml vials. Store at 4 °C.

2. *5 × 5 mm coverslips* with thickness between 0.06 and 0.08 mm (Wagner & Munz GmbH, Munich, Germany, http://www.wagnermunz.com/).

3. *Sharp angled-tip precision forceps* (e.g., Excelta SKU 50-SA, http://www.excelta.com/).

4. Bent coverglass forceps with enlarged rectangular tips (e.g., Leica Biosystems 38DI11102, http://www.leicabiosystems.com).

5. *Clear transparent nail polish.*

6. *Disposable scalpel.*

7. *Laboratory pipettes (P200, 20–200 μl, yellow tips).*

2.2 P. anserina Strains and Culture Media

1. *P. anserina Gfp::PaAtg8 strain* constructed from the wild-type strain 's' [5].

2. *Standard cornmeal agar* (BMM) [6].

3. *M2 agar* [9].

2.3 Custom Equipment

2.3.1 Sample Holder for the LSFM

The function of the LSFM holder is to provide a stable support for the sample and mechanically connect it with the xyzθ translational/rotational stage of the microscope. We describe a basic sample holder design that can be adapted to the LSFM stage available to the user. Our holder has been designed for the *monolithic Digitally Scanned Light Sheet Microscope* used in our laboratory (mDSLM, *see* Fig. 1c and [24]).

The holder consists of a stainless steel rod carved at one edge in order to support a coverslip, as shown in Fig. 2. The holder can be fabricated by any mechanical workshop. An alternative fabrication method is 3D printing, which is a reasonable approach when testing various holder configurations (*see* **Notes 1–3** for tips and tricks). In any case, the material hast to be biocompatible and endure repeated autoclaving. For machined holders we recommend stainless steel or a hard plastic material such as Delrin™ (polyoxymethylen, POM).

The 5 mm × 5 mm glass coverslips that supports the *P. anserina* sample is glued to the specimen holder by a droplet of transparent

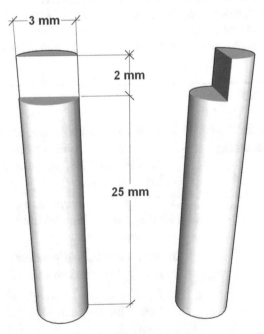

Fig. 2 Custom sample holder for LSFM. The LSFM holder connects the sample with the xyzθ translational/rotational stage of the light sheet microscope. The holder is custom built in a mechanical workshop or 3D-printed (*see* **Note 1–3**). Possible materials are stainless steel or hard plastic, such as POM

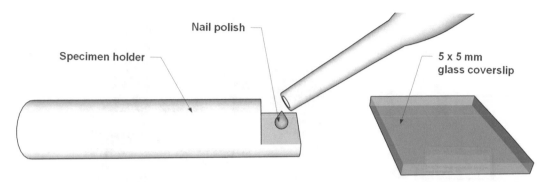

Fig. 3 Attachment of the glass substrate on the sample holder. A tiny droplet of nail polish is deposited on the carved part of the holder with a pipette and a 5 mm × 5 mm glass coverslip is firmly attached for a few seconds

nail polish. Nail polish is an effective, cheap, and quickly hardening glue for mounting samples in light microscopy. Once dried it has no harmful effects on biological specimens immersed in common culture media.

As shown in Fig. 3, a tiny amount of nail polish is deposited on the carved part of the LSFM holder by using a pipette or a brush. Next, the coverslip is rapidly but gently attached to the holder by using flat-tip coverslip forceps. The nail polish is allowed to dry for at least 30 min while the holder lies horizontally with the sample pointing upwards, to ensure a positioning parallel to the holder's longitudinal axis.

The appearance of the assembled holder, ready for mounting the sample, is shown in Fig. 4.

2.4 Imaging Equipment

1. Various suitable LSFM implementations are described in detail in [19, 32, 33] (SPIM), [20] (DSLM), [24] (monolithic DSLM, mDSLM). Commercial LSFMs are now available from the companies Zeiss (LightSheet Z.1, http://www.zeiss.com/microscopy/en_us/products/imaging-systems/lightsheet-z-1.html), Luxendo (http://luxendo.eu/), and 3i (https://www.intelligent-imaging.com/index.php).

2. Long working-distance water-dipping objective lenses with high numerical aperture (e.g., Carl Zeiss Plan-Apochromat 63x/1.0 W, 421,480–9900-000).

2.5 Software for Image Processing

Image processing software package (e.g., Fiji—Fiji is Just ImageJ, a distribution of ImageJ, http://fiji.sc/).

3 Methods

3.1 P. anserina Cultivation

The *P. anserina Gfp::PaAtg8* strain expresses an N-terminal fusion of the GFP protein to PaATG8, the fungal homologue to mammalian LC3, a well-known marker of autophagy. Labeling of ATG8

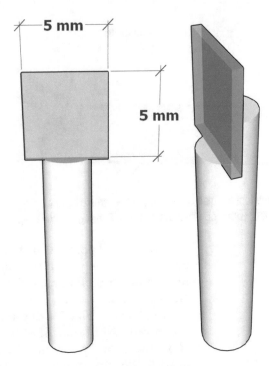

Fig. 4 Assembled sample holder. The final holder ready for mounting the sample

allows the observation of the translocation of the fusion protein from the cytosol to the autophagosome to the vacuole, where the final degradation of the autophagosome takes place in fungi. For the cloning procedure *see* [13].

1. Isolate monokaryotic spores from asci of a *Gfp::PaAtg8* cross.

2. Germination of isolated spores takes place by cultivation on standard cornmeal agar (BMM) supplemented with 60 mM ammonium acetate.

3. Incubate the spores at 27 °C in the dark for 2 days.

4. Culture freshly isolated *P. anserina* strains on M2-agar. See for the exact composition of the M2-medium.

3.2 Sample Mounting

A 2 ml low-melting point agarose is put in a heater at 65 °C–70 °C until the agarose is completely liquid. Shortly before imaging, a 5 mm × 5 mm slab of M2-agarose with the cultured mycelium growing is cut with a sharp-tip scalpel (Fig. 5). In our setup, the mycelium is grown on a thin layer (<1 mm) of M2-agarose deposited on a glass slide. The glass slide is placed inside a 100 mm petri dish also containing water-soaked tissue paper. This avoids drying of the agarose during the culture.

Next, the square slab is gently removed with a sharp angled-tip forceps and placed on the sample holder coverslip, on which a

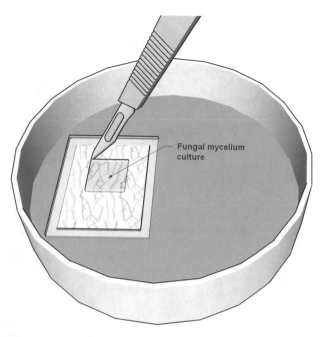

Fig. 5 Cutting the mycelium sample from the fungal culture on agar gel. A roughly 5 mm × 5 mm square slab is cut from the fungal culture by using a sterile scalpel

droplet of liquid low-melting agarose is deposited (Fig. 6a, b). The agarose ensures a stable adhesion between the glass substrate and the sample.

Figure 6c displays the real sample observed under a stereomicroscope.

3.3 LSFM Imaging

Figure 7 shows the position of the sample holder in the LSFM chamber. For imaging it is essential that the coverslip surface with the sample is oriented at an angle of 45° with respect to the illumination axes of both the illumination and the detection paths of the light sheet microscope, as depicted in Fig. 7a, b.

An illumination/detection angle of 45° ensures an optimal imaging of the nearly flat coverslip-mounted sample in the LSFM. In order to record a three-dimensional image stack, the sample is translated stepwise along the z-axis, parallel to the detection optical axis (Fig. 7a, arrow). A typical z-axis step size for the imaging of *P. anserina* is 0.5 μm. The stack recording procedure is schematically shown in Fig. 8.

In order to resolve subcellular structures in the hyphae, high-numerical aperture (NA) water-dipping objectives are recommended. We employed a Carl Zeiss Plan-Apochromat 63×/1.0 water dipping lens, which resolves tiny organelles such as individual autophagosomes. Objective lenses with low magnification and high NA (e.g., Nikon N16XLWD-PF, 16×, NA 0.80) are ideal,

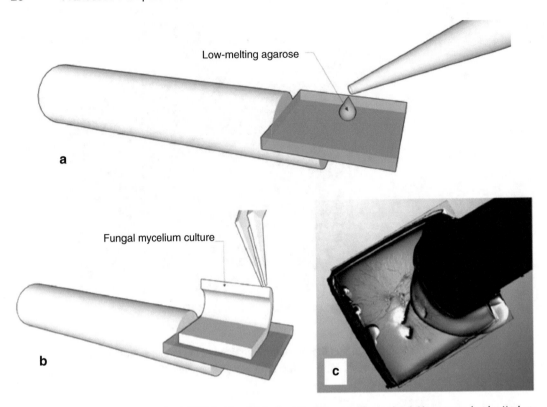

Fig. 6 Mounting the sample on the LSFM-holder. (**a**) A droplet of low-melting point 1 % agarose is pipetted on the glass coverslip. (**b**) The fungal culture cut slab is placed on the coverslip with a forceps. (**c**) A photograph of the real mounted sample recorded with a stereomicroscope (from Ref. [13]). The mycelium and hyphae are visible on the coverslip (magnification 10×)

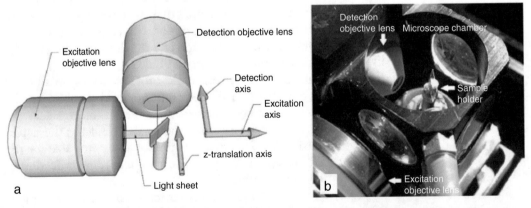

Fig. 7 Positioning the mounted sample in the LSFM. The mounted sample is inserted in the light sheet microscope (in this case an mDSLM). (**a**) Note that the coverslip surface is oriented at an angle of 45° with respect to the illumination and detection optical axes (*arrows*). (**b**) An actual implementation, including the microscope chamber, the excitation objective lens, the detection objective lens and the mounted sample. During imaging, the chamber is filled with culture media

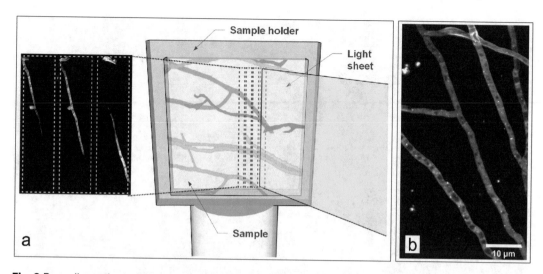

Fig. 8 Recording a three-dimensional stack of the sample. The sample, positioned at 45° is translated along the *z*-axis. (**a**) Left, *z*-slices of isolated hyphae are shown. The slices are recorded with a 0.5 µm step size. (**b**) Maximum projection of 15 slices showing the mycelium hyphae

since they combine high spatial resolution, long working distance and a large field-of-view. As illumination lens we used a Carl Zeiss Plan-Neofluar 5×/0.16, which produces a light sheet with a thickness of ~2 µm.

3.4 Results

The montage in Fig. 9 shows the individual slices of a stack, recorded at increasing depth in the sample with 0.5 µm steps. A single hypha in the mycelium is imaged.

By taking advantages of the high scanning speed of LSFM, the shape and spatial orientation of the hyphae is directly obtained (Fig. 10a–c). This provides new insights into fungal growth patterns. Moreover, the high resolution of the 63×/1.0 objective lens allows the detection of single autophagosomes. Due to the high signal-to-noise ratio and the high dynamic range of a camera, the autophagosomes can be readily segmented by applying the segmentation algorithms available, e.g., in the image processing software *Fiji* (Fig. 10b).

The light sheet microscope's high recording speed is exploited for the time-lapse imaging of rapid subcellular events. In the example shown in Figs. 11 and 12, the displacements of one individual autophagosomes are tracked in three-dimensions.

4 Notes

1. 3D printing (aka additive manufacturing) is a suitable alternative to conventional machining for the production of custom LSFM holders. It is particularly useful for prototyping and

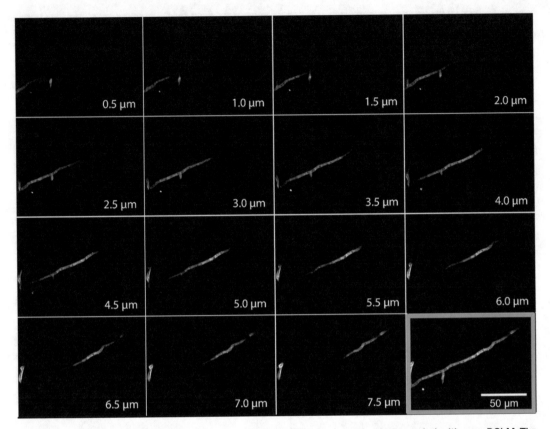

Fig. 9 Three-dimensional image stack of a single hyphae of *Podospora anserina* recorded with an mDSLM. The recording depth is shown in each slice. The highlighted image at the bottom right is a maximum projection of the stack slices and shows the entire hyphae. Acquisition parameters: detection lens CZ Plan-Apochromat 63×/1.0 W, excitation lens Plan-Neofluar 5×/0.16, laser line 488 nm, laser intensity 2.5 mW, exposure time 100 ms, emission filter 525/50. Marker: GFP-tagged Atg8

testing different configurations of a holder. A further advantage of 3D printing is that it allows the construction of shapes that are not achievable with a conventional milling machine or a lathe. Professional printing services are available (e.g., Shapeways, www.shapeways.com). CAD-files can be uploaded on the website of the 3D printer service and the printed parts are usually shipped within few days.

2. The 3D parts can be designed with CAD software packages that are downloadable for free under determined license restrictions. Examples are Inventor 2014 and Autodesk 123Design (both from Autodesk, San Rafael, CA), or Sketchup (https://www.sketchup.com). The CAD files of the designed parts can be converted to a file format that is interpretable by the 3D printer (a typical file format is .stl).

3. The biocompatibility of the material should be tested before using 3D-printed parts in experiments. Studies assessing this issue have been performed, see for instance [34].

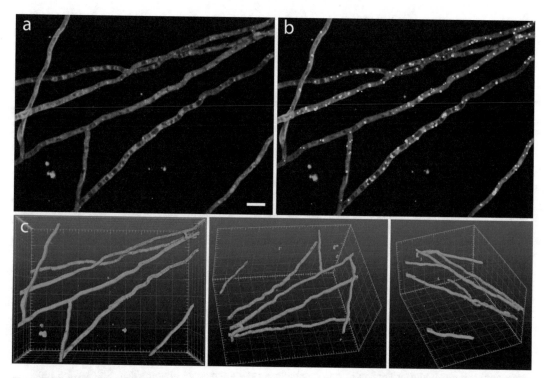

Fig. 10 Three-dimensional imaging of individual hyphae of *Podospora anserina* with a light sheet microscope (mDSLM) The specimen is a 20-day-old wild-type *P. anserina* culture, expressing Gfp-tagged Atg8. (**a**) Maximum projection of the image stack. Scale bar 10 μm. (**b**) Segmented autophagosomes (*yellow dots*) superimposed to the maximum projection. (**c**) Three-dimensional spatial orientation of the hyphae from three different points of view, showing the highly entangled architecture. The squares are 10 μm × 10 μm. The 3D rendering has been performed with the "3D Viewer" plugin of Fiji. Imaging parameters: the stack was composed by 192 slices. The slice spacing was 0.5 μm. Acquisition parameters: detection lens CZ Plan-Apochromat 63×/1.0 W, excitation lens Plan-Neofluar 5×/0.16, laser line 488 nm, laser intensity 2.5 mW, exposure time 100 ms, emission filter 525/50

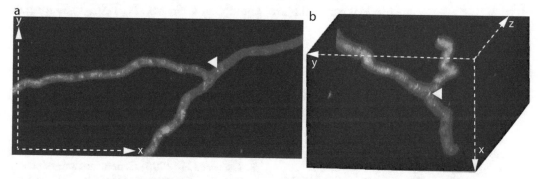

Fig. 11 Three-dimensional time-dependent localization of autophagosomes in the hyphae. (**a**) Maximum projection of one stack. The *white arrow* points at one single autophagosome within the hypha. (**b**) The same stack as a maximum projection rotated in space to highlight the shape of the hyphae from another point of view. The *white arrow* points to the same autophagosome in (**a**). The look-up table "blue orange icb" (In Fiji: Image/Lookup Tables/blue orange icb) was applied to highlight the autophagosomes. The acquisition parameters are the same as in Fig. 10. The data was processed with the "3D project" command of Fiji

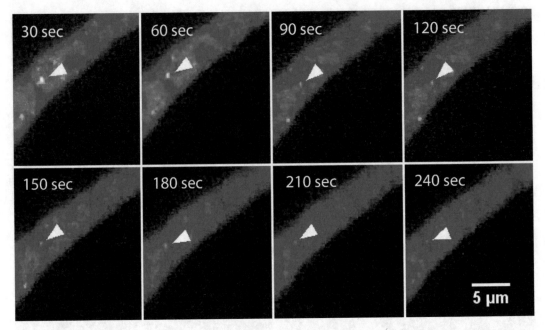

Fig. 12 Time-dependent localization of autophagosomes in the hyphae. Zoom-in of the region around the autophagosome in Fig. 11a. The time sequence shows the movements of the autophagosome. Each frame represents the maximum projection of one complete three-dimensional image stack. Stack were recorded every 30 s. The look-up table "blue orange icb" was applied to better highlight the autophagosomes. Acquisition parameters as in Fig. 10

Acknowledgments

The authors thank the LOEWE initiative of the Federal State of Hessen (Ub-Net, speaker Ivan Dikic) and the Deutsche Forschungsgemeinschaft (DFG, Os75/15-1, and Excellenzcluster für Makromolekulare Komplexe, CEF-MC II, EXC 115, speaker Volker Doetsch) for financial support.

References

1. Hickey, P. C., Swift, S. R., Roca, M. G. & Read, N. D. (2004) Microbial imaging. Methods Microbiol 34, Elsevier, p. 63–87

2. Hickey PC, Read ND (2009) Imaging living cells of *Aspergillus* in vitro. Med Mycol 47(Suppl 1):S110–S119

3. Dahms, T. E. S., Czymmek, K. J. (eds) (2015) Advanced microscopy in mycology. Springer. doi: 10.1007/978-3-319-22437-4

4. Stelzer EHK (2015) Light-sheet fluorescence microscopy for quantitative biology. Nat Methods 12:23–26

5. Rizet G (1953) Impossibility of obtaining uninterrupted and unlimited multiplication of the ascomycete *Podospora anserina*. C. R. Hebd Seances Acad Sci 237:838–840

6. Esser K (1974) *Podospora anserina*. In: King, RC (ed) Handbook of Genetics. Plenum Press, New York, 531–551

7. Osiewacz H (1996) Genetic analysis of senescence in *Podospora anserina*. In: Bos CJ (ed) Fungal Genetics. Marcel Dekker, New York, 317–335

8. Hamann A, Krause K, Werner A, Osiewacz HD (2005) A two-step protocol for efficient deletion of genes in the filamentous ascomycete *Podospora anserina*. Curr Genet 48:270–275

9. Osiewacz HD, Hamann A, Zintel S (2013) Assessing organismal aging in the filamentous fungus *Podospora anserina*. Methods Mol Biol 965:439–462

10. Wiemer M, Grimm C, Osiewacz HD (2016) Molecular control of fungal senescence and longevity. In: Wendland J (ed) The Mycota I, growth, differentiation and sexuality, 3rd edn. Springer, Switzerland, 155–181

11. Knuppertz L, Osiewacz HD (2016) Orchestrating the network of molecular pathways affecting aging: Role of nonselective autophagy and mitophagy. Mech Ageing Dev 153:30–40

12. Silar P, Lalucque H, Vierny C (2001) Cell degeneration in the model system *Podospora anserina*. Biogerontology 2:1–17

13. Knuppertz L, Hamann A, Pampaloni F, Stelzer E, Osiewacz HD (2014) Identification of autophagy as a longevity-assurance mechanism in the aging model *Podospora anserina*. Autophagy 10(5):822–834

14. Gitai Z (2009) New fluorescence microscopy methods for microbiology: sharper, faster, and quantitative. Curr Opin Microbiol 12:341–346

15. Kentner D, Sourjik V (2010) Use of fluorescence microscopy to study intracellular signaling in bacteria. Annu Rev Microbiol 64:373–390

16. Thorn K (2016) A quick guide to light microscopy in cell biology. Mol Biol Cell 27:219–222

17. Toomre D, Pawley J (2006) Disk-scanning confocal microscopy, Handb Biol confocal Microsc. Springer, New York, pp. 221–238

18. Carlton PM, Boulanger J, Kervrann C, Sibarita JB, Salamero J, Gordon-Messer S et al (2010) Fast live simultaneous multiwavelength four-dimensional optical microscopy. Proc Natl Acad Sci 107(37):16016–16022

19. Huisken J, Swoger J, Del Bene F, Wittbrodt J, Stelzer EHK (2004) Optical sectioning deep inside live embryos by selective plane illumination microscopy. Science 305:1007–1009

20. Keller PJ, Schmidt AD, Wittbrodt J, Stelzer EHK (2008) Reconstruction of zebrafish early embryonic development by scanned light sheet microscopy. Science 322:1065–1069

21. Keller PJ, Stelzer EH (2008) Quantitative in vivo imaging of entire embryos with digital scanned laser light sheet fluorescence microscopy. Curr Opin Neurobiol 18(6):624–632

22. Liu Z, Keller PJ (2016) Emerging Imaging and Genomic Tools for Developmental Systems Biology. Dev Cell 36:597–610

23. Keller PJ et al (2010) Fast, high-contrast imaging of animal development with scanned light sheet-based structured-illumination microscopy. Nat Methods 7:637–642

24. Maizel A, von Wangenheim D, Federici F, Haseloff J, Stelzer EHK (2011) High-resolution live imaging of plant growth in near physiological bright conditions using light sheet fluorescence microscopy. Plant J 68:377–385

25. Strobl F, Schmitz A, Stelzer EHK (2015) Live imaging of *Tribolium castaneum* embryonic development using light-sheet-based fluorescence microscopy. Nat Protoc 10:1486–1507

26. Strobl F, Stelzer EHK (2014) Non-invasive long-term fluorescence live imaging of *Tribolium castaneum* embryos. Development 141:2331–2338

27. Pampaloni F, Ansari N, Stelzer EHK (2013) High-resolution deep imaging of live cellular spheroids with light-sheet-based fluorescence microscopy. Cell Tissue Res 352:161–177

28. Pampaloni F, Berge U, Marmaras A, Horvath P, Kroschewski R, Stelzer EH (2014) Tissue-culture light sheet fluorescence microscopy (TC-LSFM) allows long-term imaging of three-dimensional cell cultures under controlled conditions. Integr Biol 6(10):988–998

29. Pampaloni F, Chang B-J, Stelzer EHK (2015) Light sheet-based fluorescence microscopy (LSFM) for the quantitative imaging of cells and tissues. Cell Tissue Res 360:129–141

30. Pampaloni, F., Richa, R., Ansari, N., & Stelzer, E. H. (2015). Live spheroid formation recorded with light sheet-based fluorescence microscopy. Advanced fluorescence microscopy: methods and protocols. 43–57.

31. Pampaloni F, Reynaud EG, Stelzer EHK (2007) The third dimension bridges the gap between cell culture and live tissue. Nat Rev Mol Cell Biol 8:839–845

32. Greger K, Swoger J, Stelzer EHK (2007) Basic building units and properties of a fluorescence single plane illumination microscope. Rev Sci Instrum 78(2):023705

33. Huisken J, Stainier DYR (2007) Even fluorescence excitation by multidirectional selective plane illumination microscopy (mSPIM). Opt Lett 32(17):2608

34. Hyde J, MacNicol M, Odle A, Garcia-Rill E (2014) The use of three-dimensional printing to produce in vitro slice chambers. J Neurosci Methods 238:82–87

Chapter 3

Light-Sheet Fluorescence Microscopy: Chemical Clearing and Labeling Protocols for Ultramicroscopy

Nina Jährling, Klaus Becker, Saiedeh Saghafi, and Hans-Ulrich Dodt

Abstract

Light-sheet microscopy is an effective technique in neuroscience, developmental biology, and cancer research for visualizing and analyzing cellular networks and whole organs in three dimensions. Because this technique requires specimens to be translucent they commonly have to be cleared before microscopy inspection. Here, we provide 3DISCO based protocols for preparing cleared samples of immuno-stained neural networks, lectin-labeled vascular networks, and Methoxy-X04 labeled beta-amyloid plaques in mice. 3DISCO utilizes the lipophilic solvents tetrahydrofuran (THF) and dibenzylether (DBE) for dehydration and successive clearing. Crucial steps for obtaining transparent tissues and preserving the fragile endogenous GFP are the transcardial perfusion, as well as the proper implementation of the 3DISCO clearing process using peroxide free chemicals. We further provide a protocol for resin embedding of 3DISCO cleared specimens that allows long term archiving of samples for years with virtually no loss in signal quality.

Key words Chemical clearing, Whole-mount immune-labeling, Vascular networks, Light-sheet microscopy, 3D reconstruction, 3DISCO, Peroxide elimination, Alzheimer disease

1 Introduction

In the last decade novel developments in light-sheet microscopy gave new impulses to biological sciences [1]. One implementation of light sheet microscopy is ultramicroscopy (UM), which allows 3D reconstructions of up to centimeter-sized specimens with micrometer resolution [2]. In UM the specimens are illuminated perpendicular to the observation pathway by two opposed sheets of laser light, which are formed by optical elements (*see* Fig. 1). This allows very large fields of views together with excellent optical sectioning capabilities. It has been demonstrated that via UM neuronal and vascular networks in entire mouse brains can be imaged with cellular resolution, including their far ranging axonal connections of up to several millimeters length [2, 3].

Since it is essential for light sheet microscopy that the specimens are transparent, chemical clearing of the samples usually is required. One of the first tissue clearing approaches was developed

Yolanda Markaki and Hartmann Harz (eds.), *Light Microscopy: Methods and Protocols*, Methods in Molecular Biology, vol. 1563,
DOI 10.1007/978-1-4939-6810-7_3, © Springer Science+Business Media LLC 2017

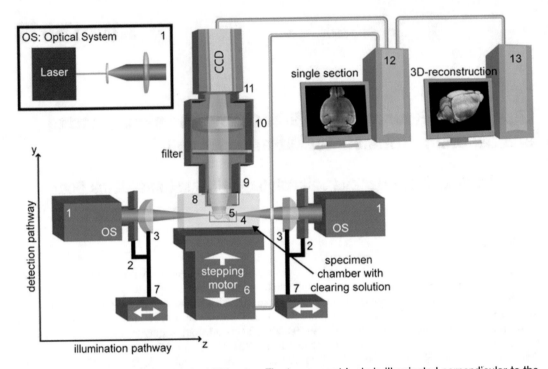

Fig. 1 UM-setup. Principle of a standard UM-setup. The transparent brain is illuminated perpendicular to the observation pathway by a thin sheet of light formed by a laser and cylindrical lenses placed left and right from the specimen container. The fluorescence light that is exited in the specimen is projected to a camera target via an objective. Scattered excitation light is blocked by a matched optical band-pass filter. By stepwise moving the specimen through the light sheet a stack of images is recorded. *1*. Optical system (OS), which generates an expanded laser beam with a truncated Gaussian intensity profile. *2*. Rectangular-slit aperture. *3*. Cylindrical lens, *4*. Clamp for holding the specimen, *5*. Sample. *6*. computer-controlled z-stage *7*. Computer-controlled linear stages for adjusting the position of the cylinder lenses. *8*. Immersion cap. *9*. Objective. *10*. Tube lens. *11*. Camera target. *12*, Computer for controlling the setup. *13* Computer for 3D image reconstruction. Published in Jährling et al. (2015), Cerebral β-amyloidosis in mice investigated by ultramicroscopy. PLoS ONE 10(5): e0125418. doi:10.1371/journal.pone.0125418

about 100 years ago by the German anatomist Werner Spalteholz [4]. Spalteholz discovered that the incubation of biological tissues in a medium of similar refractive index than proteins (usually between 1.5 and 1.6 if the samples are dehydrated) markedly reduces light scattering and leads to translucent, or even fully transparent samples assumed that the light absorption by chromophores is not too high. Spalteholz systematically screened various organic solvents for their potential to make isolated organs from humans and animals transparent. He developed a mixture containing about five volume parts methyl salicylate and three volume parts benzyl benzoate, which he successfully applied for the clearing of even very large anatomical samples, as the human heart. However, due to the lack of powerful 3D microscopy techniques, as confocal or light sheet microscopy, during this time Spalteholz clearing never became common in the field of microscopy.

Later BABB, also termed "Murray's clear," became a standard for clearing biological samples in the field of microscopy [5, 6]. It consists of a mixture of 1 vol. part benzyl alcohol (BA) and 2 vol. parts benzyl benzoate (BB). BABB clearing generally provides good specimen transparency at moderate incubation times of usually not more than several days [2]. However, highly depending on the incubation times, it can cause severe bleaching of GFP and other endogenous marker proteins, especially if it is not free of peroxides [7]. This is a severe drawback, since GFP is one of the most important labeling tools in light microscopy, which allows highly specific fluorescence staining of anatomical structures that are expressed under the control of a distinct reporter gene. However, if the GFP expression rates are high enough, and the exposure times are kept as short as possible, it nevertheless can be used for clearing of GFP expressing mouse brains or embryos [2].

Due to the limited compatibility of BABB with endogenous fluorescence markers as GFP, Becker et al. [7] and Ertürk et al. [8] developed the 3DISCO (*3-D*imensional *I*maging of *S*olvent-*C*leared *O*rgans) clearing approach. In 3DISCO benzyl alcohol and benzyl benzoate are replaced by dibenzylether (DBE). Furthermore, the standard dehydration medium ethanol that also significantly impairs the fluorescence of GFP is substituted by the cyclic ether tetrahydrofuran. With $n = 1.561$ DBE has a slightly higher refractive index than BABB ($n = 1.559$). Additionally to the improved GFP preservation, DBE provides a somewhat faster tissue penetration compared to BABB, and last but not least is cheaper and less toxic [7].

The transcardial perfusion and fixation with phosphate buffered saline (PBS) followed by 4 % formaldehyde is a crucial step during animal preparation having a major effect on the quality of the cleared samples. Typical sources of errors during the fixation perfusion that can be avoided with some practice are uncomplete flushing out the blood volume, formation of air bubbles, or insufficient perfusion times.

Although in the recent years several water based clearing solutions, e.g., Sca/e [9], CLARITY [10], or CUBIC [11], have been developed, which require no tissue dehydration step, solvent based clearing methods still are a good choice for many applications since they are fast, uncomplicated to handle and usually provide excellent clearing results even with large and/or highly myelinated tissues as entire brains or spinal cords from mice. Especially for such samples the clearing results obtained by hydrophilic (water based) clearing solutions often are poor.

It is important that DBE used for clearing of fluorescence labeled samples is free from contaminations with peroxides and aldehydes, since both compounds efficiently quench fluorescence already in minute concentrations (>1 mg/L) [12]. Ether peroxides are formed by exposure to oxygen. Under the influence of light they react further to benzaldehyde [13] being also a fluorescence quencher for GFP. Benzaldehyde contaminations in DBE being stored for a prolonged time can be detected by a characteristic bitter-almond like odor, or using Brady's test for aldehydes [14]. Depending on the manufacturer and the lot number, DBE can contain significant peroxide concentrations >1 mg/l already at time of purchase, making it unsuitable for clearing GFP expressing samples without prior purification. Peroxides can be easily detected for example using Quantofix 25 test stripes (Sigma-Aldrich Austria, Order no. Z249254). The test stripes are briefly dipped into the clearing solution and shortly rinsed under a water tap. Peroxides are indicated by a blue coloration appearing after a few seconds.

To remove peroxide and aldehyde contaminations in DBE and BABB absorption column chromatography with activated basic aluminum oxide (basic activated Brockman 1, Sigma-Aldrich, Order no. 199443) can be applied as described in [7]. The generation of peroxides in purified DBE can be slowed down by using brown bottles that are filled with an inert gas as argon.

Here we present clearing protocols for 3DISCO clearing of murine tissues, whole-mount immunostaining of the neuronal networks in mouse embryos [15], lectin-labeling of vascular networks [16], and staining of beta-amyloidosis using methoxy-X04 labeling [17].

For long term archiving of the cleared samples we describe a protocol for resin embedding allowing a virtually unlimited storage of these samples with virtually no fluorescence bleaching [18]. For comfortably mounting specimens for UM inspection custom made clamps made from polyoxymethylene (POM) that prevent them from moving in the specimen chamber have been proofed to be useful. We present some technical drawings describing the fabrication of such clamps that have been proved to work well in practice.

2   Materials

Prepare and store all reagents at room temperature unless indicated otherwise.

2.1   Intra-Cardiac Perfusion and Fixation of Mice (Quantity per Mouse)

1. 40 ml phosphate buffered saline (PBS) containing 1000 units/ml heparin pH 7.4 (*see* **Note 1**).

2. 100 ml 4 % freshly prepared paraformaldehyde solution (PFA), pH 7.4 (*see* **Note 1**).

3. 30 ml 4 % ice-cold (4 °C) paraformaldehyde solution, pH 8.2 (*see* **Note 1**).

2.2   Peroxide Elimination in THF

Chemicals

1. Tetrahydrofuran (THF, Sigma-Aldrich, 186562).

2. Aluminum oxide Brockmann I, basic-activated (Sigma-Aldrich, 199443).

3. Butyl hydroxyl toluene (BHT), (Sigma-Aldrich, W218405).

4. Calcium chloride, water free (Sigma-Aldrich, C1016).

5. Quantofix Peroxide 25 test stripes (Sigma-Aldrich, Z249254).

6. Argon gas.

Lab Equipment

1. Storage bottles from brown glass.

2. Dropping funnel with pressure compensation.

3. Chromatography column (30–50 cm long).

4. Two-necked round bottom flask.

5. Drying tube from plastic.

6. Rubber and glass joints.

7. Silicon tubes.

2.3 Peroxide Elimination in DBE

Chemicals

1. Aluminum oxide (basic-activated, Brockmann I grade, Sigma-Aldrich 19,943)

2. Dibenzylether (DBE, Sigma-Aldrich, 108014).

3. Molecular sieve (3 Å mesh, Sigma-Aldrich, 208582).

4. Quantofix peroxide 25 test stripes (Sigma-Aldrich, Z249254).

Lab Equipment

1. Storage bottles from brown glass.

2. Büchner funnel with filter plate of 16–40 μm pore width.

3. Vaccum-tight filtering flask.

4. Silicon tubes and joints.

5. Vacuum pump (e.g., Laboport, KNF, USA).

2.4 Chemicals for Clearing of Mouse Brains and Hippocampi

1. PBS 10 mM (Dulbecco, Biochrom AG, Germany, L182).

2. Peroxide-free tetrahydrofuran.

3. Peroxide-free DBE.

2.5 Chemicals for Clearing of Mouse Spinal Cord/Brain Stem

1. PBS 10 mM (Dulbecco, Biochrom AG, Germany, L182).

2. 4 % freshly prepared paraformaldehyde (PFA).

3. Peroxide-free tetrahydrofuran.

4. Peroxide-free DBE.

5. Dichloromethane (DCM) (Sigma-Aldrich, 270997).

2.6 Chemicals for Clearing of Drosophila melanogaster

1. 4 % freshly prepared PFA.
2. Ethanol puriss., absolute 99.5 % (Sigma-Aldrich, Germany, 0274380).
3. Benzylalcohol (Sigma-Aldrich, Germany, 24122).
4. Benzylbenzoate (Sigma-Aldrich, Germany, B6630).

2.7 Whole-Mount Immunohisto-chemistry of Mouse Embryos

1. DENT's Fix: 80 % methanol and 20 % dimethyl sulfoxide (DMSO) [5].
2. DENT's Bleach: 1 part 30 % hydrogen peroxide H_2O_2 and two parts DENT's Fix [5].
3. Tris-buffered saline (TBS).
4. Anti-neurofilament-160 antibody (monoclonal, clone NN18, Sigma-Aldrich, Germany) diluted 1:200 in blocking serum consisting of four parts calf serum and one part dimethyl sulfoxide (v/v).
5. Goat anti-mouse antibodies conjugated to Alexa 488 (Invitrogen, USA) diluted in 1:200 in blocking serum.
6. Ethanol puriss. Absolute, 99.5 % (Sigma-Aldrich, Germany, 0274380) (see **Note 2**).

2.8 Lectin-Labeling of Murine Tissues (See Note 3)

1. 5 ml PBS containing 20 μl/ml heparin.
2. 10 ml 1 % PFA in PBS.
3. 10 ml PBS containing 10 μg FITC from *Lycopersicon esculentum* (Sigma-Aldrich, Germany, L0401) per ml PBS.
4. PBS (Dulbecco, Biochrom AG, Germany, L182).
5. 4 % freshly prepared PFA in PBS.
6. Ethanol or peroxide-free THF.

2.9 Methoxy-X04-Labeling

1. 75 μl of 10 mg/ml methoxy-X04 [19] in dimethyl sulfoxide.
2. PBS.
3. 4 Vol% fresh paraformaldehyde PFA in PBS.
4. Peroxide-free THF.
5. Peroxide-free DBE.

2.10 Resin Embedding of Cleared Samples

1. Silastic E-RTV silicone rubber (Dow Corning, Germany).
2. Custom made casting frames from acrylic glass (Acrylic Glass GS, Senova GmbH, Austria) [18].
3. Resin Component A: 11.5 ml D.E.R. 332 (bisphenol-A diglycidyl ether, Sigma Aldrich Austria, 31185) at 50 °C.
4. Resin Component B: 3.5 ml D.E.R. 736 (polypropylene glycol diglycidyl ether, Sigma-Aldrich Austria, 31191).
5. Resin Component C: 3 ml isophorone diamine (IPDA, 5-amino-1,3,3-trimethylcyclohexanemethylamine, Sigma-Aldrich, Austria, 118184) (see **Note 4**).

2.11 Custom-Made Clamps Specimen Fixation Clamps

1. Block of polyoxymethylene (POM) (*see* **Note 5**).
2. 2× screws (plastic material or made of steel with plastic heads).

3 Methods

3.1 Perfusion and Fixation Procedure (See Fig. 2)

1. Kill mice with carbon dioxide and immediately fix them in dorsal position (*see* **Note 6**).
2. Open the chest and excise the diaphragm.
3. Expose the heart.
4. Make a small incision in the cardiac apex using fine scissors.
5. Insert a blunt cannula into the left heart ventricle.
6. Move the cannula carefully into the *aorta ascendens*. Fix the position of the needle using fine hemostatic forceps. Connect the cannula with a flexible tube.
7. Insert the tube to the rolls of peristaltic pump (e.g., ISM796B, Ismatec, Germany)
8. Insert the other end of the tube into to a container filled with PBS plus heparin.
9. Make a cut in the right auricle appendage.
10. Start the pump to drain the blood out of the mouse body (*see* **Note 7**).
11. Perfuse at least 30 ml PBS pH 8.2 to rinse out the blood, completely.
12. Perfuse 100 ml 4 % PFA pH 8.2 for fixation.

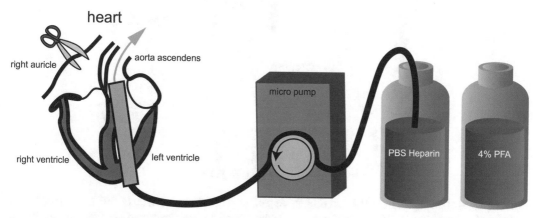

Fig. 2 Transcardial perfusion fixation. A fine cannula is inserted from the cardiac apex into the heart and then carefully pushed into the *aorta ascendens*. After cutting the right auricle appendage using fine scissors, the blood is drained out of the mouse body via a peristaltic pump. Afterwards, fixation is started by perfusion of to 4 Vol% PFA

3.2 Dissection and Post Fixation

1. Carefully remove the organs of interest from the body. For removing the brain first expose the calvarial bone by carefully cutting along the sagittal suture.

2. Immediately post-fix the organs in 4 % PFA at 4 °C overnight. For better diffusion of the fixation medium place the sample tubes on a shaker.

3.3 Removing Peroxides from Clearing Chemicals

Peroxide removal in THF is done by column absorption chromatography with basic activated aluminum oxide activity grade Brockman I (Sigma-Aldrich, Austria, Order no. 199443, about 250 g per liter THF) (*see* Fig. 3 *left*). The stabilizer, which is contained in commercially distributed THF is also removed during chromatography. This stabilizer is required to prevent the generation of dangerous amounts of peroxides by sunlight or exposure to oxygen. Therefore, it is essential by safety reasons to substitute it, e.g., by adding 250 mg/l butyl hydroxyl toluol (BHT) into the receiver flask (Sigma-Aldrich, Austria, Order no. W218405). THF which is insufficiently stabilized can explode after prolonged exposure to oxygen and/or sunlight and may be life threatening!

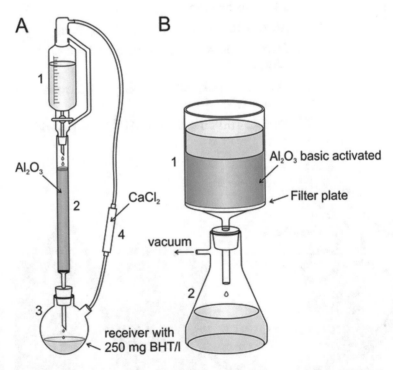

Fig. 3 Removal of peroxides from THF and DBE. (**a**) Apparatus for peroxide cleaning of THF *1*: Dropping funnel with pressure compensation. *2*. Chromatography column filled with basic activated aluminum oxide. *3*. Two necked round bottom flask. *4*. Drying tube filled with calcium chloride. (**b**) Apparatus for peroxide removal in DBE and BABB *1*: Filter unit with filter plate (16–40 μm pore size). *2*. Vacuum tight filtering flask. Figure from Becker K et al. (2012), Chemical clearing and dehydration of GFP expressing mouse brains. PLoS ONE 7(3): e33916. doi:10.1371/journal.pone.0033916

Due to their higher viscosity and boiling points, removal of peroxides in BABB and DBE can be done by vacuum filtering. The filter funnel is filled with ~250 g activated aluminum oxide per liter and suction is applied to the receiver flask (*see* Fig. 3 *right*).

3.4 Chemical Clearing of Mouse Organs

1. Wash the brains 3× in PBS for 30 min each.

2. If required, split the fixed brains along the median line into hemispheres.

3.4.1 Entire Mouse Brains

3. Incubate the entire brains/brain hemispheres in an ascending row of THF concentrations (50, 70, 80, 96 Vol%, 3× 100 Vol, 12 h each step) (*see* **Note 8**).

4. Incubated the samples 1–2 days in peroxide free DBE until they become transparent. To improve the diffusion of the clearing medium place the samples on a shaker.

3.4.2 Entire Mouse Brains (Short Protocol) [8]

1. Incubate the brains successively in 50, 70, 80, 100 Vol% peroxide free THF for 12 h each.

2. The next day incubate them in 100 Vol% peroxide free THF for 1 h.

3. Incubate the brains for 3 h in peroxide free DBE.

3.4.3 Dissected Mouse Hippocampi [7]

1. Prepare mouse brains as described in Subheading 3.1.

2. Dissect the hippocampi under a binocular and store them in 4 Vol% PFA for post fixation overnight.

3. Incubate them 3 times in PBS, 15 min each step.

4. Dehydrate them using 50, 80, 96, 100 Vol% THF (1 h each step, last step overnight).

3.4.4 Brain Stem

1. Incubate brain stems in 50, 70, 80 Vol%, 2× 100 % THF for 1 h each.

2. Incubate the brain stems for 45 min in dichloromethane.

3. Incubate the brain stems for at least 30 min in peroxide free DBE until they become clear.

3.4.5 Spinal Cord (See Fig. 4)

1. Incubate spinal cords in 50, 70, 80 Vol%, 3× 100 Vol%.THF (30 min each step).

2. Incubate spinal cords in dichloromethane for 20 min.

3. Incubate spinal cords for at least 30 min in peroxide free DBE until they become clear.

3.5 Fixation and Chemical Clearing Procedure for Drosophila a melanogaster [20] (See Fig. 5)

1. Kill adult white eyed *Drosophila* with ether and fix them in 4 % PFA overnight (*see* **Note 9**).

2. Dehydrate the flies in a graded ethanol series (50, 70, 96, 100 %, 1 h each step, last step overnight).

3. Incubate the flies in BABB for at least 4 h until they are transparent.

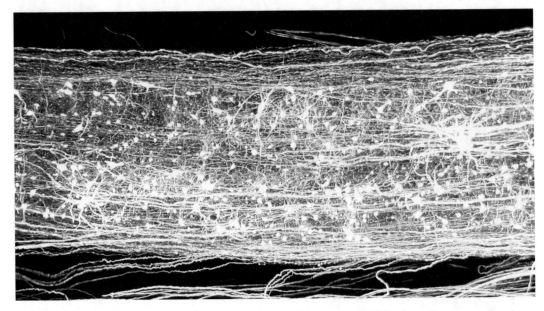

Fig. 4 3D reconstruction from spinal cord (GFP-mouse line). Spinal cord of a GFP expressing mouse. Specimen was cleared using 3DISCO and recorded by UM using a 4× objective, NA 0.28

3.6 Whole-Mount Immunohisto-chemistry of Mouse Embryos [21]

1. Fix mouse embryos in DENT's fix overnight.
2. Bleach them in DENT's Bleach overnight.
3. Wash them three times in TBS.
4. Rinse them in the primary antibody solution for 2 days at room temperature.
5. Wash the embryos three times in TBS for 1 h each. Then transfer them into the secondary antibody solution.
6. Dehydrate the embryos in an ascending ethanol series (50, 70, 80, 96 %, 3× 100 %, 2 h each, last step overnight). To enhance diffusion of the dehydration medium place the vials on a shaker.
7. Incubate them for at least 2 days in BABB or DBE until they become transparent.

3.7 Lectin-Labeling for Staining of Vascular Networks [16] (See Note 3) (See Fig. 6)

1. Kill mice and perfuse them transcardially with 5 ml PB plus heparin until the fluid becomes clear (*see* **Note 7**).
2. Perfuse them with 1 % PFA for pre-fixation.
3. Perfuse 10 ml PBS with 20 μl/ml FITC-Lectin.
4. After 2 min incubation perfuse further 30 ml 4 % PFA.
5. Remove the brains from the scull and incubate them in 4 % PFA at 4 °C for 4 h.
6. Rinse the brains three times with PBS.
7. Dehydrate and clear the brains according to Subheading 3.4.1.

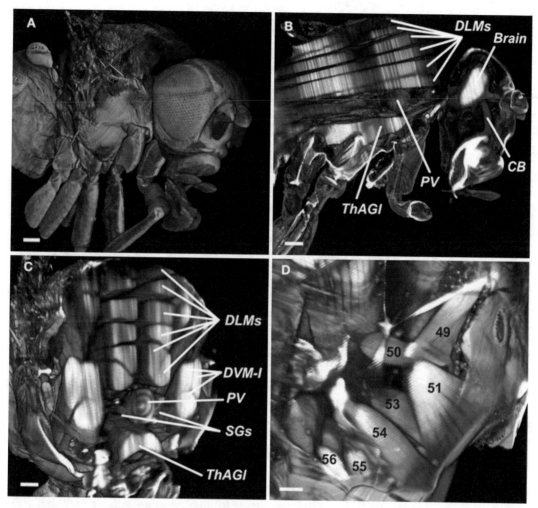

Fig. 5 3D reconstruction from Drosophila. (**a**) Reconstructed surface of an entire fly. Scale bar 100 μm. (**b**) Sagittal view of the fly's inner anatomy, showing parts of the flight muscles, the nervous, and the cardiac system. *DLMs* dorsal longitudinal muscles, *ThAGl* thoracico-abdominal ganglion, *PV* proventriculus, *CB* cibarium. Scale bar: 100 μm. (**c**) Detail of the fly virtually sectioned along a transversal plane through the thorax. *DVM-I* dorsal–ventral muscles, *SGs* salivary glands. Scale bar: 100 μm. (**d**) Detail showing the direct flight muscles DFM49–DFM56. DFM52 is only rudimentarily visible, because it is clipped by the viewing plane. Scale bar 40 μm. Figure as originally published in Jährling et al. 2010, Three-dimensional reconstruction and segmentation of intact *Drosophila* by ultramicroscopy. Front Syst Neurosci 8; 4: 1, doi: 103,389/neuro.06.001.210

3.8 Methoxy-X04-Labeling for Amyloid Plaque Staining [17] (See Fig. 7)

1. Intraperitoneally inject mice with methoxy-X04 in solved in dimethyl sulfoxide. Repeat the injection after 24 h (*see* **Note 6**).

2. Two hours after the last injection animals deeply anesthetize the animals by intraperitoneal injection with ketamine/xylazine (*see* **Note 6**).

3. Transcardially perfused the mice with PBS followed by 4 % PFA in PBS (for details *see* Subheading 3.1).

4. Remove and fix the brains according to Subheading 3.2.

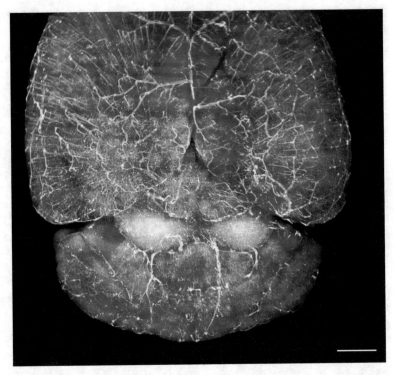

Fig. 6 Lectin Labeling. 3D-reconstruction vascular networks in a lectin-labeled mouse brain using maximum intensity projection. The reconstruction was obtained from 567 images deconvolved with Huygens software. Scale bar 1000 μm. Reprinted from Jährling et al. (2009), Organogenesis 5:4, 227–230; October/November/December 2009; © 2009 Landes Bioscience

5. Wash the brains three times in PBS for 1 h each.

6. Dehydrated the brains in an ascending series of ethanol (50, 70, 80 %, 96 for 24 h, 4×, each step for 24 h).

7. Incubate the brains in BABB until they became transparent.

3.9 Resin Embedding of Cleared Samples for Long Time Storage [18]

3.9.1 Fabrication of Embedding Molds

Fabricate embedding molds from silicone rubber (e.g., Silastic E-RTV, Dow Corning, Germany [22]) using custom made casting frames made from Plexiglas (*see* Fig. 8). Cure the silicone rubber for 2 h at 80 °C. Remove the molds from the casting frames on the next day.

3.9.2 Resin Embedding of Specimens

1. Mix the resin components (A + B + C) carefully in a 50 ml falcon cube. Component should be heated at 50 °C before use since it crystallizes at room temperature.

2. Degas the resin mixture in a vacuum chamber at about 100 mbar for 60 min for degassing (*see* **Note 10**).

3. Take the specimen out of the clearing solution and remove the liquid from the surface by gently dabbing on a sheet of soft tissue.

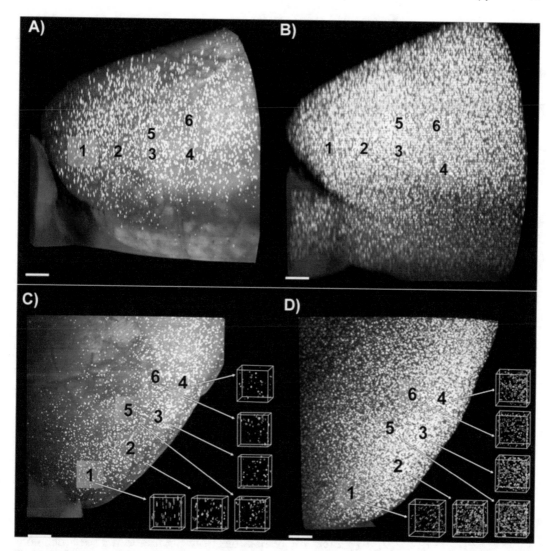

Fig. 7 Cerebral beta-amyloidosis (*yellow dots*) in the left hemisphere of the frontal cortex of two age groups of the APPPS 1 mouse model. Comparison between a young (2.3-month-old) and an adult (7.5-month-old) APPPS1 brain. 3D reconstructions demonstrate an age-related increase in β-amyloid plaques. The maximum intensity projections of reconstructed images confirm a higher plaque density with increasing age. (**a**) Typical image obtained from a young mouse (2.7-month-old). (**b**) Typical image obtained from an adult mouse (7.8-month-old). Six probing cubes (*purple color*) were virtually placed in the frontal cortex for measuring the β-amyloid plaque numbers and volumes via a threshold segmentation technique. (**c, d**) Top view of the frontal cortex: example from the young group (**c**) and old group (**d**). After segmentation amyloid plaque volumes of the six cubed shaped areas are represented in various *colors*. Scale bar 500 μm. Published in Jährling et al. (2015), Cerebral β-amyloidosis in mice investigated by ultramicroscopy. PLoS ONE 10(5): e0125418. doi:10.1371/journal.pone.0125418

4. Incubate the specimens in a small volume of the degassed resin mixture for about 15 min.

5. Fill the molds (*see* **Note 11**) to about one third with the resin mixture and embed the specimens.

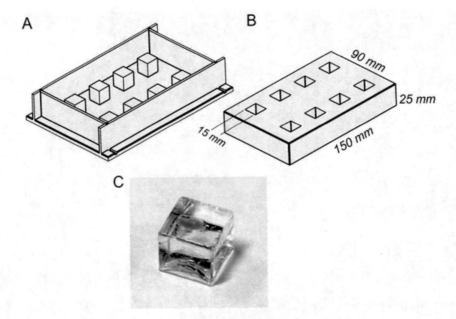

Fig. 8 Fabrication of resin embedding molds. (**a**) Casting frame made from acrylic glass. (**b**) Silicon rubber mold. (**c**) Cured resin block with an embedded cleared mouse brain hemisphere. Figure from Becker et al. (2014), Reduction of photo bleaching and long term archiving of chemically cleared GFP-expressing mouse brains. PLoS ONE 9(12): e114149. doi:10.1371/journal.pone.0114149

6. Fill up the molds completely with resin mixture.

7. If necessary carefully adjust the specimens position using an injection cannula.

8. Cure the resin blocks in the dark at room temperature for at least 2 days.

9. To protect the resin cubes from floating in the specimen container used for light sheet microscopy glue them on little metal plates using silicone glue.

3.10 Custom-Made Clamps for Fixing the Samples

A mechanic workshop can produce custom-made clamps from POM according to the technical drawings presented in Fig. 9 (*see* **Note 12**). Unlike for example PVC, POM is resistant against DBE or BABB.

4   Notes

1. To improve fluorescence preservation of GFP the pH of the buffer and fixation solutions can be adjusted to more basic values of about 8.2 [23, 24].

2. Instead of ethanol also THF can be used as a dehydration medium.

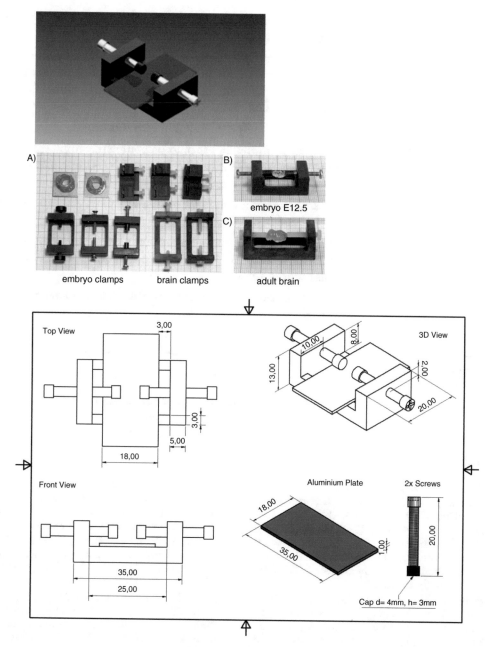

Fig. 9 Custom-made sample clamp. Photos and technical drawings from custom-made specimen clamps. The clamps can be made from POM by a mechanical workshop

3. This protocol is for young mice (6-week-old). For older animals the volume of all reagents should be twice.

4. The resin component C should be stored under an inert gas as argon to protect it from oxygen.

5. POM should be used since it is resistant to DBE and BABB.

6. All animal preparation must be performed according to the animal protection regulations of your country.

7. By controlling the stiffness of the tail and the increasing discoloration of the liver the progress of fixation can be controlled. Further signs of successful perfusion are the white discolorations of ears and nose.

8. In Ertürk et al. [8] the 96 % Vol step is omitted.

9. During fixation the flies should be completely immersed in the fixation medium. This can be achieved by adding a few drops of ethanol to the fixation medium.

10. This step is essential to achieve best possible optical properties of the cured resin block.

11. Square molds of 15 mm × 15 mm are recommended for mouse brains and 10 × 10 mm are recommended for embedding mouse hippocampi.

12. In order to avoid light reflections black plastic material should be used.

Acknowledgment

We thank Massih Foroughipour for preparing the technical drawings of the custom-made specimen clamps.

References

1. Keller PJ, Dodt HU (2012) Light sheet microscopy of living or cleared specimens. Curr Opin Neurobiol 22:138–143

2. Dodt H-U, Leischner U, Schierloh A et al (2007) Ultramicroscopy: three-dimensional visualization of neuronal networks in the whole mouse brain. Nat Methods 4:331–336. doi:10.1038/nmeth1036

3. Ertürk A, Mauch CP, Hellal F et al (2011) Three-dimensional imaging of the unsectioned adult spinal cord to assess axon regeneration and glial responses after injury. Nat Med 18:166–171. doi:10.1038/nm.2600

4. Spalteholz W (1911) Über das Durchsichtigmachen von menschlichen und tierischen Präparaten 48

5. Dent JA, Polson AG, Klymkowsky MW (1989) A whole-mount immunocytochemical analysis of the expression of the intermediate filament protein vimentin in Xenopus. Development 105:61–74

6. Klymkowsky MW, Hanken J (1991) Whole-mount staining of Xenopus and other vertebrates. Methods Cell Biol 36:419–441

7. Becker K, Jährling N, Saghafi S, et al. (2012) Chemical clearing and dehydration of GFP expressing mouse brains. PLoSOne 7:e33916–. doi: 10.1371/journal.pone.0033916

8. Ertürk A, Becker K, Jährling N et al (2012) Three-dimensional imaging of solvent-cleared organs using 3DISCO. Nat Protoc 7:1983–1995. doi:10.1038/nprot.2012.119

9. Hama H, Kurokawa H, Kawano H, Ryoko A et al (2011) Sca/e: a chemical approach for fluorescene imaging and reconstruction of transparent mouse brain. Nat Neurosci 14:1481–1488

10. Chung K, Wallace J, Kim S-Y et al (2013) Structural and molecular interrogation of intact biological systems. Nature 497:332–337. doi:10.1038/nature12107

11. Susaki EA, Tainaka K, Perrin D et al (2014) Whole-brain imaging with single-cell resolution using chemical cocktails and computational analysis. Cell 157:726–739. doi:10.1016/j.cell.2014.03.042

12. Alnuami AA, Zeedi B, Qadri SM, Ashraf SS (2008) Oxyradical-induced GFP damage and

loss of fluorescence. Int J Biol Macromol 43:182–186

13. Eichel FG, Othmer DF (1949) Benzaldehyde by Autoxidation by Dibenzyl Ether. Ind Eng Chem 41:2623–2626. doi:10.1021/ie50479a054

14. Brady OL, v.Elsmie G (1926) The use of 2 : P-Dinitrophenylhydrazine as a reagent for aldehydes and ketones. Analyst 51:77–78.

15. Becker K, Jahrling N, Kramer ER et al (2008) Ultramicroscopy: 3D reconstruction of large microscopical specimens. J Biophotonics 1:36–42

16. Jährling N, Becker K, Dodt H (2009) 3D-reconstruction of blood vessels by ultramicroscopy. Organogenesis 5(4):227–230

17. Jährling N, Becker K, Wegenast-braun BM, Grathwohl SA (2015) Cerebral β -Amyloidosis in Mice Investigated by Ultramicroscopy. pp 1–13. doi: 10.1371/journal.pone.0125418

18. Becker K, Hahn CM, Saghafi S, Ja N (2014) Reduction of photo bleaching and long term archiving of chemically cleared GFP-expressing mouse brains. pp 1–11. doi: 10.1371/journal.pone.0114149

19. Klunk WE, Bacskai BJ, Mathis CA et al (2002) Imaging Abeta plaques in living transgenic mice with multiphoton microscopy and methoxy-X04, a systemically administered Congo red derivative. J Neuropathol Exp Neurol 61:797–805

20. Jährling N, Becker K, Schönbauer C et al (2010) Three-dimensional reconstruction and segmentation of intact Drosophila by ultramicroscopy. Front Syst Neurosci 4:1. doi:10.3389/neuro.06.001.2010

21. Jährling N, Becker K, Kramer ER, Dodt H-U (2008) 3D-Visualization of nerve fiber bundles by ultramicroscopy. Med Laser Appl 23:209–215. doi:10.1016/j.mla.2008.06.001

22. Cavey MJ, Wong GK-S (1993) Custom silicone rubber molds for epoxy resin embedding. Trans Am Microsc Soc 112:81–84

23. Enoki S, Saeki K, Maki K, Kuwajima K (2004) Acid denaturation and refolding of green fluorescent protein. Biochemistry 43:14238–14248. doi:10.1021/bi048733+

24. Schwarz MK, Scherbarth A, Sprengel R et al (2015) Fluorescent-protein stabilization and high-resolution imaging of cleared, intact mouse brains. PLoS One 10:e0124650. doi:10.1371/journal.pone.0124650

Chapter 4

Two-Photon Intravital Microscopy Animal Preparation Protocol to Study Cellular Dynamics in Pathogenesis

Erinke van Grinsven*, Chloé Prunier*, Nienke Vrisekoop*, and Laila Ritsma*

Abstract

Two-photon intravital microscopy (2P-IVM) is an advanced imaging platform that allows the visualization of dynamic processes at subcellular resolution in vivo. Dynamic processes like cell migration, cell proliferation, cell–cell interactions, and cell signaling have an interactive character and occur in complex environments. Hence, it is of pivotal importance to study these processes in living animals, using for example 2P-IVM. 2P-IVM can be performed on a variety of tissues, from the skin of the animal to internal organs, and a variety of methods can be utilized to perform 2P-IVM on these tissues. Here, we discuss the protocols and considerations for four of those 2P-IVM methods, namely tissue explant imaging, skin imaging, surgical exposure imaging, and multi-day window imaging. We carefully compare and explain in depth how to set up each method. Lastly, in the notes section we mention some alternative solutions for the 2P-IVM methods described. In conclusion, this protocol can be used as a guide towards deciding which 2P-IVM method to use and to enable the setup of this method.

Key words Two-photon intravital microscopy, Explant, Skin, Surgical exposure, Imaging window

1 Introduction

1.1 Opportunities for Two-Photon Intravital Microscopy

The body is a complex system of dynamic interconnected biological processes like cell migration, cell proliferation, cell–cell interactions, and cell signaling. Due to the interactive character of these processes in complex environments it is of pivotal importance to study these in living animals. Some research questions can be addressed by ex vivo analysis using for instance immunohistochemistry, FACS assays, protein analysis, or mRNA characterization. However, even when performing these analyses at multiple time points, they nevertheless represent snapshots of dynamic processes. Intravital microscopy (IVM), microscopy inside a living animal, is

---

* These authors contributed equally to this work.

Yolanda Markaki and Hartmann Harz (eds.), *Light Microscopy: Methods and Protocols*, Methods in Molecular Biology, vol. 1563, DOI 10.1007/978-1-4939-6810-7_4, © Springer Science+Business Media LLC 2017

an exciting method to capture truly dynamic processes in real time. A variety of IVM platforms exists, offering whole body, to macroscopic, to microscopic resolution.

In this chapter two-photon IVM (2P-IVM) is discussed. Two-photon IVM allows for fluorescence imaging at microscopic resolution, deep into living tissues [1]. In conventional fluorescence microscopy, single photons continuously excite fluorophores above and below the focal plane [2]. With 2P-IVM two photons need to simultaneously hit the fluorophore for excitation, which will only occur at the focal plane [2, 3]. Therefore, two-photon microscopy results in less phototoxicity and less photobleaching than regular single-photon microscopy. In addition, the use of longer wavelengths, characteristic for two-photon microscopy, has the advantage of deeper tissue penetration [2]. Another benefit of two-photon excitation is Second Harmonic Generation (SHG). Due to their specific structure certain biological components, like type I collagen or microtubules, are subjective to this optical phenomenon, generating a signal at half the wavelength used for excitation [4, 5]. Without the need for labeling, this signal can provide structural detail of the imaged site. Hence, 2P-IVM is an extremely useful tool to image cellular dynamics deep into living tissues for prolonged periods of time. A few of those dynamic processes are discussed below.

1.2 Migration

It goes without saying that the dynamic migratory behavior of cells has been a major focus of 2P-IVM studies. The migration of many different cell types can be and have been studied using this technique (*see* Fig. 1a). Two well-known examples are tumor cells and leukocytes, as reviewed by [6, 7], respectively. The time interval and duration of a 2P-IVM experiment clearly depends on the research question and the speed of the cell of interest. When studying slow cell migration over a couple of days, photoconvertible proteins such as Kaede or Dendra2 offer a great tool [8, 9]. In the first imaging session, cells at a specific location are marked by changing their color. In subsequent imaging sessions these differently colored cells can be traced. This tool is also used to study the redistribution of cells to other parts of the body [10]. Speed, displacement, and directionality of migrating cells are parameters which are regularly determined using 2P-IVM. Additionally, the localization of migrating cells can be of interest. Finally, the different modes of migration, namely mesenchymal, amoeboid, collective migration and migration in streams can be defined using 2P-IVM.

1.3 Proliferation

Proliferation, or cell division, is one of the hallmarks of cancer [11]. Moreover, it also plays a major role during development and tissue homeostasis. Due to its dynamic nature, 2P-IVM is the ideal tool for studying proliferation. Using this technique, cell division has been studied by real-time visualization and by lineage tracing. The Fucci cell cycle reporter or Histone 2B tagged with a

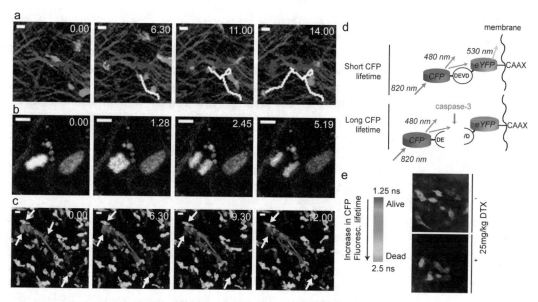

Fig. 1 Intravital microscopy examples. (**a**) OTI-GFP CD8+ T cell (*green*) migration in a murine spleen, imaged through an abdominal imaging window. Seven days earlier, the mouse was challenged with the ovalbumin peptide SIINFEKL in the presence of incomplete Freud's adjuvant and CpG. SHG signal is displayed in *magenta*. Migration tracks are indicated in *blue* and *white*. (Data of L. Ritsma) (**b**) Proliferation of C26 tumor cells in a murine liver metastasis, imaged through an abdominal imaging window. The tumor cells express Histone 2B-Dendra (*green*), and SHG signal is displayed in *magenta*. Maximum intensity projection of z-stack. (Data of L. Ritsma) (**c**) Interaction between neutrophils (*green*) and C26 (*red*) tumor cells in murine liver, imaged through an abdominal imaging window. DsRed-expressing tumor cells were injected in the mesenteric vein of LysM-GFP mice. One interacting cell is tracked, others are pointed out by *arrows*. Maximum intensity projection of z-stack. (Data of N. Chen and N. Vrisekoop) (**d**) Schematic illustration of a FRET-probe used to detect induction of apoptosis in vivo. The biosensor consists of caspase-3 with a donor fluorophore (CFP) and acceptor fluorophore (eYFP) attached. When apoptosis is induced, caspase-3 will be cleaved at the DEVD motif, leading to separation between the fluorophores and loss of FRET signal. Simultaneously, the lifetime of the CFP signal will increase. Figure adapted with permission from [30]. (**e**) FRET-FLIM images of a C26 tumor, imaged through an abdominal imaging window. The tumor cells, expressing the FRET-probe explained in (**d**), are shown before (*upper panel*) and 20 h after (*lower panel*) docetaxel (DTX) treatment. The *colors* indicate the relative donor fluorescence lifetime and therefore the extent of apoptosis, as illustrated in the *bar on the left*. Figure adapted with permission from [30]. Scalebars, 10 μm. Time, in minutes

fluorophore are effective methods for real-time visualization of proliferation (*see* Fig. 1b) [12–15]. The second method to study tumor cell proliferation, lineage tracing, measures proliferation indirectly. During lineage tracing, genetic expression of a fluorophore is inherited by the daughter cell upon cell division. Thus, by counting the number of cells that express the inherited fluorophore, one can make inferences about cell division. This method has been used effectively to study stem cell homeostasis in the small intestine [16]. Lineage tracing has also been applied to study proliferation of cancer cells [17] and cancer stem cells [18], among others.

1.4 Cell–Cell Interactions

Visualizing interactions between cells in vivo is another important application of 2P-IVM. For instance in immunological research, where T cell activation by interactions with dendritic cells in secondary lymphoid organs has been extensively studied [19–21]. Other examples include interactions between B and T cells, T cells interacting with the stromal lymph node network and effector T cells killing target cells [22, 23]. In tumor biology the interactions between expanding or migrating tumor cells as well as between tumor cells and different cells of the tumor microenvironment (*see* Fig. 1c), including immune cells, have been subjects of particular interest, as reviewed by [24–26].

1.5 Signaling Molecules

2P-IVM can be used to perform high-resolution microscopy at subcellular resolution. This makes it possible to visualize signaling molecules and protein activities inside a living animal. Molecular biosensors, often developed to report intracellular signaling events in vitro, can also be used in 2P-IVM studies [27–31]. Many of these biosensors are Förster resonance energy transfer (FRET) sensors that contain two fluorophores that transfer energy when placed in the right orientation and when in close proximity to one another [32, 33]. The efficiency of FRET is calculated from the intensity of the fluorescence emitted by the acceptor fluorophore, quantifying for example proximity or binding of two molecules [33]. However, intensity-based measurements can be obscured by photobleaching, scattering, etc. These problems can be overcome by combining FRET with Fluorescence Lifetime Imaging (FLIM) in 2P-FLIM-FRET (*see* Fig. 1d, e) [31]. FLIM is based on the fluorescence lifetime of the donor fluorophore, i.e., the time that the donor fluorophore will reside in the excited state. If FRET occurs, the fluorescence lifetime of the donor fluorophore will be shortened. FLIM systems detect this and calculate FRET efficiency based on the lifetime of the unbound donor [34]. Hence, FLIM-FRET is especially advantageous when imaging deep into tissues.

Non-FRET-based sensors often use activation of a fluorescent biomolecule, like the calcium sensor Fluo-3. Calcium sensors have been used to study calcium dynamics in renal podocytes during injury and disease [35], and during B cell response to dendritic antigen presentation in the lymph node [36], among others. With more sensors being developed and fluorescence intensities of current sensors being improved, we anticipate an increase in their use in 2P-IVM studies.

1.6 Pharmacology

2P-IVM has mainly been used to study dynamic biological processes as described above. In addition, it is now emerging as a powerful tool to evaluate drug distribution and action at the single cell level [37]. For example, IVM can be used to study the effect of antimitotic drugs on spindle assembly, subsequent mitotic arrest, slippage, multinucleation, and apoptosis in individual cancer cells

[13]. Moreover, this technique allows studying the impact of drugs on cell migration and invasion in vivo [38]. Finally, with the development of a new generation of fluorescent probes, it is now possible to follow drugs across several cellular compartments and to assess their pharmacokinetics using IVM (*see* Fig. 1e) [39, 40]. These approaches will be advantageous to understand the real impact of drugs in vivo but also to develop new therapeutic strategies to adapt patient treatment to avoid the development of drug resistance [41, 42].

1.7 Comparison of Various Intravital Microscopy Techniques

A variety of IVM techniques have been developed to study the mechanisms mentioned above. Of them, (1) the ex vivo intravital imaging of explants, and the in vivo intravital imaging of an organ through: (2) the skin, (3) a surgical exposure, and (4) a window are presented here (*see* Table 1).

For 2P-IVM of explants, the organ of interest will be removed from the animal, submerged in oxygenated media resembling physiological conditions, and then imaged (*see* Fig. 2). The animal itself is sacrificed upon organ harvesting. Whole organs, part of organs, but also tissue slices can be explanted and imaged [43, 44]. Explants can be imaged for up to 4–8 h.

In vivo imaging of the skin is relatively easy because it does not require surgery to expose the tissue. After hair removal, the animal can immediately be prepared for 2P-IVM [45]. This is in contrast to the surgical exposure and imaging window techniques. For the first technique, a surgical procedure exposes the tissue/organ of interest [46–50], either by making an incision in the skin/muscles above the organ of interest, or by creating a skinflap with the tissue of interest attached. For the latter technique, a surgical procedure is required to implant an imaging window in front of the organ of interest [51–56]. After implantation of the imaging window the animal can be awake in between imaging sessions, enabling multi-day 2P-IVM.

In conclusion, IVM is a powerful tool to study dynamic processes in vivo. There is not a single right way to perform IVM and the best technique depends on the research question. Each technique has its own characteristics and Table 1 recites the advantages and disadvantages regarding the method, the IVM settings and the animal ethics issues. In the protocols below, we describe in detail how to set up intravital microscopy for the four imaging techniques.

2 Materials

2.1 General

1. Multi-photon imaging system.

2. Anesthetics machine.

3. Induction cage.

Table 1
Characteristics, advantages, and disadvantages of the different 2P-IVM methods

		Explant	Skin	Surgical exposure	Window
Generic	Surgery	No	No	Yes	Complex
	Hydration necessary	Animal: No Tissue: Yes	Animal: Yes Tissue: No	Animal: Yes Tissue: Yes	Animal: Yes Tissue: No
	Temperature control necessary	Animal: No Tissue: Yes	Animal: Yes Tissue: No	Animal: Yes Tissue: Yes	Animal: Yes Tissue: No
Procedure	Blood circulation intact	No	Yes	Yes	Yes
	Wound repair reaction	No	No	Yes, open wound	Yes, after surgery
Imaging	Fluorescence	Genetic, Injected	Tattooing, Genetic, Injected	Genetic, Injected	Genetic, Injected
	Anesthesia during imaging	No	Yes	Yes	Yes
	Ex vivo processing	Yes	No	No	No
	Multiple organs	Yes	Limited to skin	Yes	Yes
	Accessibility	Whole organ	na	Large part of organ	Limited part of organ
	Breathing artifacts	No	No	Some	Yes
	Time	Hours	Weeks	Hours	Weeks
	Time points	Single	Multiple	Single	Multiple
Animal ethics	Anesthesia	1x	Repeated	1x	Repeated
	Solitary housing	No	No	No	Yes
Examples of applications		Motor axon dynamics; Immune cell dynamics in lymph node, lung and thymus	Skin stem cell dynamics; Skin resident T cells dynamics; Neutrophil dynamics in the skin after damage or infection	Tumor cell migration; Cell division; Cell trafficking; Cell-cell interactions; Drug response	Tumor cell colonization; Stem cell homeostasis; Chemotherapies mechanism of action
References		[43, 44, 57, 67–69]	[58, 60, 70]	[71–75]	[16, 18, 30, 41, 42, 76–80]

Summary of the different characteristics, advantages, and disadvantages of the ex vivo intravital imaging of explants and the in vivo intravital imaging of an organ through the skin, a surgical exposure, and a window. *na* = not applicale

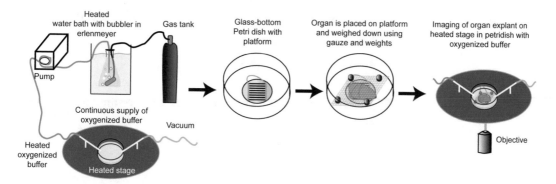

Fig. 2 Explant setup for 2P-IVM. A cartoon depicting the setup for explant imaging. First, the system is calibrated and set up. Oxygenized medium at 37 °C is continuously provided to the dish by a peristaltic pump. Once the setup is done, the organ is harvested and then positioned and fixed in the glass bottom petri dish. Lastly, the petri dish is placed in the heated perfusion chamber and filled with oxygenized medium

4. Ventilator.

5. Face mask.

6. Medical air (O_2 21.5 % vol/vol, N_2 78.5 % vol/vol).

7. Microdissection scissors.

8. Scissors.

9. Graefe forceps curved serrated.

10. Buprenorphine hydrochloride (0.3 mg/ml).

11. Autoclave or glass bead sterilizer.

12. Heating pad.

13. 3M Vetbond, super glue, tissue tape or play dough for mouse/organ fixation.

14. Mouse monitoring system (optional).

15. Surgical tape.

2.2 Explant

1. Appropiate perfusion chamber + peristaltic pump system.

2. Imaging platform to ensure oxygenation underneath tissue.

3. Mice.

4. Phenol-free medium.

5. Airstone (aquarium bubbler).

6. Tubing.

7. Thermometer.

8. Tank of 95 % O_2, 5 % CO_2 mixed gas.

9. 37 °C water bath.

10. When imaging tissue slices generated by a vibratome, ice-cold PBS and low melting agarose are additionally needed.

2.3 Skin

1. Appropiate stage insert or imaging box with coverslip.
2. Mice, preferably albino.
3. Rectal temperature probe.
4. 25 G needle + syringe.
5. Subcutaneous catheter + syringe infusion pump.
6. Saline solution.
7. Tail vein catheter (optional).
8. Eye ointment.
9. Clipper.
10. Depilation cream.

2.4 Surgical Exposure

1. Appropriate stage insert or imaging box with coverslip.
2. Mice.
3. Rectal temperature probe.
4. 25 G needle + syringe.
5. Subcutaneous catheter + syringe infusion pump.
6. Saline solution.
7. Tail vein catheter (optional).
8. Eye ointment.
9. Razor.
10. Depilation cream.
11. Betadine scrub.
12. Sterile gauze.
13. Parafilm.

2.5 Window

1. Appropriate stage insert or imaging box that fits an imaging window.
2. Mice, preferable aged 10 weeks or older.
3. Rectal temperature probe.
4. 25 G needle + syringe.
5. Subcutaneous catheter + syringe infusion pump.
6. Saline solution.
7. Tail vein catheter (optional).
8. Eye ointment.
9. Razor.
10. Depilation cream.
11. Betadine scrub.

3 Methods

3.1 Explant

1. Oxygenize phenol-free medium (*see* **Note 1**) by submersing an airstone (aquarium bubbler) connected to concentrated O_2 gas (95 % O_2, 5 % CO_2 mix) (*see* Fig. 2). Pre-warm the phenol-free medium to 37 °C in a water bath. Since the bubbling of gas tends to decrease the temperature of the buffer, the water bath generally needs to be set higher in order to reach 37 °C.

2. Set up a peristaltic pump that continuously provides fresh oxygenized media to a heated perfusion chamber (*see* **Note 2**). The overflowing media can be discarded through another end of the peristaltic pump or via a vacuum system (*see* Fig. 2). Check the temperature of the buffer in the dish. If lower than 37 °C adjust the temperature of the water bath and heated perfusion chamber accordingly.

3. Anesthetize the mouse in an induction chamber using 2.5 % (vol/vol) isoflurane (*see* **Note 3**).

4. Ensure the mouse is properly anesthetized by performing a toe pinch (*see* **Note 4**).

5. Place the unconscious mouse with its nose in a face mask connected to the anesthetics machine and lower the isoflurane to 1.5 % (vol/vol). Ensure the mouse is on a heating pad to maintain its body temperature (*see* **Note 5**).

6. Fix all four legs of the mouse using tape and excise the organ of interest.

7. Sacrifice the mouse based on the institutional guidelines. Methods to be used include cervical dislocation, or a mixture of O_2 and CO_2.

8. When imaging the complete organ, rinse the organ of interest once or twice in pre-warmed oxygenized media before proceeding to **step 9**. When imaging a slice of an organ prepare 4 % low melting agarose in PBS and cool down to 40 °C in a water bath. Then place the organ in a 6 or 12 well plate and cool down the agarose further until 38–39 °C and fill the well with agarose. Let cool in fridge until agarose is solid. Then cut out a square of the agarose containing the organ of interest and glue the square of agarose to the specimen disk of the vibratome using 3M Vetbond. For some organs it is necessary to support the agarose square containing the tissue by gluing a large wall of agarose behind it. Make a thick slice of tissue using the vibratome. Ensure using ice cold PBS to surround the tissue as the vibrations of the vibratome can quickly heat up the buffer.

9. Fixation of the tissue is performed in an empty dish (*see* Fig. 2). For an inverted microscope (*see* **Note 6**), place the tissue on an imaging platform to ensure oxygenation underneath the tissue [57] and fix the tissue (*see* **Note 7**).

10. Fill the dish with oxygenized medium (*see* Fig. 2).

11. Image the organ of interest (*see* **Note 8**).

3.2 Skin

1. Preferably use albino mice, since melanin-containing cells in the skin are very light-sensitive and upon death these cells subsequently trigger immune cell recruitment. If albino mice cannot be used care should be taken with the laser power and phototoxicity and immune cell recruitment should be ruled out in control experiments.

2. Anesthetize the mouse in an induction chamber using 2.5 % (vol/vol) isoflurane (*see* **Note 8**).

3. Ensure the mouse is properly anesthetized by performing a toe pinch (*see* **Note 4**).

4. Place the unconscious mouse with its nose in a face mask connected to the anesthetics machine and lower the isoflurane to 1.5 % (vol/vol) (*see* Fig. 3a). Ensure the mouse is on a heating pad to maintain its body temperature (*see* **Note 5**).

5. Now, a tail vein catheter can be inserted in order to inject fluorescent probes to image for example the vasculature.

6. Lubricate both eyes with eye ointment (*see* **Note 9**).

7. Shave the total area you want to image (*see* **Note 10**). When imaging the ear, the area is not shaved but long hairs are cut with scissors instead.

8. Ensure proper hydration of the mouse by placing a catheter subcutaneously. Fix tubing from a syringe infusion pump to an over-the-needle catheter (22 G). Fill tubing and syringe with saline and inject the mouse subcutaneously by lifting the skin between two fingers while holding the needle parallel to the mouse and by subsequently sticking the needle in the space between your fingers. Next, remove the needle and leave the catheter inside the mouse. Fix the catheter by taping the outside of the needle to the skin of the mouse using surgical tape. Set the machine to provide a continuous flow of saline. For mice, set at 100 µl per hour (*see* **Note 11**).

9. Monitor respiration (*see* **Notes 12** and **13**) by looking at the chest of the mouse for at least 10 s. A breath rate between 50 and 100 breaths per minute is advisable.

10. The mouse body temperature must be maintained to 37 °C during imaging (*see* **Note 5**). To maintain the body temperature, you can use a heated chamber. Body temperature monitoring can be realized with a rectal probe (*see* **Note 14**).

11. Place the mouse onto the microscope stage (*see* **Notes 6** and **15**). When using an inverted microscope, a variety of platforms have been described to immobilize the ear. Among them, the aluminum clamp that immobilizes the ear during imaging [58] and an

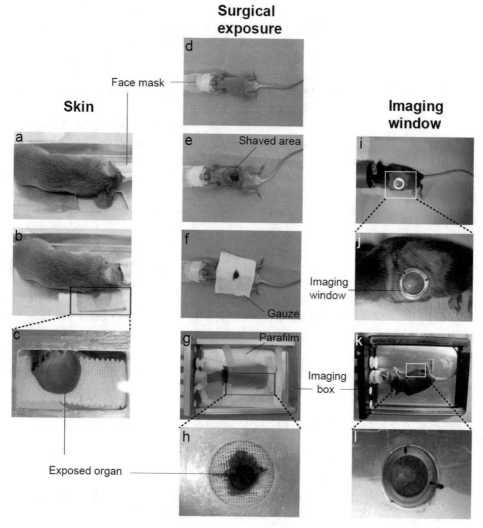

Fig. 3 Illustrated procedure for skin, surgical exposure, and imaging window techniques. On the left, pictures illustrating the setup for the skin method: (**a**) the mouse is placed in the imaging box and continuous anesthesia is ensured through a face mask, (**b**) the skin area that will be imaged is immobilized on the cover glass at the bottom of the customized imaging box and gently covered with tape, (**c**) the exposed skin is lying on the cover glass and is ready to be imaged. In the middle, pictures illustrating the setup for the surgical exposure method: (**d**) the mouse is placed under continuous anesthesia through a face mask, (**e**) the mouse is shaved and the organ of interest surgically exposed, (**f**) the organ is kept hydrated by placing wet sterile gauze around it, (**g**) the mouse is transferred to the imaging box and gently covered with parafilm, (**h**) the organ is lying on the cover glass at the bottom of the customized imaging box and is ready to be imaged. On the right, pictures illustrating the setup for the imaging window method: (**i**) the mouse is placed under continuous anesthesia through a face mask, (**j**) the organ of interest is surgically exposed and the window inserted, (**k**) the mouse is transferred to the imaging box, (**l**) the window is inserted in a circular hole at the bottom of the customized imaging box and the organ is ready to be imaged

association of spatulas that hold a coverslip placed onto the mouse's ear [59]. Alternatively, the ventral side of the ear pinna can be spread out on a thin layer of PBS on a cover glass at the bottom of a custom stage insert or imaging box. To immobilize the ear it can be gently covered by a piece of Durapore 3M tape, but care should be taken to avoid pressure on the ear (*see* Fig. 3b, c). The anterior half of the ear pinna is most suitable for imaging as the amount of hair follicles and melanin containing cells is sparse in this area [60]. A similar stage insert or imaging box can be used to image other parts of the skin. In that case, the mouse needs to be placed with the desired part of the skin on top of the coverslip and fixed to minimize movement [61].

12. Image for a few hours or over multiple days (*see* **Notes 8** and **16**).

13. Once the imaging is done, the mouse needs to be housed properly. First, remove the anesthesia but keep the mouse heated to maintain its body temperature (*see* **Note 17**). If the mouse regains consciousness, place the mouse back into its cage and monitor the mouse until it is back to its normal behavior. Keep monitoring the mouse's behavior at least once a week.

14. Sacrifice the mouse after imaging based on the institutional guidelines. Methods to be used include cervical dislocation, or a mixture of O_2 and CO_2.

3.3 Surgical Exposure

1. Pre-sterilize instruments using an autoclave or a glass bead sterilizer.

2. Provide the mouse with analgesics to reduce pain during surgery (*see* **Note 18**).

3. Anesthetize the mouse in an induction chamber using 2.5 % (vol/vol) isoflurane (*see* **Note 3**).

4. Ensure the mouse is properly anesthetized by performing a toe pinch (*see* **Note 4**).

5. Place the unconscious mouse with its nose in a face mask connected to the anesthetics machine and lower the isoflurane to 1.5 % (vol/vol) (*see* Fig. 3d). Ensure the mouse is on a heating pad to maintain its body temperature (*see* **Note 5**).

6. Now, a tail vein catheter can be inserted in order to inject fluorescent probes to image for example the vasculature.

7. Shave and depilate the mouse (*see* **Note 10**) (*see* Fig. 3e).

8. Apply betadine scrub to avoid infections.

9. Lubricate both eyes with eye ointment (*see* **Note 9**).

10. Fix all four legs of the mouse using surgical tape and expose the organ of interest.

11. Keep tissue hydrated (*see* **Notes 19** and **20**) by placing wet sterile gauze around imaged tissue (*see* Fig. 3f).

12. Transfer the mouse to the stage insert/imaging box containing a cover glass at the bottom (*see* **Note 7**).

13. If necessary fix the skinflap or tissue by using 3M Vetbond, super glue, tissue tape or play dough. Make sure not to use glue on the area you want to image.

14. Fix the mouse to the stage insert/imaging box to minimize movement and cover with parafilm (*see* Fig. 3g, h).

15. Ensure proper hydration of the mouse by placing a catheter subcutaneously. Fix tubing from a syringe infusion pump to an over-the-needle catheter (22 G). Fill tubing and syringe with saline and inject the mouse subcutaneously by lifting the skin between two fingers while holding the needle parallel to the mouse and by subsequently sticking the needle in the space between your fingers. Next, remove the needle and leave the catheter inside the mouse. Fix the catheter by taping the outside of the needle to the skin of the mouse using surgical tape. Set the machine to provide a continuous flow of saline. For mice, set at 100 µl per hour (*see* **Note 11**).

16. Mouse temperature during imaging should be maintained near 37 °C (*see* **Note 5**). To maintain the body temperature, you can use a heated chamber. Body temperature monitoring can be realized with a rectal probe (*see* **Note 14**).

17. Monitor respiration (*see* **Notes 12** and **13**) by looking at the chest of the mouse for at least 10 s. A breath rate between 50 and 100 breaths per minute is advisable.

18. Image up to 40 h (*see* **Note 8**).

19. Sacrifice the mouse after imaging based on the institutional guidelines. Methods to be used include cervical dislocation, or a mixture of O_2 and CO_2.

3.4 Imaging Windows

1. Pre-sterilize instruments using an autoclave or a glass bead sterilizer.

2. Provide the mouse with analgesics to reduce pain during surgery (*see* **Note 18**).

3. Anesthetize the mouse in an induction chamber using 2.5 % (vol/vol) isoflurane (*see* **Note 3**).

4. Ensure the mouse is properly anesthetized by performing a toe pinch (*see* **Note 4**).

5. Place the unconscious mouse with its nose in a face mask connected to the anesthetics machine and lower the isoflurane to 1.5 % (vol/vol). Ensure the mouse is on a heating pad to maintain its body temperature (*see* **Note 5**).

6. Now, a tail vein catheter can be inserted in order to inject fluorescent probes to image for example the vasculature.

7. Shave and depilate the mouse (*see* **Note 10**).

8. Apply betadine scrub to avoid infections.

9. Lubricate both eyes with eye ointment (*see* **Note 9**).

10. Fix all four legs of the mouse using surgical tape and implant the imaging window (*see* **Note 21**).

11. Fix the window for imaging (*see* **Notes 6** and **22**) (*see* Fig. 3i, j). For an inverted microscope use a stage insert/imaging box mount that fits/fixes the window. For the abdominal imaging window or certain cranial imaging windows, use an insert with a central hole that tightly fits the window (14.5 mm) (*see* Fig. 3k, l). For the dorsal skinfold chamber, use an insert with a large central hole (>12 mm) for imaging and three smaller holes for the bolts.

12. Ensure the window is fixed in a similar position over multiple days to allow retracing based on microscope coordinates (*see* **Note 23**).

13. Ensure proper hydration of the mouse by placing a catheter subcutaneously. Fix tubing from a syringe infusion pump to an over-the-needle catheter (22 G). Fill tubing and syringe with saline and inject the mouse subcutaneously by lifting the skin between two fingers while holding the needle parallel to the mouse and by subsequently sticking the needle in the space between your fingers. Next, remove the needle and leave the catheter inside the mouse. Fix the catheter by taping the outside of the needle to the skin of the mouse using surgical tape. Set the machine to provide a continuous flow of saline. For mice, set at 100 µl per hour (*see* **Note 11**).

14. Mouse temperature during imaging should be maintained near 37 °C (*see* **Note 5**). To maintain the body temperature, you can use a heated chamber. Body temperature monitoring can be realized with a rectal probe (*see* **Note 14**).

15. Monitor respiration (*see* **Notes 12** and **13**) by looking at the chest of the mouse for at least 10 s. A breath rate between 50 and 100 breaths per minute is advisable.

16. Image for a few hours or over multiple days (*see* **Notes 8** and **16**).

17. In between the imaging sessions, house the mouse individually as it requires recovery time after surgery. Moreover, other mice might bite the window which can cause it to dislodge. After the imaging session, remove the anesthesia but keep the mouse heated to maintain its body temperature (*see* **Note 5**). When the mouse regains consciousness, place the mouse back into its cage and monitor the mouse until it is back to its normal behavior. Keep monitoring the mouse's behavior at least once

a week. Lastly, water and food should be available ad libitum, and a food pellet should be provided on the cage bedding the first day after surgery.

18. Sacrifice the mouse after imaging based on the institutional guidelines. Methods to be used include cervical dislocation, or a mixture of O_2 and CO_2.

4 Notes

1. The color of phenol can interfere with imaging.

2. A variety of heated perfusion chambers are commercially available.

3. An alternative method of anesthesia is the use of injection anesthesia, of which the most commonly used is a combination of ketamine and xylazine. The recommended dose for imaging window surgery is: 100 mg/Kg ketamine and 10 mg/Kg xylazine. It will induce a surgical plane for about half an hour. Injection anesthesia is an alternative to inhalation anesthesia, but is not preferred because it provides limited control over depth and length of anesthesia. Moreover, when additional anesthesia is required overdosing happens easily. For longer surgeries (>1.5 h), the combination of Hypnorm (Fluanison (neuroleptic) + Fentanyl (opioid) (0.4 ml/Kg) + Midazolam (benzodiazepine sedative) (2 mg/Kg)) at a dose of 1:1:2 in sterile water is advised. It will induce a surgical plane for about 4 h. The combination of Hypnorm and Midazolam can be easily reverted by injecting 100 μg/Kg of buprenorphine.

4. To ensure proper anesthesia, the mouse should have a breath rate between 50 and 100 breaths per minute. The mouse should not be gasping for air (anesthesia too deep), nor should it still show toe twitches (anesthesia too superficial).

5. A mouse is not able to maintain its body temperature during anesthesia which can lead to hypothermia or hyperthermia. Hence, proper regulation and monitoring of the mouse body temperature is essential. Ensure not to overheat the mouse, as this enhances the depth of the anesthetic and might be lethal owing to respiratory failure. In the absence of a heated chamber, a heated circulating water blanket, chemical heat pad or an electrical blanket can be used.

6. It is possible to convert an upright microscope into an inverted microscope and vice versa using objective inverters.

7. Fix the tissue by weighing it down with small weights, by using playdough, or by using 3M Vetbond to glue only the corners of the tissue with small amounts of glue. For an upright microscope, use a dipping lense for imaging.

8. Care should be taken when performing 2P-IVM to prevent tissue destruction. A laser power that is too high can result in (two- or three-) photon absorption of endogenous molecules, which might lead to the creation of reactive oxygen species (ROS) or ionization of those molecules, ultimately leading to tissue destruction and recruitment of immune cells [62, 63].

9. Dehydration of the eyes can cause permanent damage.

10. Hair is strongly autofluorescent; therefore, it is essential to remove as much hair as possible to prevent hampering imaging.

11. If no syringe infusion pump is available, an alternative option is to inject the mouse with a bolus of saline. Take the skin of the neck of the mouse between two fingers, and use a 25 G needle to inject 100 µl saline subcutaneously by sticking the needle in the space between your fingers. This will keep the mouse hydrated for about 1 h, and needs to be repeated when imaging for multiple hours.

12. Breath rate is the easiest parameter to monitor because no equipment is necessary (*See* **Note 4**).

13. Monitoring of the heart rate and/or oxygen saturation is optional. Monitoring devices can be used to measure the heart rate of a mouse. Place the tail or foot clip at the right location. Wait until the monitor picks up the signal. Sometimes the clip needs to be adjusted a few times before a strong signal is picked up. Interference between the infrared signals of the device and 2P-IVM lasers can be observed. It is therefore necessary to cover the device with a light-proof drape. A heart rate between 300 and 400 bpm is advisable, and oxygen saturation should be above 95 % [64].

14. In some systems it is possible to have the mouse body temperature (as measured by the rectal probe) regulate the heating platform to maintain a constant body temperature.

15. When using an upright microscope (*see* **Note 6**), an aluminum clamp [58], a brass stage that holds the ear of the mouse during imaging [45] and an association of spatulas [59] can also be used to image the skin. For imaging other parts of the body such as nerves in the foot, a metal fixator constituted of two fixator wings associated to a metal ring can be used [65].

16. Imaging can be performed for a few hours or over multiple days. When properly hydrated, mice can be imaged for up to 40 h. However, when imaging multiple days in a row, do not image the mouse for more than 3 h per day. If possible, try to give the mouse as much time in between the imaging sessions as possible, preferably >24 h.

17. The mouse wake-up time should take between 10 s and 1 min. If it takes longer, the mouse can be provided with pure oxygen for approximately 1 min.

18. For mice under inhalation anesthesia, subcutaneous or intra-muscular administration of an opioid analgesic such as buprenorphine (100 μg/Kg), 30 min prior to surgery is rec-ommended. Postoperative administration of buprenorphine will provide additional pain relief for 12 h. Ketamine/Xylazine and hypnorm already contain an analgesic component that will exert its effect during surgery, so additional pain relief is not recommended.

19. Given that the mouse is kept at 37 °C, dehydration of the sur-gically exposed organ is a serious threat.

20. An alternative method is to use a pump to generate a continu-ous flow of PBS over the tissue.

21. Various imaging windows are available such as the dorsal skin-fold chamber, mammary imaging window, dorsal imaging and the cranial imaging. Detailed protocols for each can be found here [51–55].

22. In case of an upright microscope, fix the window using holders that hover above the mouse and fix the window. For the cranial imaging window use a stereotactic frame to secure the head of the mouse.

23. In case of an upright microscope, use a window design with extensions so that the clamps fix the mouse in a similar way over multiple time points [66]. In case a window is completely symmetrical and has no protrusions anywhere, use marks on the window and insert and align the marks before imaging (*see* Fig. 3l) [51]. In case of a cranial imaging window, stereotactic coordinates may be used, or the rotation angle of the mouse head can serve as a guide. In case bolts protrude from the win-dow (dorsal skinfold chamber), use an insert with holes for the bolts to place the window in the exact same position over mul-tiple imaging sessions [52].

Acknowledgments

We apologize in advance to those authors whose contributions are omitted due to space restrictions. L.R. was supported by a Rubicon grant from the Netherlands Organization for Scientific Research (NWO: 825.13.016), a postdoctoral fellowship from the Susan G. Komen foundation (PDF15329694), and a Gisela Thier Fellowship from the Leiden University Medical Center (LUMC).

References

1. Condeelis J, Weissleder R (2010) In vivo imaging in cancer. Cold Spring Harb Perspect Biol 2:a003848. doi:10.1101/cshperspect.a003848

2. Ritsma L, Ponsioen B, Rheenen J (2012) Intravital imaging of cell signaling in mice. IntraVital 1:2–10. doi:10.4161/intv.20802

3. Denk W, Strickler J, Webb W (1990) Two-photon laser scanning fluorescence microscopy. Science 248(80):73–76

4. Campagnola PJ, Millard AC, Terasaki M et al (2002) Three-dimensional high-resolution second-harmonic generation imaging of endogenous structural proteins in biological tissues. Biophys J 82:493–508

5. Freund I, Deutsch M, Sprecher A (1986) Connective tissue polarity. Optical second-harmonic microscopy, crossed-beam summation, and small-angle scattering in rat-tail tendon. Biophys J 50:693–712

6. Fein MR, Egeblad M (2013) Caught in the act: revealing the metastatic process by live imaging. Dis Model Mech 6:580–593. doi:10.1242/dmm.009282

7. Lämmermann T, Germain RN (2014) The multiple faces of leukocyte interstitial migration. Semin Immunopathol 36:227–251. doi:10.1007/s00281-014-0418-8

8. Kedrin D, Gligorijevic B, Wyckoff J et al (2008) Intravital imaging of metastatic behavior through a mammary imaging window. Nat Methods 5:1019–1021

9. Victora GD, Schwickert TA, Fooksman DR et al (2010) Germinal center dynamics revealed by multiphoton microscopy with a photoactivatable fluorescent reporter. Cell 143:592–605

10. Chtanova T, Hampton HR, Waterhouse L A et al (2014) Real-time interactive two-photon photoconversion of recirculating lymphocytes for discontinuous cell tracking in live adult mice. J Biophotonics 7:425–433. doi:10.1002/jbio.201200175

11. Hanahan D, Weinberg RA (2011) Hallmarks of cancer: the next generation. Cell 144:646–674

12. Alexander S, Weigelin B, Winkler F, Friedl P (2013) Preclinical intravital microscopy of the tumour-stroma interface: invasion, metastasis, and therapy response. Curr Opin Cell Biol 25:659–671. doi:10.1016/j.ceb.2013.07.001

13. Orth JD, Kohler RH, oijer F F et al (2011) Analysis of mitosis and antimitotic drug responses in tumors by in vivo microscopy and single-cell pharmacodynamics. Cancer Res 71:4608–4616. doi:10.1158/0008-5472.CAN-11-0412

14. Rompolas P, Deschene ER, Zito G et al (2012) Live imaging of stem cell and progeny behaviour in physiological hair-follicle regeneration. Nature 487:496–499. doi:10.1038/nature11218

15. Chittajallu DR, Florian S, Kohler RH et al (2015) In vivo cell-cycle profiling in xenograft tumors by quantitative intravital microscopy. Nat Methods 12:577–585. doi:10.1038/nmeth.3363

16. Ritsma L, Ellenbroek SIJ, Zomer A et al (2014) Intestinal crypt homeostasis revealed at single-stem-cell level by in vivo live imaging. Nature 507:362–365. doi:10.1038/nature12972

17. Coffey SE, Giedt RJ, Weissleder R (2013) Automated analysis of clonal cancer cells by intravital imaging. IntraVital. doi:10.4161/intv.26138

18. Zomer A, Inge Johanna Ellenbroek S, Ritsma L et al (2013) Brief report: intravital imaging of cancer stem cell plasticity in mammary tumors. Stem Cells 31:602–606. doi:10.1002/stem.1296

19. Mempel TR, Henrickson SE, Andrian UH (2004) T-cell priming by dendriticcells in lymph nodes occurs in three distinct phases. Nature 427:154–159

20. Bousso P (2008) T-cell activation by dendritic cells in the lymph node: lessons from the movies. Nat Rev Immunol 8:675–684. doi:10.1038/nri2379

21. Shakhar G, Lindquist RL, Skokos D et al (2005) Stable T cell-dendritic cell interactions precede the development of both tolerance and immunity in vivo. Nat Immunol 6:707–714. doi:10.1038/ni1210

22. Germain RN, Robey EA, Cahalan MD (2012) A decade of imaging cellular motility and interaction dynamics in the immune system. Science 336:1676–1681. doi:10.1126/science.1221063

23. Lee W-Y, Sanz M-J, Wong CHY et al (2014) Invariant natural killer T cells act as an extravascular cytotoxic barrier for joint-invading Lyme Borrelia. Proc Natl Acad Sci U S A 111:13936–13941

24. Tanaka K, Toiyama Y, Okugawa Y et al (2014) In vivo optical imaging of cancer metastasis using multiphoton microscopy: a short review. Am J Transl Res 6:179–187

25. Zal T, Chodaczek G (2010) Intravital imaging of anti-tumor immune response and the tumor microenvironment. Semin Immunopathol 32:305–317. doi:10.1007/s00281-010-0217-9

26. Phan TG, Bullen A (2010) Practical intravital two-photon microscopy for immunological research: faster, brighter, deeper. Immunol Cell Biol 88:438–444. doi:10.1038/icb.2009.116

27. ank M M, Santos AF, Direnberger S et al (2008) A genetically encoded calcium indicator for chronic in vivo two-photon imaging. Nat Methods 5:805–811

28. Bogdanov AA, Lin CP, Simonova M et al Cellular activation of the self-quenched fluorescent reporter probe in tumor microenvironment. Neoplasia 4:228–236

29. Timpson P, McGhee EJ, Morton JP et al (2011) Spatial regulation of RhoA activity during pancreatic cancer cell invasion driven by mutant p53. Cancer Res 71:747–757

30. Janssen A, Beerling E, Medema R, Rheenen J (2013) Intravital FRET imaging of tumor cell viability and mitosis during chemotherapy. PLoS One 8:e64029. doi:10.1371/journal.pone.0064029

31. Nobis M, McGhee EJ, Morton JP et al (2013) Intravital FLIM-FRET imaging reveals dasatinib-induced spatial control of src in pancreatic cancer. Cancer Res 73:4674–4686. doi:10.1158/0008-5472.CAN-12-4545

32. Förster T (1948) Zwischenmolekulare Energiewanderung und Fluoreszenz. Ann Phys 437:55–75

33. Hochreiter B, Garcia AP, Schmid JA (2015) Fluorescent proteins as genetically encoded FRET biosensors in life sciences. Sensors 15:26281–26314. doi:10.3390/s151026281

34. Lakowicz JR (2006) Principles of Fluorescence Spectroscopy, 3rd edition, third edit. Springer

35. Burford JL, Villanueva K, Lam L et al (2014) Intravital imaging of podocyte calcium in glomerular injury and disease. J Clin Invest 124:2050–2058. doi:10.1172/JCI71702

36. Qi H, Egen JG, Huang AYC, Germain RN (2006) Extrafollicular activation of lymph node B cells by antigen-bearing dendritic cells. Science 312(80):1672–1676. doi:10.1126/science.1125703

37. Conway JRW, Carragher NO, Timpson P (2014) Developments in preclinical cancer imaging: innovating the discovery of therapeutics. Nat Rev Cancer 14:314–328. doi:10.1038/nrc3724

38. Prunier C, Josserand V, Vollaire J, et al. (2016) LIM kinase inhibitor pyr1 reduces the growth and metastatic load of breast cancers. Cancer Res 0008–5472.CAN–15–1864–. doi:10.1158/0008-5472.CAN-15-1864

39. Budin G, Yang KS, Reiner T, Weissleder R (2011) Bioorthogonal probes for polo-like kinase 1 imaging and quantification. Angew Chem Int Ed Engl 50:9378–9381. doi:10.1002/anie.201103273

40. Reiner T, Earley S, Turetsky A, Weissleder R (2010) Bioorthogonal small-molecule ligands for PARP1 imaging in living cells. Chembiochem 11:2374–2377. doi:10.1002/cbic.201000477

41. Laughney AM, Kim E, Sprachman MM et al (2014) Single-cell pharmacokinetic imaging reveals a therapeutic strategy to overcome drug resistance to the microtubule inhibitor eribulin. Sci Transl Med 6:261ra152. doi:10.1126/scitranslmed.3009318

42. Hirata E, Girotti MR, Viros A et al (2015) Intravital imaging reveals how BRAF inhibition generates drug-tolerant microenvironments with high integrin β1/FAK signaling. Cancer Cell 27:574–588. doi:10.1016/j.ccell.2015.03.008

43. Dzhagalov IL, Melichar HJ, Ross JO, et al. (2012) Two-photon imaging of the immune system. Curr Protoc Cytom Chapter 12:Unit12.26. doi: 10.1002/0471142956.cy1226s60

44. Kerschensteiner M, Reuter MS, Lichtman JW, Misgeld T (2008) Ex vivo imaging of motor axon dynamics in murine triangularis sterni explants. Nat Protoc 3:1645–1653

45. Li JL, Goh CC, Keeble JL et al (2012) Intravital multiphoton imaging of immune responses in the mouse ear skin. Nat Protoc 7:221–234. doi:10.1038/nprot.2011.438

46. Donndorf P, Ludwig M, Wildschütz F et al. (2013) Intravital microscopy of the microcirculation in the mouse cremaster muscle for the analysis of peripheral stem cell migration. J Vis Exp e50485

47. Masedunskas A, Porat-Shliom N, Tora M et al. (2013) Intravital microscopy for imaging subcellular structures in live mice expressing fluorescent proteins. J Vis Exp e50558

48. Ewald AJ, Werb Z, Egeblad M (2011) Preparation of mice for long-term intravital imaging of the mammary gland. Cold Spring Harb Protoc 2011:pdb.prot5562. doi: 10.1101/pdb.prot5562

49. Liou HLR, Myers JT, Barkauskas DS, Huang AY (2012) Intravital imaging of the mouse popliteal lymph node. J Vis Exp e3720

50. Sellers SL, Payne GW (2011) Intravital microscopy of the inguinal lymph node. J Vis Exp e2551

51. Ritsma L, Steller EJ a, Ellenbroek SIJ, et al. (2013) Surgical implantation of an abdominal imaging window for intravital micros-

copy. Nat Protoc 8:583–594. doi: 10.1038/nprot.2013.026

52. Palmer GM, Fontanella AN, Shan S et al (2011) In vivo optical molecular imaging and analysis in mice using dorsal window chamber models applied to hypoxia, vasculature and fluorescent reporters. Nat Protoc 6:1355–1366

53. Yang G, Pan F, Parkhurst CN et al (2010) Thinned-skull cranial window technique for long-term imaging of the cortex in live mice. Nat Protoc 5:201–208

54. Holtmaat A, Bonhoeffer T, Chow DK et al (2009) Long-term, high-resolution imaging in the mouse neocortex through a chronic cranial window. Nat Protoc 4:1128–1144. doi:10.1038/nprot.2009.89

55. Alieva M, Ritsma L, Giedt RJ et al (2014) Imaging windows for long-term intravital imaging: General overview and technical insights. IntraVital 3:e29917. doi:10.4161/intv.29917

56. Farrar MJ, Schaffer CB (2014) A procedure for implanting a spinal chamber for longitudinal in vivo imaging of the mouse spinal cord. J Vis Exp e52196. doi:10.3791/52196

57. Torabi-Parizi P, Vrisekoop N, Kastenmuller W et al (2014) Pathogen-related differences in the abundance of presented antigen are reflected in CD4+ T cell dynamic behavior and effector function in the lung. J Immunol 192:1651–1660

58. Chan KT, Jones SW, Brighton HE et al (2014) Intravital imaging of a spheroid-based ortho-topic model of melanoma in the mouse ear skin. IntraVital 2:e25805. doi:10.4161/intv.25805

59. Pineda CM, Park S, Mesa KR et al (2015) Intravital imaging of hair follicle regeneration in the mouse. Nat Protoc 10:1116–1130

60. Peters NC, Egen JG, Secundino N et al (2008) In vivo imaging reveals an essential role for neutrophils in leishmaniasis transmitted by sand flies. Science 321:970–974. doi:10.1126/science.1159194

61. Ariotti S, Beltman JB, Chodaczek G et al (2012) Tissue-resident memory CD8+ T cells continuously patrol skin epithelia to quickly recognize local antigen. Proc Natl Acad Sci U S A 109:19739–19744

62. Débarre D, Olivier N, Supatto W, Beaurepaire E (2014) Mitigating phototoxicity during multiphoton microscopy of live Drosophila embryos in the 1.0-1.2 μm wavelength range. PLoS One 9:e104250. doi:10.1371/journal.pone.0104250

63. Ritsma L, Vrisekoop N, Rheenen J (2013) In vivo imaging and histochemistry are com-bined in the cryosection labelling and intravital

microscopy technique. Nat Commun 4:2366. doi:10.1038/ncomms3366

64. Verhoeven D, Teijaro JR, Farber DL (2009) Pulse-oximetry accurately predicts lung pathol-ogy and the immune response during influenza infection. Virology 390:151–156

65. Yuryev M, Molotkov D, Khiroug L (2014) In vivo two-photon microscopy of single nerve endings in skin. J Vis Exp e51045

66. Bochner F, Fellus-Alyagor L, Kalchenko V et al (2015) A novel intravital imaging window for longitudinal microscopy of the mouse ovary. Sci Rep 5:12446

67. Stoll S, Delon J, Brotz TM, Germain RN (2002) Dynamic imaging of T cell-dendritic cell interactions in lymph nodes. Science 296:1873–1876

68. Miller MJ, Wei SH, Parker I, Cahalan MD (2002) Two-photon imaging of lymphocyte motility and antigen response in intact lymph node. Science 296:1869–1873

69. Bousso P, Robey E (2003) Dynamics of CD8+ T cell priming by dendritic cells in intact lymph nodes. Nat Immunol 4:579–585

70. Lämmermann T, Afonso PV, Angermann BR et al (2013) Neutrophil swarms require LTB4 and integrins at sites of cell death in vivo. Nature 498:371–375. doi:10.1038/nature12175

71. Patsialou A, Bravo-Cordero JJ, Wang Y et al. (2013) Intravital multiphoton imaging reveals multicellular streaming as a crucial compo-nent of in vivo cell migration in human breast tumors IntraVital 2:e25294

72. Zomer A, Maynard C, Verweij FJ et al (2015) In vivo imaging reveals extracellular vesicle-mediated phenocopying of metastatic behavior. Cell 161:1046–1057

73. Nakasone ES, Askautrud HA, Kees T et al (2012) Imaging tumor-stroma interac-tions during chemotherapy reveals contribu-tions of the microenvironment to resistance. Cancer Cell 21:488–503. doi:10.1016/j.ccr.2012.02.017

74. Engelhardt JJ, oldajipour B B, Beemiller P et al (2012) Marginating dendritic cells of the tumor microenvironment cross-present tumor antigens and stably engage tumor-specific T cells. Cancer Cell 21:402–417

75. Arnon TI, Horton RM, Grigorova IL, Cyster JG (2013) Visualization of splenic marginal zone B-cell shuttling and follicular B-cell egress. Nature 493:684–688

76. Ritsma L, Steller EJA, Beerling E, et al. (2012) Intravital microscopy through an abdominal imaging window reveals a pre-micrometastasis stage during liver metastasis. Sci Transl Med 4:158ra145–158ra145

77. Beerling E, Seinstra D, de Wit E, et al. Plasticity between epithelial and mesenchymal states unlinks emt from metastasis-enhancing stem cell capacity. Cell Rep. doi: 10.1016/j.celrep.2016.02.034

78. Manning CS, Jenkins R, Hooper S, et al. (2013) Intravital imaging reveals conversion between distinct tumor vascular morphologies and localized vascular response to Sunitinib. pp 1–12.

79. Lai CP, Kim EY, Badr CE et al (2015) Visualization and tracking of tumour extracellular vesicle delivery and RNA translation using multiplexed reporters. Nat Commun 6:7029. doi:10.1038/ncomms8029

80. Snuderl M, Batista A, Kirkpatrick ND et al (2013) Targeting placental growth factor/neuropilin 1 pathway inhibits growth and spread of medulloblastoma. Cell 152:1065–1076. doi:10.1016/j.cell.2013.01.036

Chapter 5

Imaging of Brain Slices with a Genetically Encoded Voltage Indicator

Peter Quicke, Samuel J. Barnes, and Thomas Knöpfel

Abstract

Functional fluorescence microscopy of brain slices using voltage sensitive fluorescent proteins (VSFPs) allows large scale electrophysiological monitoring of neuronal excitation and inhibition. We describe the equipment and techniques needed to successfully record functional responses optical voltage signals from cells expressing a voltage indicator such as VSFP Butterfly 1.2. We also discuss the advantages of voltage imaging and the challenges it presents.

Key words Voltage imaging, Fluorescence imaging, Brain slices, Voltage indicators, Fluorescence microscopy, Voltage sensitive fluorescent proteins

---

1 Introduction

A key goal of neuroscience is to understand how spatiotemporal patterns of membrane voltage in sets of neurons can encode and compute neuronal information. Classical electrophysiology has enabled great advances in our understanding of cellular functions; however, as an essentially one-dimensional technology recording a single time course per electrode, it suffers from a trade-off between recording fidelity, cell number, and spatial localization. Patch clamp electrophysiology can monitor and perturb membrane voltage from a single cell exquisitely accurately [1]; multi-electrode arrays are able to record extracellular potentials from many cells simultaneously but with limited spatial resolution [2]. Optical imaging offers an increase in dimensionality compared to electrical recordings with much improved spatial field of view and resolution at the cost of relying on indicators to transduce neuronal activity into an optical signal. These can be organic fluorescent dye or genetically encoded fluorescent protein-based indicators of membrane voltage or calcium concentration [3]. The indicator kinetics and optical properties determines the type of activity monitored and the achievable spatiotemporal resolution [4].

Yolanda Markaki and Hartmann Harz (eds.), *Light Microscopy: Methods and Protocols*, Methods in Molecular Biology, vol. 1563, DOI 10.1007/978-1-4939-6810-7_5, © Springer Science+Business Media LLC 2017

Calcium indicators are often simpler to use than voltage indicators for a variety of reasons. It is possible to fit a greater number of indicator molecules into the cytosol rather than into the plasma membrane where voltage indicators must be located, increasing the signal brightness. The underlying signal transduced by calcium indicators, transient calcium influx following action potentials (APs), has slower dynamics than voltage signals, giving the indicators longer to respond and relaxing the lower bound on the required sampling rate. AP-related calcium signals also essentially consist of all-or-nothing events that are easier to extract from noisy data than graded voltage signals. This feature reduces the constraints on the quality of the imaging system.

Calcium signals convey less of the richness of neuronal activity compared to voltage signals. Calcium transients following APs do not occur in all neurons [5], and in some neurons calcium signals are not well correlated with AP firing [6]. Calcium indicators are effectively second order indicators of the neural signal of interest; they transduce a proxy for neuronal activity into an optical signal. Using voltage and calcium indicators in concert could allow large scale analysis of neuronal populations as "black box" computational groupings, with the indicators showing postsynaptic potentials (inputs to neurons) and APs (output of neurons) respectively.

Optical imaging is limited in depth by scattering in tissue. One photon wide-field imaging can image cell-size structures not deeper from the tissue surface than 100 μm while two-photon imaging can resolve cells as deep as 1 mm [7]. To study subcortical structures in the mouse it is therefore necessary to either image through an implanted device (e.g., a fiber bundle [8], GRIN lens [9], or prism [10]) or turn to imaging of ex vivo brain slices. Imaging of brain slices not only offers an opportunity to investigate specific neural circuits that are not easily accessible to in vivo imaging methods but also offers manipulations that are difficult under in vivo conditions (e.g., addition of pharmacological agents, mechanical cutting of connections). In the context of the approaches described here (development of genetically encoded indicator imaging), slices are also a valuable test bed due to the lack of haemodynamic signals and movement artefacts associated with in vivo recordings which have to be accounted for in postprocessing [11].

While two-photon imaging is intrinsically optically sectioning and so can image with cellular resolution deep in scattering tissue [12], in its standard implementation it suffers from the fact that by design a single small volume of tissue is imaged at each time point. This volume is then scanned through the sample to build up a 2- or 3-dimensional image point by point. In order to image at rates high enough to resolve neural activity the dwell time at each pixel must be very short (or the number of pixels must be very few).

This limits the number of photons that can be collected, reducing the achievable signal-to-noise ratio (R, *see* **Note 1**). For calcium imaging, acceptable R values can be more readily achieved due the typically larger $\Delta F/F$ values; for voltage imaging, where $\Delta F/F$ is typically small, maximizing R is a major challenge. One-photon imaging is limited in its ability to resolve single cells in scattering tissues except in special cases. This is because fluorescence excited outside of the focal plane is collected at the camera. This problem can be minimized by sparse labeling of cells, reducing the fluorescence contributed by unfocussed sources.

One-photon wide field imaging is able to collect many more signal photons than two-photon point-scan imaging as photons are collected for all pixels simultaneously. Moreover, one-photon excitation cross sections are typically much larger than two-photon cross sections. For these reasons, one-photon wide field imaging is more suitable to resolve small changes in indicator brightness. This feature suits imaging of population activity with indicators such as VSFP Butterfly [13].

In this chapter we describe the equipment and methods needed to image optical voltage signals in mouse brain slices using VSFPs. The protocol we describe is designed to enable imaging of large areas of brain slices at high (100 Hz or greater) frame rates and is mainly used to characterize the performance of genetically encoded voltage indicators (GEVIs). It is also well suited to studying communication between different brain regions by imaging the spread of population activity. In conjunction with sparsely expressed indicators activity at the level of single cells could also feasibly be resolved. The setup is based on commercially available components with custom-written Matlab scripts for data acquisition and analysis.

2 Materials

2.1 Microscope

1. THT Macroscope (Brainvision Inc.) with the following components:
   - 10×/0.3NA water dipping objective (Nikon).
   - 2× Planapo 1× objectives (Leica).
   - 580 nm long pass emission dichroic (Semrock).
   - 495 nm long pass excitation dichroic (Brainvision).
   - 542/27 nm emission filter (Semrock).
   - 594 nm long pass emission filter (Semrock).
   - 482/18 nm excitation filter (Semrock).
   - 2× Orca flash 4.0 sCMOS cameras (Hamamatsu).
2. LEX2 blue LED excitation source (Brainvision).

3. MSG10-1100S-SD Fibre optic light guide (Moritex).

4. ML-50 Condenser lens (Moritex).

2.2 Slicing

1. Tools for perfusion surgery: rough forceps, fine forceps, scissors, hemostat (Fine Science Tools).

2. 27G needles, 10 ml syringe, insulin syringe.

3. Ketamine 100 mg/ml and xylazine 20 mg/ml.

4. Ice and ice box.

5. Slicing ACSF (108 mM choline chloride, 3 mM KCl, 26 mM $NaHCO_3$, 1.25 mM NaH_2PO_4, 25 mM glucose, 3 mM sodium pyruvate, 1 mM $MgCl$ and 2 mM $CaCl_2$).

6. Bath ACSF (120 mM NaCl, 3 mM KCl, 23 mM $NaHCO_3$, 1.25 mM NaH_2PO_4, 10 mM glucose, 1 mM $MgCl$, and 2 mM $CaCl_2$).

7. VT1000S Vibratome (Leica).

8. 250, 100, and 1000 ml beakers.

9. Slice incubation chamber consisting of a 1 l measuring cylinder with the base removed and replaced with fine netting such that it fits into the 1 l beaker.

10. Cyanoacrylate glue.

11. Filter paper.

12. 95 % O_2/5 % CO_2 gas cylinder.

13. Vapro 5520 Vapor Pressure Osmometer (Wescor).

2.3 Imaging Chamber

1. Minipuls 3 peristaltic pump (Gilson).

2. Tubing for delivery of ACSF and O_2/CO_2.

3. Vibration damping table.

4. SHD 42/15 Slice harp (Warner Instruments).

5. TC 324b Bath temperature controller (Warner Instruments).

2.4 Data Acquisition

1. Digidata 1322A Digitizer (Molecular Devices).

2. 2× PCs with at least 32GB RAM to run the cameras. 1× PC capable of running pClamp software.

3. Matlab 2015a software including Image Acquisition and Image Processing packages (Mathworks).

4. pClamp Electrophysiology software (Molecular Devices).

2.5 Ephys

1. Electrode glass (World Precision Instruments).

2. PC-10 Electrode puller (Narishige).

3. Axopatch 200b patch clamp amplifier and CV 203BU headstage (Molecular Devices).

4. Isoflex Stimulus Isolator (A.M.P.I).

5. Master 8 (A.M.P.I).

6. MRE Micromanipulators and controller (Luigs and Neumann).

2.6 Misc

1. Bayonet Neill–Concelman (BNC) to BNC cables & SubMiniature version A (SMA) to BNC cables.

3 Methods

The microscope images slices through a 10×/0.3NA water dipping objective and uses a Brainvision dichroic to split the emitted fluorescence into two channels corresponding to the fluorophores in the FRET pair of the dual differential emission GEVI (VSFP Butterfly 1.2 [13]). The emitted light is then focussed onto the active areas of two sCMOS cameras using inversely mounted 1× Planapo Leica objectives. The use of the Brainvision splitting optics leads to a very wide light path, reducing aperture losses relative to "dual view" systems [14, 15] allowing large FOVs and a wide range of objectives to be accommodated. The microscope is mounted on a stage that can be moved relative to the slice chamber so that different locations within the brain slice can be imaged while stimulation electrodes are already placed into the slice. The microscope needs to be set up on a vibration isolation table with a frame and curtain that can block out ambient light that would contaminate the recordings. The table needs to be big enough to comfortably accommodate micromanipulators for electrodes and it is also useful to have a frame surrounding the air table but isolated from it which can be used for equipment such as peristaltic pumps for ACSF perfusion.

Each camera is controlled by a single computer; timing is controlled by a third computer that also records any electrophysiological traces using pClamp. For an acquisition the cameras are initialized by their respective computer and they wait for a trigger from pClamp which also controls the excitation shutter, stimulus isolator, and via a Master 8, a synchronization LED and the peristaltic pump. Frame out pulses from the cameras, if available, can also be read into pClamp to ensure the timing of the images for post processing.

3.1 Setting Up the Rig

1. Connect the cameras to their computers and configure the drivers and control software. This can be commercially available software that comes with the cameras such as Hokawo (Hamamatsu), or custom written software in Matlab. It is essential that the software supports hardware triggering for the cameras. It is also useful at this stage to perform tests to ensure that the cameras are exactly synchronized frame-by-frame.

This can be done by imaging an LED flashing at a fixed rate and ensuring that the light and dark frames appear at the same time points for both cameras (*see* **Note 2**).

2. Select the filters and dichroics required for the indicator to be imaged and install the filters into their mounts. Ensure that filters are clean, free of dust, and mounted in the correct orientation.

3. Install the microscope optics into the z-stage on the air table above the slice chamber. The optics with the cameras mounted can be prone to toppling and so it can be useful to use long springs to secure the setup to screws attached to the air table.

4. Connect the digitizer to the control computer. Using BNC cables connect the digitizer's digital control lines to the two camera's triggers using a splitter, to the excitation source shutter, the stimulus isolator and the Master 8 external in input triggering channel 1. Connect the Master 8 channel 1 to an LED on the air table and channel 2 to control the peristaltic pump. Internally connect channel 1 and 2 in the Master 8.

5. Configure the pClamp protocol so that the different outputs are triggered at the correct times. The cameras should be triggered first, then the Master 8, then the excitation source. The control flow is illustrated in Fig. 1. This can be checked again by imaging a fluorescent target and ensuring that the system operates as expected.

6. Connect the O_2/CO_2 gas tubing to the regulator so that the perfusion bath ACSF can be oxygenated before being pumped to the imaging chamber. Set up the peristaltic pump and perfusion system such that a flow rate of a minimum of 3 ml/min of oxygenated ACSF is pumped through the imaging chamber. It is useful to use larger bore tubing on the outflow line so that flooding is avoided.

7. Attach the cameras to the optics and align them. To do this image a suitable flat target such as a black cross on a light background. First adjust the path lengths so that the two cameras are focussed in the same position. As an alignment tool it is useful to take an image of a flat target with both cameras and take the difference of the images. When displayed in false color this will show misalignment clearly. Rotate one camera to fix rotation misalignments and use the dichroic adjusting knobs on the side of the dichroic housing to adjust translations. Iterate the process until satisfied.

3.2 Slice Experiments

Experiments with transgenic mice tend to involve older animals, and a detailed discussion of the challenges and techniques to overcome them can be found in reference [16]. It is important to ensure a good supply of well oxygenated ACSF when the slice is in

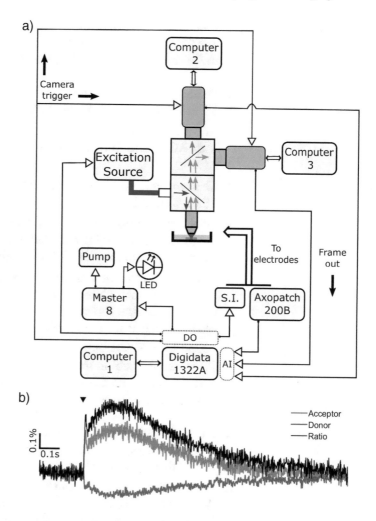

Fig. 1 (**a**) A diagram showing the control flow and light paths for the setup. *DO* digital out, *A.I* analogue input, *S.I* stimulus isolator. The acquisition is synchronized by the digitizer, which triggers the cameras, Master 8, excitation source, and stimulus isolator. The electrophysiological and frame out signal from the cameras, if required, can be recorded simultaneously. (**b**) An example trace recorded from a region of interest in cortical layer 2/3 expressing VSFP Butterfly 1.2. *Black arrow* shows stimulus point

the imaging chamber; however, fluid movement can introduce artefacts into the image time courses and so it is useful to set up the peristaltic pump such that it transiently halts during acquisition of an image sweep. In our setup a Gilson Minipuls 3 Peristaltic Pump can be directly switched on and off via a hardware input and is controlled by pClamp via a Master 8. The stock bath and dissection ACSF prepared will keep at 4 °C for 3 days; the required amount for the number of experiments planned for the week can be made up by scaling the quantities below.

3.2.1 Preparation: Day Before Experiment

1. Prepare 1 l of 2× bath ACSF and 1 l of 1× dissection ACSF. Do not add any Mg or Ca as these can precipitate out of solution, so it is best to add them just before use.

3.2.2 Preparation: Day of Experiment

1. Dilute 500 ml of 2× bath ACSF to 1× with distilled H_2O to make 1 l and measure out 200 ml of dissection ACSF into a beaker.

2. Add 2 ml and 1 ml of 1 M $CaCl_2$ and $MgCl_2$ respectively to the bath ACSF and 400 and 200 μl of the same to the dissection ACSF.

3. Measure and adjust the osmolality of both solutions to be 285 ± 5 mmol/Kg

4. Fill a large ice box with ice and place the dissection ACSF into the ice. Fill slice holding chamber with room temperature ACSF leaving ~300 ml for perfusion through the imaging chamber.

5. Using 70 % ethanol clean and prepare the area where the procedure is to take place, laying out all the equipment needed, clean the surgical tools and the vibratome chamber, blade, and blade holder. Place the vibratome parts in a freezer at −20 °C. Lay out the glue and filter paper.

6. Place cleaned tubing from the carbogen cylinder into the bath and dissection ACSF and bubble the solutions gently for at least 20 min prior to the procedure.

3.2.3 Slicing

1. Deeply anesthetize the mouse expressing the indicator with at least 100 mg/kg 10 mg/kg ketamine/xylazine IP injection [17]. Check that the mouse is anesthetized using the pedal reflex.

2. Perfuse the mouse transcardially with 10–20 ml of dissection ACSF. Once perfused, decapitate the mouse and remove the brain from the skull and place into ice cold dissection ACSF.

3. Remove the vibratome chamber from the freezer and place a line of superglue onto the mounting plate.

4. Take the brain out of the dissection ACSF and place on a piece of filter paper. Remove the cerebellum and, depending of area of interest cut a flat surface to glue to the vibratome plate using a razor blade wetted with ACSF.

5. Glue the brain anterior down on the vibratome plate, screw into the bath, and fill the bath with dissection ACSF. Place the bath onto the vibratome and attach the vibratome blade.

6. If making coronal slices it is optional to hemisect the brain sagittally and remove the ventral white matter in two sections by making a diagonal cut below the cortex.

7. Make 300–350 μm slices at around 0.6 mm/sec and 90 Hz.

8. Transfer the slices from the vibratome bath to the recovery chamber using a 3 ml Pasteur pipette with the end cut off.

9. Leave the slices for at least 2 h to recover at room temperature.

3.2.4 While Slices Recovering

1. Wash through the imaging chamber and perfusion system with 50 ml of each of 70 % ethanol, distilled water, and bath ACSF.

2. Ensure that the two camera channels are aligned.

3. Check that all control software is working and that there is adequate hard drive space.

3.2.5 Imaging and Electrophysiology

1. Using the pipette transfer the slice into the imaging chamber. Use a slice harp to anchor the slice. It is sometimes possible to physically rotate the chamber to ensure the slice is in the same orientation to the camera.

2. Using a 1.6× objective take a transmitted/scattered light image and a fluorescence image for reference.

3. Change to a 10× objective and navigate to your section of interest. Take a scattering and fluorescence reference image again and then place your stimulating and/or field electrodes into your desired location.

4. Image the slice for a fixed duration with the same stimulus point so that trials can be averaged and compared. It is useful to stimulate approximately 1/3 of the way through the run to allow time for a baseline to be collected before the stimulus response and for the full response decay to be measured. We typically image in 3 s trials, stimulating at the 1 s point.

5. It is also useful to develop some quick analysis tools to look at ROIs after the run is complete to check for a response and get an idea its strength and the noise level (*see* **Note 3**).

4   Notes

There are a few key points that are essential for collecting useful datasets.

1. Choosing the correct filter set and excitation source for the indicator is critical and requires a compromise between collecting as many photons as possible while still rejecting as much light originating from sources other than the chosen indicator, such as autofluorescence and stray excitation light, as possible. Collection of photons is crucial for resolving the small changes in indicator brightness that arise from neuronal activity. Considering a shot-noise limited regime the signal-to-noise ratio, R, is given by

$$R \leq \frac{\Delta F}{F} \sqrt{n}.$$

[3], where $\Delta F/F$ is the fractional fluorescence change of the indicator arising from the event to be detected and $\sqrt{n}$ is the

number of collected photons. Typically not all photons collected will have been emitted by the fluorophores that indicate the signal of interest; some photons collected at the camera will have originated from nonresponsive indicator (e.g., indicator molecules not targeted to the plasma membrane in the case of GEVIs), tissue autofluorescence, stray background light and, importantly, indicator-expressing cells that do not contribute to the signal of interest. If the fraction of photons coming from these sources is f_B, then the effective achievable R will be reduced to

$$R \leq \frac{\Delta F}{F} \sqrt{n} \sqrt{1 - f_B}$$

Careful selection of emission and excitation filters and labeling only cells that contribute to the signal of interest can minimize f_B. When using a FRET-based indicator such as VSFP Butterfly 1.2 there is likely less autofluorescence emitted around the redder fluorescent protein's wavelength as the excitation light being used is generally too short to effectively excite endogenous fluorophores with similar emission spectra (e.g., with a very long Stokes shift). This allows the use of a wider emission filter for this path to maximize collected signal photons. Conversely, as the bluer fluorescent protein's emission spectrum is more likely to overlap with that of fluorophores that will be excited by the excitation source and it is also more prone to direct leakage from the excitation source itself the filter on this channel must be more tightly limited around the peak of the indicator's emission spectrum. For each individual channel in the setup and indicator type this trade-off must be optimized to maximize R.

2. A second key point that will ease subsequent data analysis and interpretation is ensuring that the cameras in a dual color acquisition setup are aligned, and are collecting synchronous and regular image frames. If the two light paths are spatially misaligned, then a suitable transform will have to be found to map the color images onto each other before any dual color analysis can be performed, which is an error prone and computationally expensive task. Non synchronous or irregular frame collection can distort the time courses of neural activity and confuse subsequent analysis. It is always best to use hardware based checks for timing issues. It is often possible to record the hardware frame out signal from the cameras and include it in the analysis as necessary. Another technique is to use an LED flash at the beginning and end of each acquisition to provide a timestamp for both cameras to compare their timing. To avoid timing issues in the first place it is important to use impedance matched

connectors and splitters such as 50 Ω BNCs when transmitting timing critical information such as camera triggers.

3. To remove any drift in baseline signal an exponential function can be fit to the fluorescence time course for each pixel, discounting the pixels showing a stimulation response (or alternatively use sweeps with no evoked responses). By dividing by this exponential the time course is corrected for signal of interest-independent components due to chromophore bleaching, photoconversion, etc. and baseline-normalized, facilitating further analysis. Depending on the noise level in the image it may be necessary to bin the image to achieve an adequate R. Depending on the magnification and NA of the objective used, this may have no effect on the resolution as the camera sensors used here are spatially oversampling.

Acknowledgments

This work was supported by the Engineering and Physical Sciences Research Council [grant number EP/L016737/1]. We would like to thank Elisa Ciglieri, Amanda Foust, Taylor Lyons, and Chenchen Song for their very helpful comments and advice on the manuscript.

References

1. Sakmann B, Neher E (1984) Patch clamp techniques for studying ionic channels in excitable membranes. Annu Rev Physiol 46:455–472

2. Obien MEJ, Deligkaris K, Bullmann T et al (2015) Revealing neuronal function through microelectrode array recordings. Front Neurosci 8:423

3. Knöpfel T, Díez-García J, Akemann W (2006) Optical probing of neuronal circuit dynamics: genetically encoded versus classical fluorescent sensors. Trends Neurosci 29:160–166

4. Knöpfel T (2012) Genetically encoded optical indicators for the analysis of neuronal circuits. Nat Rev Neurosci 13:687–700

5. Franconville R, Revet G, Astorga G et al (2011) Somatic calcium level reports integrated spiking activity of cerebellar interneurons in vitro and in vivo. J Neurophysiol 106:1793–1805

6. Antic SD, Empson RM, Knöpfel T (2016) Voltage imaging to understand connections and functions of neuronal circuits. J Neurophysiol. doi:10.1152/jn.00226.2016

7. Hoover E, Squier J (2013) Advances in multiphoton microscopy technology. Nat Photonics 7:93–101

8. Flusberg BA, Cocker ED, Piyawattanametha W et al (2005) Fiber-optic fluorescence imaging. Nat Methods 2:941–950

9. Murray TA, Levene MJ (2012) Singlet gradient index lens for deep in vivo multiphoton microscopy. J Biomed Opt 17:021106

10. Murayama M, Pérez-Garci E, Lüscher HR et al (2007) Fiberoptic system for recording dendritic calcium signals in layer 5 neocortical pyramidal cells in freely moving rats. J Neurophysiol 98:1791–1805

11. Carandini M, Shimaoka D, Rossi LF et al (2015) Imaging the awake visual cortex with a genetically encoded voltage indicator. J Neurosci 35:53–63

12. Denk W, Strickler JH, Webb WW (1990) Two-photon laser scanning fluorescence microscopy. Science 248:73–76

13. Akemann W, Mutoh H, Perron A et al (2012) Imaging neural circuit dynamics with a voltage-sensitive fluorescent protein. J Neurophysiol 108:2323–2337

14. Kinosita K, Itoh H, Ishiwata S et al (1991) Dual-view microscopy with a single camera: Real-time imaging of molecular orientations and calcium. J Cell Biol 115:67–73

15. Haga T, Takahashi S, Sonehara T et al (2011) Dual-view imaging system using a wide-range dichroic mirror for simultaneous four-color single-molecule detection. Anal Chem 83:6948–6955

16. Ting JT, Daigle TL, Chen Q et al (2014) Acute brain slice methods for adult and aging animals: application of targeted patch clamp analysis and optogenetics. Methods Mol Biol 1183:221–242

17. Holtmaat A, Bonhoeffer T, Chow DK et al (2009) Long-term, high-resolution imaging in the mouse neocortex through a chronic cranial window. Nat Protoc 4:1128–1144

Chapter 6

FRET Microscopy for Real-Time Visualization of Second Messengers in Living Cells

Axel E. Kraft and Viacheslav O. Nikolaev

Abstract

Förster Resonance Energy Transfer (FRET) microscopy is a useful tool in molecular biology and medical research to monitor and quantify real-time dynamics of protein-protein interactions and biochemical processes. Using this well-established technique, many novel signaling mechanisms can be investigated in intact cells or tissues and even in various subcellular compartments. Here, we describe how to perform FRET measurements in living cells expressing FRET-based biosensors and how to evaluate these data. This general protocol can be applied for FRET measurements with various fluorescent biosensors.

Key words FRET, Microscopy, Imaging, Fluorescence, Biosensor

1 Introduction

Förster or Fluorescence Resonance Energy Transfer (FRET) microscopy is a powerful tool for real-time monitoring of signaling events in living cells and tissues [1, 2]. Classical biochemical techniques require thousands of cells to analyze a limited number of time points without any spatial resolution at the cellular level. The great advantage of FRET microscopy is the ability to visualize temporal and spatial changes of, for example, second messengers, not only within a single cell but also in subcellular compartments [3]. This technique is widely used for, e.g., pH measurements [4], detection of disease-related molecules [5], and visualization of compartmentation of second messengers such as cyclic nucleotides in cardiomyocytes [6].

FRET microscopy became a well-established method to investigate many novel signaling mechanisms and biochemical processes in living cells. Typical unimolecular fluorescent biosensors consist of a binding domain for the molecule of interest, which is flanked between two fluorescent proteins that act as energy donor and acceptor [2, 7]. The donor protein is excited with a single-wavelength light. The emitted light energy can be partially

Yolanda Markaki and Hartmann Harz (eds.), *Light Microscopy: Methods and Protocols*, Methods in Molecular Biology, vol. 1563, DOI 10.1007/978-1-4939-6810-7_6, © Springer Science+Business Media LLC 2017

transferred to the neighboring acceptor protein, which also emits fluorescence light without being directly excited. The binding of the molecule of interest to the binding domain leads to a conformational change of the biosensor, resulting in an altered distance between donor and acceptor. With increased distance between the two fluorophores, the emitted light of the donor loses the ability to excite the acceptor, which leads to a reduction of transferred energy [2]. By monitoring the donor/acceptor fluorescence ratio, changes in concentration of the molecule of interest can be recorded and analyzed in real time. Alternatively, bimolecular sensors can consist of two interacting proteins, one fused to the donor and another one to the acceptor fluorophore to monitor changes in protein-protein interaction over time. FRET biosensors can be introduced into living cells by plasmid transfection, viral gene transfer or they can be expressed in transgenic animal models [8].

This chapter describes the method of how to perform FRET microscopy, calculate FRET ratio, and evaluate cellular dynamics of second messengers in living cells.

2   Materials

2.1   FRET Imaging System

1. Inverted fluorescent microscope (Nikon ECLIPSE T*i*-S) equipped with an oil immersion objective (Plan Apo λ 60×/1.40 oil) and a suitable filter cube (including an excitation filter for the donor fluorophore and a longpass dichroic mirror, e.g., ET436/30 and LP455, respectively, if the donor fluorophore is CFP).

2. Fluorescence light source (coolLED *p*E-100) with a wavelength similar to the maximum spectral absorbance of the donor, in our case 440 nm for the cyan fluorescence protein (CFP).

3. Beam-splitter (Photometrics Dual-View DV2) including a filter cube consisting of a dichroic mirror and two emission filters for the donor and acceptor fluorophores. For CFP and yellow fluorescent protein (YFP) as a donor-acceptor pair, the DV2-cube 05-EM is routinely used. It includes a 505dcxr dichroic mirror, D480/30m and D535/40m emission filters.

4. CMOS Camera (QIMAGING optiMOS).

5. Arduino digital input/output board.

6. Microscopy software (Micro-Manager1.4.5 together with ImageJ). Refer to a previously published protocol that describes how to connect all imaging system components and how to set up the software [9].

2.2   Materials for FRET Measurements

1. Immersion oil for microscopy.

2. FRET Buffer: 144 mM NaCl, 5.4 mM KCl, 1 mM MgCl$_2$ × 6H$_2$O, 1 mM CaCl$_2$, and 10 mM HEPES. Weigh

8.42 g NaCl, 0.40 g KCl, 2.03 g $MgCl_2 \times 6H_2O$, and 2.38 g HEPES. Add 1 ml of a 1 M $CaCl_2$ solution and water up to a volume of 1 L. Adjust pH with 1 M NaOH to 7.4, filter through a 0.22 µm filter, and store at room temperature.

3. Round glass coverslides (25 mm diameter) with adherent cells expressing FRET biosensor.

4. Attofluor cell chamber for microscopy (Invitrogen) or similar.

2.3 Materials for Calculation of the Spectral Bleedthrough Correction Factor

1. 6-well plate with adherent cells (HEK293 cell line) plated on autoclaved glass coverslides in Dulbecco's Modified Eagle Medium (DMEM) supplemented with 10 % fetal calf serum, L-glutamine, and antibiotics.

2. Donor fluorescence protein expression plasmid, e.g., pECFP-N1.

3. Lipofectamine 2000 transfection reagent.

3   Methods

3.1 FRET Measurements in Living Cells

1. Place a coverslide with adherent cells into a cell chamber for microscopy.

2. Wash the cells with 400 µL of FRET buffer to remove nonadherent and dead cells (*see* **Note 1**).

3. Add 400 µL of fresh FRET buffer.

4. Put a small drop of immersion oil onto the objective and place the measuring chamber onto the microscope.

5. Focus on the cell layer using transillumination light and search a cell that is nicely attached to the coverslide (*see* **Note 2**).

6. Switch to the fluorescent light and check whether the biosensor is homogeneously expressed in the cell. If not the case, search for another cell.

7. Start imaging software and adjust the settings to reach a good signal-to-noise ratio of the cell (*see* **Note 3**).

8. Select the time interval between the individual images (e.g., 5–10 s) (*see* **Note 4**).

9. Start data acquisition.

10. Run a plugin that splits the image into donor and acceptor channels and calculates the ratio for each pixel (*see* **Note 5**).

11. Mark the region of interest and run the plugin that calculates the acceptor to donor ratio over time and displays a graph (*see* **Note 5**).

12. Wait until a stabile baseline is reached (*see* Fig. 1). We suggest waiting at least for 15 frames. Make sure that the starting FRET ratio values of each individual experiment are in a similar

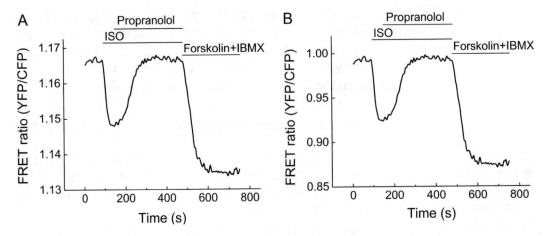

Fig. 1 Representative real-time FRET measurement of an adult mouse cardiomyocyte expressing a FRET bio-sensor for 3′,5′-cyclic adenosine monosphosphate (cAMP). The cell was sequentially stimulated with the β-adrenergic agonist isoprenaline (ISO, 100 nM, 90 s), the β-blocker propranolol (10 μM, 170 s), and the adenylyl cyclase activator forskolin (10 μM) plus the phosphodiesterase inhibitor 3-Isobutyl-1-methylxanthin (IBMX, 100 μM, 470 s). An uncorrected FRET ratio (YFP/CFP) is presented in (**a**), while (**b**) shows a corrected and normalized ratio trace obtained as described in Subheading 3.2. Decrease of FRET ratio corresponds to an increase of intracellular cAMP

range; otherwise variable spectral bleedthrough correction factors are needed.

13. Add the pharmacological compound of interest by carefully pipetting 400 μL of solution to the measuring chamber. This step can be repeated with further compounds as often as necessary (*see* Fig. 1).

14. Stop the experiment and save the images for offline data evaluation. Clean both the cell chamber and the objective of the microscope and start a new experiment.

3.2 Data Evaluation

1. Open the recorded images using the "Open Micromanager File" function and run a plugin that splits the acquired images into donor and acceptor channels.

2. Select the region of interest for which the average intensity should be calculated. Determine the individual values for donor and acceptor intensities for all frames.

3. Calculate the FRET Ratio: $\text{FRET} = \dfrac{\text{average acceptor intensity}}{\text{average donor intensity}}$.

4. To correct for the spectral bleedthrough effect, subtract the correction factor b (*see* Subheading 3.3) from the FRET ratio resulting in the corrected FRET ratio.

$$\text{FRET}_{\text{corr}} = \text{FRET} - b$$

5. Normalize the corrected FRET ratios to the average value of the baseline.

3.3 Calculating Spectral Bleedthrough Factor

The emission spectrum of the donor and acceptor overlap in the region of the maximum emission of the acceptor, which leads to a detection of the donor fluorescence in the acceptor channel [9]. It is necessary to calculate a spectral bleedthrough factor (b) to account for this phenomenon. The bleedthrough of the acceptor into the donor channel is usually negligible. For the determination of this correction factor, HEK293 cells are transfected with a plasmid that encodes only for the donor fluorophore.

1. Take 300 μL of DMEM without additives.
2. Add 3 μg of the donor fluorophore plasmid DNA. Mix.
3. Add 7 μL of Lipofectamine 2000. Mix well.
4. Incubate for 20 min (up to 40 min is possible).
5. Add 50 μL of transfection mix per well to the cells.
6. Incubate the cells for at least 24 h before measuring.
7. Perform FRET measurements as described in Subheading 3.1. Finish the experiment when a stable baseline is reached. Save the images and stop the experiment (*see* **Note 6**).
8. For determination of the correction factor proceed **steps 1–3** of Subheading 3.2. The calculated FRET ratio corresponds to the correction factor b.
9. Calculate the mean of at least ten cells to obtain a reliable correction factor.

4 Notes

1. Make sure to remove most of the dead and not adherent cells before starting the measurements since those could overlay the measured cells, making an experiment unusable. If necessary, wash several times.

2. By gently tapping with the fingers on the side of the microscope, it can be checked whether the cell is attached nicely to the coverslide.

3. To reach a good signal-to-noise ratio, the intensity of the LED and the exposure time can be varied. By increasing the light intensity and exposure time, better pictures are obtained but the propensity for photobleaching is increased as well. If photobleaching occurs (recognized by a rundown of the measured FRET ratio), the intensity of the LED and (or) the exposure time should be reduced. If these steps are not helpful, pick another cell.

4. Shorter time steps between the images lead to a more detailed trace but can also result in cell damage and photobleaching. Consider also that FRET measurements require a large amount

of image data storage (one experiment with 300 images requires approximately 300 MB).

5. ImageJ plugins are available online and easily customizable. Several tutorials on how to modify those plugins are available. *See* also our published plugins [9].

6. The exposure time and LED intensity should be chosen in a similar way as in real FRET experiments.

Acknowledgments

The work in authors' laboratory is supported by the Deutsche Forschungsgemeinschaft (grants NI 1301/1, FOR 2060), DZHK, and the Gertraud und Heinz Rose-Stiftung.

References

1. Herbst KJ, Ni Q, Zhang J (2009) Dynamic visualization of signal transduction in living cells: from second messengers to kinases. IUBMB Life 61:902–908

2. Zaccolo M (2004) Use of chimeric fluorescent proteins and fluorescence resonance energy transfer to monitor cellular responses. Circ Res 94:866–873

3. Sprenger JU, Nikolaev VO (2013) Biophysical techniques for detection of cAMP and cGMP in living cells. Int J Mol Sci 14:8025–8046

4. Chan YH, Wu C, Ye F et al (2011) Development of ultrabright semiconducting polymer dots for ratiometric pH sensing. Anal Chem 83:1448–1455

5. Busch C, Schroter T, Grabolle M et al (2012) An in vivo spectral multiplexing approach for the cooperative imaging of different disease-related biomarkers with near-infrared fluores-cent forster resonance energy transfer probes. J Nucl Med 53:638–646

6. Froese A, Nikolaev VO (2015) Imaging alterations of cardiomyocyte cAMP microdomains in disease. Front Pharmacol 6:172

7. Börner S, Schwede F, Schlipp A et al (2011) FRET measurements of intracellular cAMP concentrations and cAMP analog permeability in intact cells. Nat Protoc 6:427–438

8. Sprenger JU, Perera RK, Steinbrecher JH et al (2015) In vivo model with targeted cAMP biosensor reveals changes in receptor-microdomain communication in cardiac disease. Nat Commun 6:6965

9. Sprenger JU, Perera RK, Gotz KR et al (2012) FRET microscopy for real-time monitoring of signaling events in live cells using unimolecular biosensors. J Vis Exp:e4081

Chapter 7

Imaging the Dynamics of Cell Wall Polymer Deposition in the Unicellular Model Plant, *Penium margaritaceum*

David Domozych, Anna Lietz, Molly Patten, Emily Singer, Berke Tinaz, and Sandra C. Raimundo

Abstract

The unicellular green alga, *Penium margaritaceum*, represents a novel and valuable model organism for elucidating cell wall dynamics in plants. This organism's cell wall contains several polymers that are highly similar to those found in the primary cell walls of land plants. *Penium* is easily grown in laboratory culture and is effectively manipulated in various experimental protocols including microplate assays and correlative microscopy. Most importantly, *Penium* can be live labeled with cell wall-specific antibodies or other probes and returned to culture where specific cell wall developmental events can be monitored. Additionally, live cells can be rapidly cryo-fixed and cell wall surface microarchitecture can be observed with variable pressure scanning electron microscopy. Here, we describe the methodology for maintaining *Penium* for experimental cell wall enzyme studies.

Key words Live-cell immunolabeling, *Penium margaritaceum*, Cell wall, Monoclonal antibodies, CLSM, VP-SEM, Enzymes

1 Introduction

The deposition of cell wall polymers during expansion, division, and development of a plant cell requires a highly coordinated sequence of events that encompass components of the endomembrane system, cytoskeletal network, plasma membrane, and extracellular milieu [1–4]. This activity is carefully regulated by genetic controls and modulated through the plant cell's life by both internal prompts and external environmental signals that are, in turn, perceived by complex, cross-talking signal transduction mechanisms [5]. The plant cell wall is comprised of a highly structured mosaic of polymers, primarily polysaccharides and proteins, along with various ions, enzymes, and water [6, 7]. In the cell wall of expanding and dividing cells, the primary cell wall, microfibrillar cellulose forms the load-bearing foundation that is tethered by, and embedded in, a matrix of hemicelluloses, pectins, and highly

Yolanda Markaki and Hartmann Harz (eds.), *Light Microscopy: Methods and Protocols*, Methods in Molecular Biology, vol. 1563, DOI 10.1007/978-1-4939-6810-7_7, © Springer Science+Business Media LLC 2017

glycosylated proteins. Precise geographic and temporal deposition/ secretion of these components at the cell surface followed by their insertion into the preexisting wall architecture represent the basis of cell wall development. Despite recent technological advances in the biochemical and structural analyses of cell wall dynamics, we know surprisingly little about the deposition and post-deposition modulation of specific polymers during wall development. Several major problems are responsible for this. Most plants used in cell wall studies are multicellular. Consequently, high-resolution imaging of specific cell wall constituents and the wall deposition events occurring around a single cell surrounded by other cells in a tissue are exceptionally challenging. Likewise, in microscopy-based imaging of multicellular plants, common fixation protocols and sectioning often alter cell wall architecture and lead to removal of key wall components and/or the appearance of confounding artifacts. Live cell labeling of specific components of a single plant cell wall and subsequent analysis of their modulations over time and in response to environmental signals would greatly benefit our understanding of cell wall dynamics. Recently, the utilization of the unicellular charophyte, *Penium margaritaceum*, has provided novel and detailed views of polymer deposition mechanism in a living green plant [8–10]. *Penium* possesses many wall polymers similar to those found in the primary cell wall of land plants. This alga can be easily grown and maintained in culture. Quite robust, it can withstand somewhat harsh culturing variations, such as pH, temperature, and the presence of exogenous compounds, such as enzymes, subcellular inhibitors, or hormones. Furthermore, it can be live labeled with antibodies specific for cell wall polymers and returned to culture where subsequent imaging and experimentation can be performed. These features make *Penium* a valuable model in studying cell wall dynamics.

Here, we describe the methods for live cell labeling of *Penium*, monitoring dynamic events during cell expansion and division and using enzyme treatments to compromise cell wall structure and subsequently to analyze effects on cell and wall development.

2   Materials

2.1 Growth and Maintenance of Penium margaritaceum

1. *Penium margaritaceum* is available from the Skidmore College Algal Culture Collection (contact lead author of this chapter).

2. 55 mL or 200 mL Nunc tissue culture flasks, noncoated (Fisher Scientific 55 mL # 12-562-002; 200 mL # 12-575-200).

3. 15 mL sterile centrifuge tubes (Fisher Scientific # 05-527-90).

4. 10 mL sterile plastic pipettes (Fisher Scientific # 12-567-603).

5. Woods Hole Soil (WHS) medium: To 750 mL of deionized water (18 MΩ) add 1 mL of the stock solutions described on Table 1, and 50 mL of Soil Water Extract (2.1.6). Mix, adjust

Table 1
Stock solutions used to prepare Woods Hole Medium (WHM)

Solutions	Mol. weight (g/mol)	Stock in 1 L dH$_2$0 (g)	Stock concentration (mM)	Per liter media (mL)	Media concentration (μM)
Macronutrients					
CaCl$_2$.2H$_2$O	147.02	36.76	250	1	250
MgSO$_4$.7H$_2$O	246.47	36.97	150	1	150
NaHCO$_3$	84.01	12.60	150	1	150
K$_2$HPO$_4$.3H$_2$O	228.20	11.40	50	1	50
NaNO$_3$	84.99	85.01	1000	1	1000
Vitamin stock					
Thiamine (vitamin B$_1$)	337.27	0.10	300 μM	1	300 pM
Biotin	244.31	0.0005	2 μM		2 pM
Cyanocobalamin (vitamin B$_{12}$)	1355.37	0.00055	0.4 μM		0.4 pM
Or use 1 mL of Gamborg's vitamin solution (Sigma #G1019)					
EDTA solution					
Na$_2$EDTA	372.24	4.36	12	1	12
Trace elements				1	
FeCl$_3$.6H$_2$O	270.30	3.15	12		12
CuSO$_4$.5H$_2$O	249.69	0.01	0.04		0.04
ZnSO$_4$.7H$_2$O	287.56	0.022	0.08		0.08
CoCl$_2$.6H$_2$O	237.93	0.01	0.04		0.04
MnCl$_2$.4H$_2$O	197.91	0.18	0.91		0.91
Na$_2$MoO$_4$.2H$_2$O	241.95	0.006	0.025		0.025
H$_3$BO$_3$	61.83	1.00	16		16
Trizma base					
Trizma-HCl	121.14	250.0	2000	1	2000

Note: All chemicals were purchased from Sigma; stock solutions should be kept refrigerated (4 °C) for up to 1 year

pH to 7.2 and bring volume to 1000 mL. The medium is dispensed in 500 mL stoppered glass bottles and autoclaved at 120 °C for 20 min (*see* **Note 1**).

6. Soil Water Extract: deposit into a 1 L glass flask, 2.5 cm of garden soil (without pesticides or fertilizers) and cover with 800 mL deionized water. Place on a hot plate and heat to boiling. Turn heat down and let simmer for 6 h. Let cool overnight

and repeat the heating process for the second day. On the third day, filter the extract through multiple layers of filter paper. The extract should be brown and clear. It may be stored for up to a year in a refrigerator (*see* **Note 2**).

2.2 Live Cell Labeling and Analysis

Prepare all solutions using ultrapure water (18 MΩ) and analytical grade reagents. Store stock solutions in a refrigerator unless otherwise stated. Follow all institutional and government waste disposal protocols for the laboratory.

1. Primary monoclonal antibodies (mAbs): JIM5, JIM7, JIM13, LM13, LM6 (Plant Probes, Leeds, UK); CCRCM-M38, CCRC-M131, CCRC-M132, CCRC-M34 (Complex Carbohydrate Research Center, Athens, Georgia).

2. Secondary antibodies: anti-rat TRITC (Sigma # T4280), anti-rat FITC (Sigma # F6258), anti-mouse TRITC (Sigma # T5393), anti-mouse FITC (Sigma # F9137) (*see* **Note 3**).

3. Other stains: Calcofluor-fluorescent brightener 2B (Sigma # F3543).

4. WHS medium.

5. WHS-BSA block: Dissolve 0.25 g of bovine serum albumin (Sigma # A2153) in 100 mL WHS (*see* **Note 4**).

6. Petri dishes 60 × 15 mm (Fisher Scientific # FB0875713A); 100 × 15 mm (Fisher Scientific # FB0875713).

7. 1.5 mL microcentrifuge tubes (Fisher Scientific # 02-681-320).

8. 15 mL sterile centrifuge tubes (Fisher Scientific # 05-527-90).

9. 10–200 μL and 100–1000 μL micropipettors and pipette tips.

10. Microtube shaker or rotator for continuous mixing of cell suspensions with labels.

11. Microcentrifuge (Fisher Scientific accuSpin Micro 17).

12. Table top clinical centrifuge (Sorvall ST8R).

13. Aluminum foil.

14. Vortex (Vortex Genie2).

15. Microscope slides (Fisher Scientific # 12-550-343) and 22 × 22 mm coverslips (Fisher Scientific # 12-541-B).

2.3 Enzymatic Treatment of Live Cells

1. Enzymes—Megazyme, Bray, Ireland: endo-arabinanase (# E-EARAB), α-L-arabinofuranosidase (# E-AFASE), α-L-arabinofuranosidase (# E-AFAM2); pectate lyase (# E-PCLYAN); ß-galactosidase (# E-BGLAN), α-L-rhamnosidase (# E-RHAMS). Sigma-Aldrich, St. Louis, MO, USA: cellulase from *Trichoderma reesei* (# C8546-5KU).

2. 0.1 M KOH solution: Dissolve 0.56 g of KOH in 100 mL deionized water.

3. WHS medium.

4. WHS pH 6.0 medium: Dissolve 0.4 g of MES (Sigma # M8250) in 100 mL of WHS and adjust pH to 5.8 with 0.1 M KOH.

5. WHS pH 8.0 medium: Adjust pH of 100 mL WHS medium to 8.0 with 0.05 M KOH.

6. 12-welled noncoated Petri dishes (Fisher Scientific # 351143).

7. 1–20 μL, 10–100 μL and 100–1000 μL micropipettors and pipette tips.

8. 15 mL sterile centrifuge tubes (Fisher Scientific # 02-681-320).

9. Table top centrifuge (with speeds to $1000 \times g$).

2.4 Observing Cell Expansion and Division Events

1. 60 × 15 mm Petri dishes (Fisher Scientific # FB0875713A).

2. WHS with 3 % (w/v) low gelling agar (Sigma # A0701) kept at 45 °C in an oven.

3. WHS medium.

4. 20–200 μL micropipettor with disposable tips.

2.5 Variable Pressure Scanning Electron Microscopy

1. 1.5 mL microcentrifuge tubes (Fisher Scientifics # 02-681-320).

2. 1–20 μL, 10–100 μL, and 100–1000 μL micropipettors and pipette tips.

3. Microcentrifuge (Fisher Scientific accuSpin Micro17).

4. Fine tip forceps.

5. Nylon membrane 0.45 μm (Thomas Scientific # 4313S12).

6. JEOL cryostub (JEOL Corp., Peabody, MA).

7. Liquid nitrogen.

2.6 Microscopy

Olympus BX60 (Olympus America Inc., Melville, NY, USA) equipped with an Olympus DP73 digital camera; Olympus IX70 Inverted Microscope equipped with an Olympus DP71 digital camera; Olympus Fluo View™ 300 or 1200 confocal laser scanning microscopes; JEOL JSM-6480LV scanning electron microscope (JEOL USA Inc., Peabody, MA, USA); Stereomicroscope Wild M3C (Heerbrugg, Switzerland) (*see* **Note 5**).

3 Methods

3.1 Culturing and Maintenance of Penium

Perform culture handling with aseptic technique and under a laminar flow hood at room temperature.

1. Fill a Nunc tissue culture flask to the recommended volume as marked on the side of the flask with sterile WHS medium (*see* **Note 6**).

2. Obtain a subculture of *Penium* that is 7–14 days old (i.e., since its last transfer) and aseptically pipette 2 mL of cell suspension into a 55 mL flask or 5 mL to a 200 mL flask.

3. *Penium* can be grown at 18–24 °C with a 16:8 light:dark cycle under cool white fluorescent light (74 µmol/m^2/s Photosynthetic Photon Flux). Subcultures will "turn" green after a few days. Cell suspensions from log-phase culture (7–14 days old) are used for subsequent labeling and experiments.

3.2 Live-Cell Immunolabeling (Fig. 1)

1. Harvest 10 mL aliquots of 7–14 day old cell cultures and place in 15 mL centrifuge tubes. For cells that will be viewed immediately after labeling, aseptic technique is not necessary at this point. For labeled cells that will be subsequently cultured, aseptic practice should be followed.

2. Centrifuge cell suspensions for 1 min at 750 × *g* using a clinical table top centrifuge.

3. Discard the supernatant and resuspend the pellet in 5 mL of fresh WHS. Cap the tube and shake vigorously for 20 s.

4. Repeat **steps 2** and **3**, Subheading 3.2 two times. These constitute cell washings and are performed to remove external mucilage or the extracellular polymeric substance (EPS) (*see* **Note 7**).

5. Resuspend the cell pellet in 5 mL WHS-BSA block and place on a laboratory shaker or rotator and gently mix cells for 30 min.

6. Repeat **steps 2** and **3**, Subheading 3.2 three times to remove the WHS-block.

7. Resuspend the pellet in 1.0 mL of WHS and transfer 250 µL aliquots of the resulting suspension into four 1.5 mL microcentrifuge tubes. 250 µL aliquots will provide a large number of labeled cells and for multiple immunolabelings, adjust the amount of harvested cells accordingly.

8. Centrifuge the tubes at 4000 rpm (1,500 × *g*) for 1 min in a microcentrifuge.

9. Remove the supernatant from the pellet using a 100–1000 µL micropipettor and discard.

10. Resuspend the pellet in 200 µL of mAb diluted 1/10 with WHS.

11. Cap the tube and vortex at highest setting for 5 s to mix.

12. Wrap the tube with aluminum foil and place on a mixer/rotator. Set the speed to a point where cells are gently mixed and incubate for 90 min.

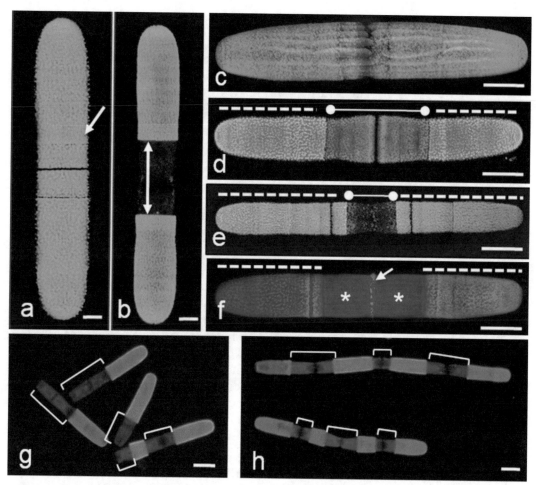

Fig. 1 Live-cell immunolabeling profiles of P. margaritaceum. (**a**) is a JIM5-labeled cell and highlights the labeling of the outer pectin layer of the cell wall (arrow). (**b**) is a JIM5-labeled cell that was returned to culture for 24 h. The dark zone (double arrow) displays the new expansion area. (**c**) is a CLSM image of a cell labeled with JIM5 overlayed with the profile of the chloroplast. The plastid often provides excellent background for cell measurements. (**d**) is a cell co-labeled with JIM5-TRITC (dotted line), placed back into culture for 24 h and then labeled with JIM5-FITC (solid line). New cell wall material is highlighted by JIM5-FITC labeling. (**e**) is a cell labeled with JIM5-TRITC (dotted line), place back in medium containing the endoarabinanase, EFAM2, for 24 h and then labeled with JIM5-FITC (solid line). The altered wall is clearly labeled at the JIM5-FITC zone. (**f**) is a cell labeled with JIM5 (dotted line) and then placed back into culture for 24 h. It was then co-labeled with JIM7 (arrow) and Calcofluor (asterisk). This profile shows the deposition of high methyl-esterified pectin (JIM7, arrow) in the cell center and the underlying layer of cellulose. (**g, h**) are profiles of cells labeled and placed back into culture for 48 h. (**g**) represents control cells and (**h**) represents cells incubated in 5 μg/mL cytochalasin E. In order to compare expansion levels in both, the unlabeled zones, i.e., the lengths of the new expansion zones and whole cell lengths are measured and surface areas (*see* Subheading 3.3) are calculated. % of expansion in control versus treated cells can then be calculated. In this experiment, cytochalasin-treated cells expanded at the same levels as control cells but did not undergo cytokinesis. Scale bars: (**a, b**) 5 μm (**c, f**) 7 μm (**d**) 10 μm (**e**) 12 μm (**g, h**) 15 μm

13. Retrieve the tubes and centrifuge at 4000 rpm for 1 min. Discard the supernatant and resuspend the pellet in fresh WHS medium. Repeat two times to wash out the mAb solution.

14. Resuspend the pellet in 1 mL of WHS-block and gently mix on laboratory shaker/mixer for 20 min.

15. Repeat the washing **step 13**, Subheading 3.2.

16. Resuspend the pellet in 200 μL of secondary antibody diluted 1/100 with WHS.

17. Cap the tube and vortex at highest setting for 5 s.

18. Wrap the tube with aluminum foil and place on a mixer/rotator. Set the speed to a point where cells are gently mixed and incubate for 90 min.

19. Retrieve the tube and repeat the washing **step 13**, Subheading 3.2.

20. The cell pellet may be: (a) resuspended in 500 μL of WHS and subsequently used for microscopy imaging; (b) resuspended in 2 mL of WHS and placed in a 60 × 15 mm Petri dish. Seal the plate with parafilm and place in culture. Aliquots of cells may be removed at time sequences thereafter and observed. New cell wall material is identified as the unlabeled zone surrounded by antibody-labeled zones; (c) resuspended in 5 mL of WHS in a 15 mL tube, covered with aluminum foil and kept at room temperature (*see* **Note 8**).

21. Microscopy imaging: Place 12–15 μL of labeled cell suspension onto a glass slide and cover with a 22 by 22 mm coverslip. Observe cells with a fluorescence microscope using the microscope specific filter for TRITC or FITC. For confocal laser scanning microscopy (CLSM), use a green laser with TRITC filter set or blue laser with FITC filter set. Cells labeled with TRITC-coupled secondary antibody may be observed as above and the chloroplast may be viewed with the blue laser and FITC filter set. The images or image sets can then be merged.

22. Co-labeling with Calcofluor: Remove a 50–100 μL aliquot of labeled cell suspension and wash as in **step 13**, Subheading 3.2.

    (a) Resuspend the cells in 1000 μL of WHS and add 1 μL of Calcofluor solution. Vortex, wrap the tube with aluminum foil, and place on a rotator for 5 min.

    (b) Wash the cells as in **step 13**, Subheading 3.2 and resuspend pellet in 500 μL of WHS. Place 12–15 μL of cell suspension on a glass slide and cover with a 22 by 22 mm coverslip. Observe the immunolabeling as in **step 21**, Subheading 3.2. Calcofluor labeling can be detected with a UV filter on a fluorescence microscope or with a 450 nm laser if using a CLSM. Calcofluor provides a bright image of the cellulose inner layer.

23. Co-labeling with a second cell wall-directed mAb: remove a 50–100 μL aliquot of cell suspension and wash as in **step 13**, Subheading 3.2. Follow **steps 10–19**, Subheading 3.2 using a second cell wall-specific mAb diluted 1/10 in WHS and a secondary antibody conjugated with a different fluorophore (i.e., if initial antibody labeling was with FITC, use TRITC for the second immunolabeling).

24. Single cell studies: place four rows of 100 μL drops of WHS on a 9 mm sterile Petri dish. Add 50 μL of labeled cell suspension to the center of the plate.

    (a) Place the Petri dish on a dissecting microscope. Take 10 μL of the labeled cell suspension and mix in one of the drops of WHS. Take 10 μL of this drop and add mix in a second drop. Repeat this serial dilution until only five to ten cells are floating in the drop.

    (b) Prepare a 48-welled Petri dish as follows. With a 1–10 μL micropipettor capture a cell from a drop and place in the center of a well. Add 5 μL of 3 % agarose-WHS to the center of a well near the cell and immediately mix. Swirl the plate to form a thin agarose sheet containing the single cell.

    - Cover the cell with a 1 mL of WHS or WHS containing an experimental agent.

    - Seal the plate with parafilm and place in culture.

    - Periodically the individual cell may be imaged with a fluorescent inverted microscope. The zones and rates of expansion in the cell and daughter cells may be obtained over several days. If a camera with time lapse capability is available, time lapse movies can be made.

3.3 Quantitative Measurements

1. Use JIM5 mAb-TRITC labeled cells for incubation in enzyme solutions. At certain time intervals, remove 100 μL of cell suspension and place in a 1.5 mL centrifuge tube.

2. Remove the supernatant and resuspend the pellet in 25 μL of WHS. Remove 12 μL of the cell suspension and place on a slide. Cover with a 22×22 mm coverslip and view with a fluorescence microscope or CLSM. New growth zones are not labeled and are surrounded by fluorescent zones.

3. Measure the length of each cell and the length of all nonlabeled zones (Fig. 1g–h). The surface area of each zone is determined by the following formula: $SA = 2(\pi \times r^2) + (2\pi \times r) \times L$ where, r = the radius of the cell (8.5 μm).

3.4 Selective Removal of Cell Wall Polymers in Live Cells Using Enzymes (Fig. 2)

1. Add 1 mL of WHS-pH 6.0 to the first 6 wells of a 12-welled Petri dish. Leave the first well with only WHS for the negative control. Add the following enzymes to each of the next five wells: 3 μL of E-EARAB, 3 μL of E-EAFASE, 3 μL of E-EAFAM2, 3 μL of E-BGLAN, and 3 μL of E-RHAMS. To another well add 1 mL of WHS-pH 6 containing 10 mg of *Trichoderma* cellulase. To another well, add 1 mL of WHS-pH 8.0 and 2 μL of E-PCLYAN (*see* **Note 9**).

2. Harvest 10 mL of 7–14 day old cell suspensions and place in a 15 mL centrifuge tube. Centrifuge at $750 \times g$ for 1 min on a table top centrifuge. Pour off the supernatant. Resuspend the pellet in 5 mL of WHS, vortex to 20 s and recentrifuge. Repeat two times to remove EPS from the cells.

3. Resuspend the pellet in 200 μL of WHS and mix. Add 20 μL of the cell suspension to each well of the enzyme plate. Swirl gently to mix the cells.

4. Seal the plate with Parafilm and place in culture. At certain time intervals chosen (hours, days), morphological changes of a certain polymer distribution within the cell wall can be observed by collecting aliquots of cells and immunolabeling with specific mAbs.

3.5 Recovery Experiments

These experiments require simple washing of the cells and return to fresh growth medium and culturing conditions.

1. Harvest 250 μL of cells from the wells and place in a 1.5 mL microcentrifuge tube. Centrifuge at 4000 rpm for 1 min. Remove the supernatant and resuspend the pellet in 500 μL of WHS. Vortex for 30 s.

2. Repeat the centrifugation and washing of the pellet two times.

3. Resuspend the pellet in 1 mL of WHS and transfer to the well of a new 12-welled plate. Seal the plate with Parafilm and place in culture.

4. After specific time periods, aliquots of cells may be collected and observed via microscopy. Cells that were labeled with an antibody may also be treated this way and new growth zones will appear as unlabeled zones when using fluorescence optics.

3.6 Cell Surface Observation with VP-SEM (Fig. 3)

1. Harvest 1 mL aliquots of the cells of interest and place them in 1.5 mL microcentrifuge tubes. Centrifuge the cells for 1 min at 4000 rpm. Discard the supernatant and resuspend the pellet in 1 mL of fresh WHS. Cap the tube and vortex for 10 s. Discard the supernatant and repeat the washing step two times. Add 50 μL of fresh WHS.

2. Place the JEOL cryostub in a shallow styrofoam box with liquid nitrogen and allow it to cool down, until the cryostub chamber fills in with liquid nitrogen (after 2–3 min a clear bubbling noise indicates that the chamber is full).

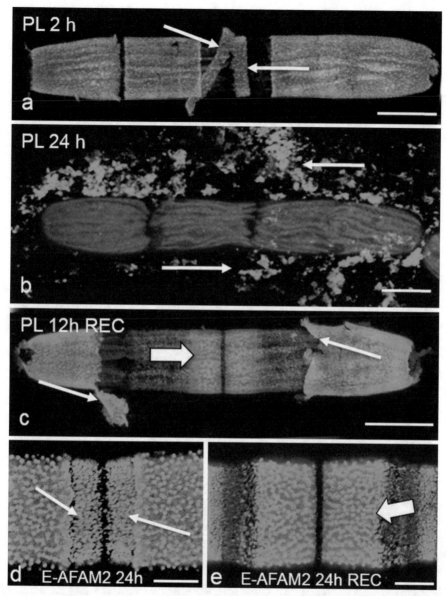

Fig. 2 Effects of exogenous enzymes on live cells. (**a**) is a cell treated with 2 U pectate lyase (PL; E-PCLYAN) for 2 h. Sheets of the outer pectin rich cell wall, as labeled by JIM5, are removed from the cell surface (arrows). (**b**) is a cell treated with pectate- lyase for 24 h. The pectin-rich outer wall, as labeled by JIM5, is removed from the wall surface (arrows). (**c**) is a cell treated with pectate lyase for 12 h, washed and allowed to recover for 12 h. New pectin is deposited in the cell center (large arrow) while sheets of old pectin (small arrows) may be observed at the polar zones. (**d**) is a cell treated with 12 U of endo-arabinanase for 24 h. The typical outer wall layer "lattice" of pectin is notably altered in the cell center (arrows). (**e**) is a cell treated with endo-arabinanase for 24 h, washed and allowed to recover in fresh medium for 24 h. New pectin is deposited in the cell center (arrow). Scale bars: (**a–c**) 15 μm (**d**) 5 μm (**e**) 4 μm

3. Place 12 μL of cells on a small piece of nylon membrane and with fine tip forceps place and secure it on the cryostub.

4. Quickly place the cryostub in the VP-SEM chamber, close it and set up the microscope to low vacuum mode. Although the

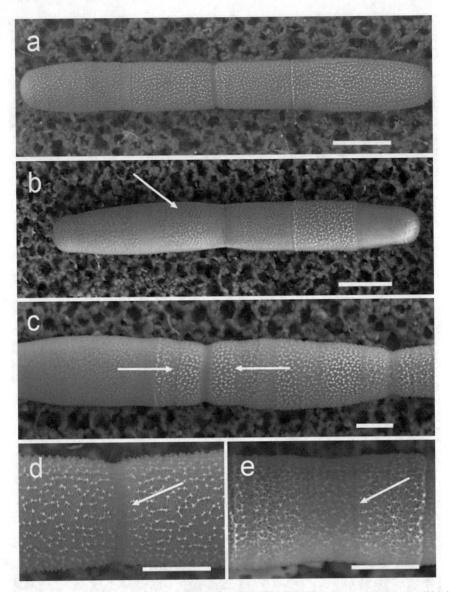

Fig. 3 Effects of exogenous enzymes on live cells generated with VP-SEM: (**a**) is a nontreated cell highlighting the typical structural appearance of Penium's cell surface. (**b**) is a cell treated for 5 days with 24 U of galacto-sidase (E-BGLAN). The typical outer wall layer lattice is clearly affected (arrow). (**c**) is a cell treated with cellulose and 24 U of galactosidase for 5 days, washed and allowed to recover in fresh medium for 48 h. New pectin is being deposited in the center of the cell (arrows), while the rest of the outer lattice of the cell is visibly affected. (**d**) is a close-up view of the center of a nontreated cell, called isthmus zone, where new cell wall material is deposited (arrow). (**e**) displays the isthmus zone of a cell treated with galactosidase for 5 days. The outer lattice is clearly affected by the effect of the enzyme (arrow). Scale bars: (**a**, **b**) 20 μm (**c–e**) 10 μm

settings may vary, usually imaging is performed using backscattered electrons signal (BEIW), with a pressure of 27 Pa, accelerating voltage of 10 kV, working distance of 6 mm, spotsize of 60 (*see* **Note 10**).

3.7 Concluding Remarks

The methods described here allow for quick and efficacious acquisition of multiple data sets of experimentally treated cells including (a) qualitative and quantitative analyses of pectin deposition during expansion; (b) a simple means of temporal assessment of cell wall expansion; (c) a conduit for multiple labelings of single live cells; and (d) a rapid way for high-resolution VP-SEM imaging for correlative analysis with immunofluorescence. In our laboratory, we have been able to thoroughly screen the effects of as many as 30 agents (e.g., enzymes) per week. The techniques described here are also adaptable to other labeling protocols including those that employ other cell wall polymer-specific antibodies, carbohydrate binding modules [11], and reciprocal probes such as labeled chitosan oligosaccharides [12].

4 Notes

1. Medium and stock reagents can be stored in a refrigerator (4 °C) for up to a year. If any stock turns cloudy, prepare a fresh supply.

2. Soil water supernatant extract may be purchased from Carolina Biological Supply Company (#153790) and used in the same quantity as "homemade" soil extracts.

3. Other fluorophore-conjugated antibodies (e.g., Alexa Fluor®-conjugates) work as well as FITC and TRITC. Also regarding secondary antibodies, extra attention must be paid before purchasing secondary antibodies, because they will bind to the primary antibodies as long as they were generated in the same mammal from which the primary antibodies were generated. If the primary antibodies were generated on rats, the secondary antibodies must also have been generated on rats. Always check the manufacturer's specifications as they will mention if the antibody is anti-rat, anti-mouse, or other.

4. Carnation Nonfat Instant Milk can be replaced by bovine serum albumin. It should be used at a concentration range of 0.5–1.0 % (w/v) in WHS. Prior to use, centrifuge the solution at $13,000 \times g$ for 2 min. Use the supernatant.

5. Our laboratory uses Olympus and JEOL microscopes. Virtually all other microscopy companies have similar microscopes that can be used for *Penium* studies. For example, an environmental SEM may be used in place of a VPSEM.

6. *Penium* also grows successfully in WHS in cotton-stoppered sterile glass flasks. We have used 125 mL and 250 mL flasks and subculturing regimes as described in this chapter.

7. *Penium* produces a fair amount of EPS even when grown on normal growth conditions; removing the EPS before any experimental procedure is a crucial step for the success of any immunolabeling or staining procedure.

8. Cells do not expand in the dark and antibody labeling remains for at least 7 days. During this time, aliquots of cell suspension can be removed, washed as in Subheading 3.2, **step 13** and cultured. Cells begin to expand and divide within 24 h. Cells labeled with mAbs may be treated with various agents to monitor effects to the cell expansion.

9. Experiments may be upscaled to 6-welled plates (e.g., 3 mL total medium per well) or down scaled to 24-welled plates (500 μL total medium per well).

10. While using VP-SEM, the cells are frozen in liquid nitrogen when they are placed on the cryostub and enter the microscope chamber. It will take around 10 min for ice crystals that cover the cells to sublimate. After that, the cells are visible and ready to be photographed; however, the user will have between 10 and 20 min before the cells thaw completely and lose the typical cell shape. After that, new sample must be prepared and the procedure has to be repeated. Settings such as kV or vacuum levels may be adjusted as needed.

Acknowledgments

This work was supported by NSF grant NSF-MCB-RUI-1517345.

References

1. Oikawa A, Lund CH, Sakuragi Y, Scheller HV (2013) Golgi-localized enzyme complexes for plant cell wall biosynthesis. Trends Plant Sci 18:49–58

2. Li S, Lei L, Yingling YG, Gu Y (2015) Microtubules and cellulose biosynthesis: the emergence of new players. Curr Opin Plant Biol 28:76–82

3. Anderson CT (2016) We be jammin': an update on pectin biosynthesis, trafficking and dynamics. J Exp Bot 67:495–502

4. Cosgrove DJ (2016) Plant cell wall extensibility: connecting plant cell growth with cell wall structure, mechanics, and the action of wall-modifying enzymes. J Exp Bot 67:463–476

5. Keegstra K (2010) Plant cell walls. Plant Physiol 154:483–486

6. Doblin MS, Pettolino F, Bacic A (2010) Plant cell walls: the skeleton of the plant world. Funct Plant Biol 37:357–381

7. Cosgrove DJ, Jarvis MC (2012) Comparative structure and biomechanics of plant primary and secondary cell walls. Front Plant Sci 3:204. http://www.frontiersin.org/Plant_Physiology/10.3389/fpls.2012.00204/full

8. Domozych DS, Sorensen I, Popper ZA, Ochs J, Andreas A, Fangel JU, Pielach A, Sachs C, Brechka H, Ruisi-Besares P, Willats WGT, Rose JKC (2014) Pectin metabolism and assembly in the cell wall of the charophyte green alga *Penium margaritaceum*. Plant Physiol 165:105–118

9. Domozych DS, Sørensen I, Sacks C et al (2014) Disruption of the microtubule network alters cellulose deposition and causes major changes in pectin distribution in the cell wall of the green alga *Penium margaritaceum*. J Exp Bot 65:465–479

10. Domozych DS, Lambiasse L, Kiemle SN, Gretz MR (2009) Cell-wall development and bipolar growth in the desmid *Penium margari-*

taceum (Zygnematophyceae, Streptophyta). Asymmetry in a symmetric world. J Phycol 45:879–893

11. Gilbert HJ, Knox JP, Boraston AB (2013) Advances in understanding the molecular basis of plant cell wall polysaccharide recognition by carbohydrate-binding modules. Curr Opin Struct Biol 23:669–677

12. Mravec JJ, Kračun SK, Rydahl MG, Westereng B, Miart F, Clausen MH, Fangel JU, Daugaard M, Van Cutsem P, De Fine LHH, Höfte H, Malinovsky FG, Domozych DS, Willats WGT (2014) Tracking developmentally regulated post-synthetic processing of homogalacturonan and chitin using reciprocal oligosaccharide probes. Development 141:4841–4850

Chapter 8

Targeted Ablation Using Laser Nanosurgery

Naga Venkata Gayathri Vegesna, Paolo Ronchi, Sevi Durdu, Stefan Terjung, and Rainer Pepperkok

Abstract

Laser-mediated dissection methods have been used for many years to micro-irradiate biological samples, but recent technological progress has rendered this technique more precise, powerful, and easy to use. Today pulsed lasers can be operated with diffraction limited, sub-micrometer precision to ablate intracellular structures. Here, we discuss laser nanosurgery setups and the instrumentation in our laboratory. We describe how to use this technique to ablate cytoskeletal elements in living cells. We also show how this technique can be used in multicellular organisms, to micropuncture and/or ablate cells of interest and finally how to monitor a successful laser nanosurgery.

Key words Laser nanosurgery, Subcellular structures, Laser ablation, Micropuncture, Photobleach

1 Introduction

Laser nanosurgery uses short laser pulses under microscopic control to enable the selective dissection of biological structures with sub-micrometer precision. It is suitable to target either subcellular structures or entire cells in an organism. The concept of targeted surgery using lasers dates back to 1965, when selective damage of the mitochondria was achieved with the help of a pulsed ruby laser [1]. Pulsed lasers at different wavelengths were also used early on to ablate stress fibers and intermediate filaments in living cells [2]. However, the setups used at the time were highly customized and only few laboratories used the method. The improvements in this technique throughout the years and finally its commercialization made it reliable, highly precise and powerful allowing its common use as a standard tool in cell and developmental biology. It has proven to be highly advantageous over the micromanipulators or needles used to dissect cells in the past, owing to its sub-micrometer precision and to the fact that no mechanical interaction with the sample is involved. Due to its capability of dissecting different

Yolanda Markaki and Hartmann Harz (eds.), *Light Microscopy: Methods and Protocols*, Methods in Molecular Biology, vol. 1563, DOI 10.1007/978-1-4939-6810-7_8, © Springer Science+Business Media LLC 2017

structures at multiple scales, laser nanosurgery has been used to perturb intracellular structures, single cells, or a subpopulation of cells in an organism, in a targeted manner. Laser surgeries have also been extensively used in medicine for various applications such as removal or damage of tissues. However, this application requires different lasers and setups and is not discussed in this chapter.

The evolution of fluorescent fusion proteins potentiated the usage of laser nanosurgery in living samples. Fluorescent proteins can be used to determine the best position for nanosurgery, to visualize the resulting process and help to gain more molecular and mechanistic insights [3]. In particular, this technique has been widely used to ablate single cytoskeletal elements to understand their functional and biophysical properties. Targeted ablation of cytoskeletal elements like actin fibers and microtubules allowed studying the contractile recoil and repair after irradiation. Indeed, severing the cytoskeletal elements allows measuring various forces, helps to simulate and model them and also to understand the mechano-sensing mechanisms in the cell [4]. Several studies have taken advantage of this method to study the forces involved in multicellular developmental processes, such as the elongation of Drosophila embryos, by dissecting actin fibers in the living organism [5]. Severing the actin stress fibers can also be used to release the cytoskeletal tension leading to a separation of the cells into two parts. This principle has been used to study the Golgi biogenesis process by removing it from cells growing on a patterned substrate [6, 7] and can be applied to cut neurites in cultured neurons [8, 9].

Laser nanosurgery has proven to be very versatile and besides the study of the cytoskeleton reported above, it has been used in a variety of applications. For instance, it proved very powerful to induce DNA breaks in order to study the molecular mechanisms for their recognition and repair [10, 11], to ablate intracellular organelles [12–14], or to create transient pores in the cell plasma membrane in order to allow the internalization of exogenous DNA, quantum dots, drugs etc. [14].

Laser ablation of a whole cell or a subpopulation in a living organism is widely used in developmental biology to study cell interactions, functions, adaptability and developmental potential [15–18]. It has been used for example to determine the function of the neurons involved in locomotion, feeding, mechano- and chemo-sensation in nematodes [19–26]. Recently, in multicellular organisms a series of experiments including laser micropuncture [27] revealed a new role for enclosed spaces that is to restrict, coordinate, and enhance signaling. It is very common to find such extracellular spaces generated by multicellular assemblies (e.g., [28–30]) in multicellular organisms. Therefore, this laser-based mechanical perturbation provides a framework to address the function of shared microenvironments in other systems as well.

Moreover, an interesting application of the method is its application for correlative light and electron microscopy experiments. Pulsed near infrared lasers can be used to create a three-dimensional marking in a tissue to identify a cell of interest for correlative light and electron microscopy applications [31, 32]. Similarly, the high peak power of pulsed lasers can also be applied to mark selective patterns on nonbiological material, such as glass [33, 34] or resin blocks [35] around the cells of interest.

In this chapter, we discuss in detail about the parameters that need to be considered and optimized to perform a laser nanosurgery experiment. We will take into consideration the suitability of different lasers and microscopy setups. Finally, we describe the procedures we use to calibrate and optimize the system in order to achieve ablation of cytoskeletal elements in cultured cells and disruption of cell contacts in a zebrafish embryo.

2 Materials

2.1 Considerations for Laser Nanosurgery Setups

2.1.1 Microscopes

In addition to application-specific custom setups for laser nanosurgery, there are several commercial systems available since recent times (*see* Table 1). Depending on the biological application in mind, they are based either on widefield fluorescence microscopes, confocal laser scanning systems (most suitable for thicker samples such as zebrafish or Drosophila embryos, where it is often necessary to acquire optical slices of the structures of interest during the ablation experiment), [37–40], or spinning disk confocal [44–46]. Custom nanosurgery systems installed on light sheet microscopes have also been reported [47, 48].

2.1.2 Lasers

A key element of the technology is the laser and the method to target it to the structure of interest. Laser pulses can induce damage to the biological material at different scales. The extent of the damage strongly depends on the power, repetition rate, and duration of the pulses. As the aim of a nanosurgery experiment is to induce a very precise ablation of the structure of interest at a submicron scale most nanosurgery applications are based on plasma-induced ablation [49], because the damage it causes remains restricted to the diffraction limited focal volume. To generate plasma in a biological sample by light, very high photon densities are needed, which are usually not achieved by continuous wave lasers. To exceed the threshold intensity for plasma formation, pulsed lasers, which achieve sufficient peak power in the femtosecond to a few nanosecond regimes are used (Table 2). Nonlinear absorption as used in 2-photon microscopy limits the plasma formation and the resulting nanosurgery to the focal volume. To ablate larger volumes or complex structures the laser can be positioned on the region of interest by a scanner or in case of a

Table 1
Examples of commercially available laser nanosurgery systems

System name	Key features	Remarks	References
Wide-field microscopy-based systems			
Leica LMD6 + LMD7	Upright widefield detection, designed for laser capture microdissection. Cut sections can be collected for further analysis. The laser is positioned by a scanner	Not optimized for nanosurgery on living samples	
Zeiss PALM microbeam	Inverted widefield detection, designed for laser catapulting microdissection. The dissection laser is positioned in the center of the imaging field and the sample has to be moved for dissection	Laser catapulting can be used to capture cells. The system can be combined with optical tweezers and with laser scanning or spinning disk confocal microscopy on special request (sequential use). Not optimized for nanosurgery on live samples	[36]
Confocal detection			
Olympus FV1200 SIM	Confocal microscope with two scanners. GaAsP detectors are available allowing more sensitive detection	Nanosurgery is possible in parallel to confocal imaging. Very flexible scan patterns are available. Multiple nanosurgery lasers can be installed in parallel	[37–40]
Bruker Opterra II	Variable pinhole linear array field scanner or high-speed line scanner with second scanner, which can be employed for nanosurgery when combined with a suitable laser	Fast optical sectioning at low photobleaching comparable to spinning disk systems. Different illumination modes available to adapt imaging conditions to experimental needs	
Zeiss LSM 780 NLO	Two-photon laser scanning system in combination with a sufficiently powerful two-photon laser, e.g., with Coherent Chameleon Ultra II	Nanosurgery can be performed during time-lapse experiments, but there is no special nanosurgery mode available	[27]
Olympus FVMPE-RS with SIM scanner	Two-photon laser scanning system with second scanner. Nanosurgery could be performed with a sufficiently powerful two-photon laser or other suitable nanosurgery laser	Nanosurgery is possible in parallel to confocal imaging. Very flexible scan patterns are available	

(continued)

Table 1
(continued)

System name	Key features	Remarks	References
Add-on solutions			
Rapp Optoelectronic (Wedel, Germany) UGA42 Firefly	Can be added to a number of commercial microscope stands	Can be combined with spinning disk microscopy systems. Detection in parallel to nanosurgery is possible	[6, 34]
Intelligent Imaging Innovations (3i, Denver, USA) Vector	Add-on for several commercial microscope stands	Can be combined with FRAP and photoactivation, simultaneous use with spinning disk microscopy is possible	[41]
MMI (Zuerich, Switzerland) CellCut	Add-on for several commercial microscope stands	Rather dedicated for isolation of cells in a fixed sample. The sample has to be moved for cutting	
Roper Scientific France (Evry Cedex, France) iPulse	Add-on for several commercial microscope stands	Can be combined with FRAP and photoactivation Can be combined with spinning disk microscopy	[42, 43]
Rowiak CellSurgeon	Add-on for several commercial microscope stands	Cutting routines to cut the surface area of three dimensional objects are available. Can be used as two-photon laser scanning microscope	

fixed laser focus position, the sample can be moved accordingly by a motorized xy-stage. The size of the induced plasma depends on the pulse energy, pulse duration, and wavelength of the employed laser as well as the focal volume determined by the numerical aperture of the objective lens [49].

In general, light of shorter wavelength can be focused into a smaller diffraction limited volume, leading to more precise nanosurgery. This is one reason why UV-A lasers (at for example $\lambda = 355$ nm) are frequently used for this purpose. Another reason is that the threshold for plasma formation depends on the employed wavelength. The energy threshold is lowest for UV light and increases towards the infrared range [49, 58]. In addition absorption of the employed nanosurgery light by the irradiated material decreases the threshold energy as well [59]. Choosing the right label for the structure to be ablated influences the ablation threshold significantly [40, 60].

The laser pulse duration is another important factor determining the efficiency of plasma formation in the focal volume. In general shorter pulses allow nanosurgery at lower energy levels. While

Table 2
Examples of laser types successfully used for laser nanosurgery

Laser type	Key features	Remarks	References
Coherent Mira 900F	Wavelength: 880 nm Pulse width: 100 fs Repetition rate: 80 MHz	Custom built system	[50]
Amplitude Systems t-Pulse 50	Wavelength: 1030 nm Pulse width: < 200 fs Repetition rate: 50 MHz Energy per pulse: 50 nJ Average power >2.5 W	Custom built system, either in combination with Zeiss Axiovert 135 m or PerkinElmer Ulraview ERS in combination with Nikon TE2000E	[44, 51]
Amplitude Systems Mikan	Wavelength: 1030 nm Pulse width <250 fs Repetition rate 50 MHz Energy per pulse: >20 nJ Average power > 1 W	Custom built system implemented on a light sheet microscope	[48]
Coherent Chameleon Ultra II Ti:Sa	Wavelength: 680–1080 nm Pulse width: 140 fs Repetition rate: 80 MHz Average power <3.5 W	Common two-photon laser as for example installed on Zeiss LSM 780 NLO microscopes	[27]
Q-switched diode pumped solid-state UV laser (e.g., JDS Uniphase, now Teem photonics)	Wavelength: 355 nm Pulse width: <500 ps Repetition rate: 1000 Hz Energy per pulse: max. 30 μJ Average power: max. 10 mW	Installed on Olympus FV1200 with SIM scanner. Also used in custom built setups	[39] (Olympus FV1200), [52, 53] (custom built)

(continued)

Table 2
(continued)

Laser type	Key features	Remarks	References
Rapp OptoElectronic diode pumped solid-state 355 nm laser	Wavelength: 355 nm Pulse width: 1 ns Repetition rate 200 Hz Energy per pulse: 150 μJ	Installed in our Rapp OptoElectronics UGA and Olympus system	[6]
Q-switched diode pumped solid-state 532 nm laser (e.g., JDS Uniphase, now Teem photonics)	Wavelength: 532 nm pulse width: <750 ps Repetition rate: 1000 Hz Energy per pulse: <40 μJ	Installed on Olympus FV1200 with SIM scanner	[37, 38]
355 nm of Roper iLasPulse	Wavelength: 355 nm Pulse width: 400 ps Repetition rate: 20,000 Hz Pulse energy: 1 μJ	Used in the Roper Scientific France iLasPulse	[42, 43]
532 nm of Roper iLasPulse	Wavelength: 532 nm Pulse width: 550 ps Repetition rate: 20,000 Hz Energy per pulse: 3.5 μJ	Used in the Roper Scientific France iLasPulse	[54]
Intelligent Imaging Innovations (3i) Ablate!	Wavelength: 532 nm Repetition rate: 200 Hz Energy per pulse > 60 μJ	Used in combination with 3i vector	[55, 56]
Diode pumped solid state	Wavelength: 349 nm Pulse width: <4 ns Repetition rate: 10–5000 Hz Energy per pulse: 120 μJ	Used in Leica LMD7	

(continued)

Table 2
(continued)

Laser type	Key features	Remarks	References
Diode pumped solid state	Wavelength: 355 nm Pulse width: <4 ns Repetition rate: 80 Hz Energy per pulse: 70 μJ	Used in Leica LMD6	
Picoquant LDH-P-C-405B	Wavelength: 405 nm Pulse width: 70 ps Repetition rate: 40 MHz		[40]
Frequency tripled solid state laser	Wavelength: 355 nm Pulse width: < 2 ns Repetition rate: 1–100 Hz Energy per Pulse: >90 μJ	Used in Zeiss PALM microbeam (current release)	
Nitrogen laser	Wavelength: 337 nm Pulse width: 3 ns Repetition rate: 30 Hz Energy per pulse: 270 μJ	Used in Zeiss PALM microbeam (older versions)	[36, 57]

up to 250 μJ are required using nanosecond pulses [49], three orders of magnitude less energy is needed when picosecond pulses are employed [61]. In the case of femtosecond pulses the energy threshold sufficient for plasma formation is in the low nJ range [62]. Most two-photon laser scanning microscopes are built with lasers delivering pulsed infrared light with a pulse width in the range of 150 femtoseconds and are used at a low attenuation level for imaging. Using these lasers at high power levels enables the user to perform nanosurgery experiments (*see* Sect. 3.2.2).

2.1.3 Objective Lenses   In general objective lenses for laser nanosurgery need to be well corrected; usually Plan Apo lenses are preferred. High transmission values especially in the wavelength range of the employed pulsed laser source are very important, not only to reach sufficient energy levels in the focus but also to prevent damage of the objective lens by the high energy deposition of the nanosurgery laser.

60× objective lenses with high numerical aperture are well suited for laser nanosurgery of cytoplasmic structures. Depending on the distance of the structure from the coverslip, the refractive index of the sample and whether the objective lens has to be changed after surgery, oil, silicon oil, glycerine, or water immersion lenses are better suited. For example we routinely use 60× water immersion objective lenses for the nanosurgery experiment and switch to 20× air lenses to follow the treated cells over time [7].

3   Methods

3.1   Nanosurgery of Cytoplasmic Structures

In this section we describe the protocol and the parameters that need to be optimized for performing the laser nanosurgery of subcellular structures. The protocol is generalized to perform laser nanosurgery of different intracellular structures and is based on an Olympus IX-81 microscope with Rapp Optoelectronic UGA (Table 1) nanosurgery setup.

3.1.1   Sample Preparation

To perform a precise ablation of subcellular structures the cells must be seeded on a dish with good optical quality. Glass is ideal for this compared to plastic, as it has a good optical quality and does not cause distortion, blur or autofluorescence during acquisition of images. The thickness of the plastic dish also makes it unsuitable for using it with high magnification and high numerical aperture (NA) objectives. Therefore, in order to perform targeted ablation of subcellular structures like actin fibers, microtubules or centrosomes the cells are usually grown on a glass bottomed dish, e.g., a typical 35 mm MatTek dish (MatTek Corporation, 35 mm petri dish, 10 mm microwell).

It is crucial to have the subcellular structure(s) that need to be ablated fluorescently labeled to visualize them while performing the laser nanosurgery. This can be achieved either by transfecting the cells with a DNA construct expressing a fluorescently tagged protein of interest or using a stable cell line expressing the same.

If actin stress fibers are the target of the nanosurgery experiment, the cell confluence is particularly important, as it influences their formation. In this case, the cells should be seeded with a 30 % confluence or lower, the day before performing the laser nanosurgery. This will allow them to have enough space to spread, which ensures formation of the stress fibers.

3.1.2   Calibration of the Nanosurgery System

To perform targeted ablation of subcellular structures, the position of the laser scanner must be controlled precisely. Therefore, the laser scanner position must be synchronized and calibrated with the x, y, and z coordinates of the monitor (user interface) using for example the Rapp UGA software.

a. Calibration of the Laser scanner in the x, y plane

The calibration of the laser scanner in the x, y plane depends on the microscopic setup and the software used. The manufacturer or the developer usually provides specific instructions depending on the system. We use a special patterned Glass slide (Rapp OptoElectronics GmbH calibration grid T1 (order number: MZ.GT1.01)) in order to visualize and manipulate the position of the UV laser precisely. One can also use a normal glass slide to find the position of the laser by etching it, but this needs higher laser power and might not be sufficiently precise and it is more difficult to find the right focal plane. The following is the protocol we use in our microscopic setup with Rapp UGA software.

1. Start the calibration mode of the software after placing the special patterned glass slide in the field of view.

2. The software first generates small circles along the four corners of the screen one after the other.

3. The laser scanner must be moved (using the keys on the keyboard) to the center of these circles indicated by the software.

4. Once the borders of the field of view are calibrated, the software moves the laser sequentially to sixteen points evenly distributed in the field of view. The software or the user determines the positions of these laser spots and uses the deviation between aimed position and actual position in the image to calibrate the scanner positioning.

This calibration can be saved and reused for several days if the system is properly maintained. Nonetheless, it is recommended to check the x, y calibration before performing an experiment.

A convenient way to do this is:

1. Select a region in the MatTek dish far from the cells of interest, to prevent unwanted damage (Fig. 1).

2. Define a pattern from the user interface of the Rapp UGA Software. The pattern can be a line, a spot (Fig. 1b) or a manually defined shape of interest.

3. Turn on the laser to etch the surface of the coverslip in this pattern (increase the laser power until you see the etching of the glass). Typically, we use 3 % of the maximum laser power to etch the glass with our laser setup (λ = 355 nm, 1 ns pulse, 150 μJ energy, and frequency 200 Hz) as shown in Fig. 1c.

4. Take an image of the etched pattern and compare it to the defined pattern (Fig. 1a). The calibration is successful if these patterns match (Fig. 1b).

5. If these two patterns do not match or if there is an offset between them (example shown in Fig. 1a), the x, y calibration as described above must be repeated.

Note: The calibration is specific for each objective lens.

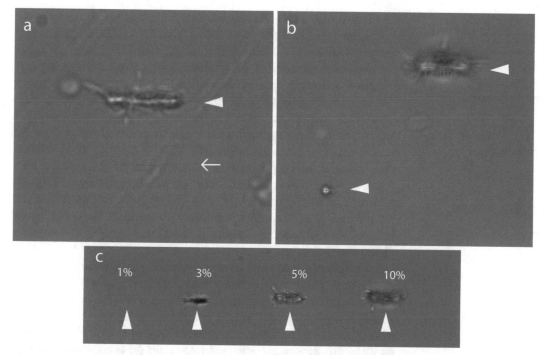

Fig. 1 Example showing the proper calibration of the laser scanner and different laser powers to etch the glass. (**a**) A region without cells was exposed to 3 % of laser power along a line pattern defined on the system's control computer (in *red* indicated with an *open arrow*). The etched pattern (*closed arrow head*) does not have the same coordinates as the defined line pattern in the software. Therefore, the laser scanner needs to be recalibrated. (**b**) The etched pattern has the same coordinates as the defined pattern. The laser scanner is properly calibrated and parameters can be saved and used for the nanosurgery. (**c**) *Arrow heads* showing a line pattern etched on a glass coverslip by exposing it to different laser powers. The minimum power needed to etch the glass is 3 %, the line pattern is confined to the selected pattern in this case compared to higher laser powers (5 % and 10 %). Using higher laser power than necessary might increase the resulting damage not confining it to the pattern and additionally generate glass fragments, cracks, or holes in the glass

b. Alignment of the z focal plane

To check the alignment of the pulsed laser in the z focal plane with respect to the imaging plane, a similar strategy is used. There might be an offset in this alignment, especially with UV and IR lasers. This is because the chromatic correction of the applied objective lens might not be sufficient in this wavelength range. The following are the steps to check the alignment of the laser in the z focal plane.

1. While having the sample in focus define any pattern as shown in Fig. 1b. Note down the z-position of the focus drive.

2. Etch the coverslip to engrave a pattern in it as shown in Fig. 1b.

3. Adjust the z-position to have the engraved pattern in focus and note down its z-position.

4. The difference between these two z-positions determines the offset of the laser in z dimension.

5. If this offset is larger than 1 μm, it is advisable to readjust the focus of the laser scanner if possible (like in our Rapp Optoelectronic UGA setup). If not, this offset must be taken into consideration while performing the laser nanosurgery. In the best case it should be modified by automatic focus adjustment during the experiment or otherwise manually.

3.1.3 Laser Nanosurgery of Actin Fibers

In the following paragraph we describe the procedures we use for nanosurgery of actin fibers (*see* Fig. 2) with our widefield microscopy based nanosurgery system (Olympus IX-81 microscope with Rapp Optoelectronic UGA (Table 1) and a 355 nm laser (Table 2) add-ons). A similar procedure, with specific adaptations in the laser power and laser scanning patterns, can be used to target other intracellular structures, and in particular other cytoskeletal elements.

The laser power to be used to selectively ablate the structure of interest must be experimentally determined. Using too high power would in fact result in an increased damaged volume or even in cell death. Too low power would on the other hand result only in photo bleaching of the structure without damage or physical ablation. In our experience the optimum laser power for nanosurgery varies from day to day or from one sample to another. Therefore, it is necessary to identify the optimal laser power for nanosurgery immediately before the experiment and ideally on the same cell culture dish as the experiment will be performed.

a. Determining the maximum possible laser power

1. Mount the cell culture dish on the microscope and secure its position. Find an area without any cells or cells of interest.

2. Define a specific pattern using the interactive software, e.g., a spot or a line or a combination of shapes (Fig. 1b).

3. Set the laser power to a minimum.

4. While having the glass surface in focus, turn on the live transmission mode and turn on the laser.

5. Increase the laser power in small steps while visualizing the glass surface, until you start to see the etching of the glass.

6. The minimum power needed to etch the glass should be noted and can be used as a reference (3 % in Fig. 1c). This power should never be reached during the nanosurgery experiment if the focus position is close to the coverslip surface, as the glass fragments generated in this way are able to damage cells in the proximity, in an unpredictable way.

Note: Fig. 1c shows different laser powers, which can etch the glass surface. 3 % of the maximum laser power is needed to etch the glass.

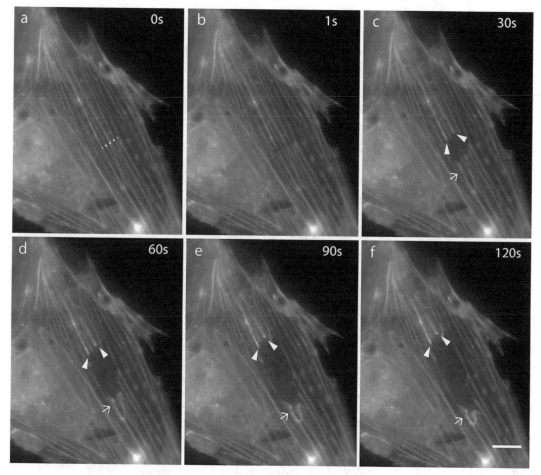

Fig. 2 Example for laser nanosurgery of actin stress fibers. HeLa cells expressing GFP-actin were exposed to 1 % of the maximum laser power (*see* Subheading 3.1.3b) and ten iterations along the line pattern shown in (**a**, *dotted line*) in order to cut the GFP-actin labeled stress fibers. (**b–f**) Time series showing images of the cell after laser ablation. The retraction (*arrow heads*) and recoil (*arrows*) of the actin fibers upon laser ablation post-laser nanosurgery can be seen by increased distance and fluorescent intensity of the structures indicated. Scale bar, 10 μm

b. Optimizing the laser power to ablate actin fibers

1. To test and optimize the laser power, prepare a dish with cells expressing GFP-actin as described earlier.

2. Set the laser power initially to one-third of the minimum power needed to etch the glass (*see* **step 6** above) and the number of iterations to 1.

3. Focus on the cell of interest and take an image before the laser nanosurgery to compare it to the image acquired immediately after ablation. Ideally a time-lapse image series before and after the nanosurgery should be acquired, as it is more informative to distinguish the ablation from photobleaching (*see* Subheading 3.3 for details).

4. Define a pattern (e.g., a line) in which the ablation should be performed.

5. While having the actin fibers of interest in focus turn on the laser with the minimum laser power (**step 2**) and minimum number of iterations.

6. Perform the laser nanosurgery in live mode while looking at the actin fibers.

7. If the actin cut is not achieved with the minimum laser power, repeat the **steps 5** and **6** by increasing the laser power in small steps until it is visibly achieved (Fig. 2).

8. Once the laser power needed to achieve the laser nanosurgery is identified, fine tune the number of iterations needed to avoid unwanted damage to the cell.

9. To ablate individual cells in multicellular organisms, the size of the defined pattern is another parameter to be optimized. This can be done in the same way as in the case of laser power, by increasing in smaller steps and by trial and error.

Typical values we use for successful nanosurgery of GFP-actin fibers in HeLa cells with our experimental setup (355 nm laser, 1 ns pulse, 150 μJ energy and frequency 200 Hz) are (Fig. 2): 1 % of the maximum laser power with ten iterations of the defined pattern (e.g., a line).

c. Laser Nanosurgery of GFP-Actin Fibers

1. Choose the cell of interest and take an image of the actin fibers.

2. Draw a line (e.g., Fig. 1b) using the Rapp UGA software in the region of interest.

3. Set the laser power and the number of iterations to the optimum values (*see* Subheading 3.1.3b, **steps 7** and **8**).

4. Scan the defined pattern with the nanosurgery laser and record the results by time-lapse microscopy with 1 s time intervals for 1–2 min after the successful laser nanosurgery.

Note: In order to obtain best results in nanosurgery of actin fibers or other cytoskeletal structures, we cut the fibers by defining a line pattern perpendicular to the cytoskeletal structure.

3.2 Nanosurgery in Multicellular Organisms

3.2.1 Sample Preparation for Zebra Fish

Every living specimen has a specific sample preparation protocol. Therefore we recommend referring to the respective model organism's guidelines for live imaging. Here we describe the preparation for zebrafish embryos.

a. Sample preparation for zebra fish embryos up to 3 days post fertilization

1. Raise the embryos in E3 buffer between 26 and 30 °C. To prevent pigmentation, 0.002 % 1-phenyl-2-thio-urea (PTU) can be added 24 h post fertilization (hpf).

2. Select the embryos based on expression of transgenes and dechorionate them with forceps or pronase.

3. Mount the embryos in 0.8 % low melting temperature agarose with 0.01 % tricaine anesthetizing agent on glass bottom MatTek dishes with the help of a needle, making sure that the target tissue is closest possible to the glass bottom.

4. Keep the samples at a stable temperature (26–30 °C).

3.2.2 Micropuncture Using 2-Photon Laser in Zebra Fish Embryo

The following protocol is based on a Zeiss LSM 780 NLO 2-Photon microscope (Table 1). Though the protocol is generalized, some steps might be slightly varied for different microscopic setups.

1. Heat the microscopic chamber (temperature depending on the sample used) prior to experiments for stability of objective focus and microscope stage.

2. Place the specimen and focus on the target cells.

3. Determine the size of the pattern, laser power, and number of iterations by trial and error as described earlier (Subheading 3.1.3b).

4. To minimize unspecific damage, the lowest possible laser power and smallest size of the defined pattern should be used. This can be achieved by gradual increase in both parameters until the perturbation is satisfactory (Subheading 3.1.3b).

5. When a large region needs to be ablated, it is better to target it with multiple small patterns instead of a single large pattern because larger patterns cause unspecific damage in *z*.

6. Perform the laser nanosurgery with the optimized parameters.

In case of zebrafish embryos, to perturb cell contacts within an assembled cell cluster (10 μm away from the embryo surface), we successfully use a maximum laser power with a single iteration (Coherent Chameleon Ultra II at 100 % laser power and at 960 nm) with 6× zoom and 4 pixel diameter circular pattern (0.43 μm) (*see* Fig. 3, [27]).

To ablate/kill whole cells require slightly larger patterns and multiple ablation cycles depending on the cell type.

3.3 Monitoring the Success of Laser Nanosurgery

In order to distinguish successful laser ablation from pure photobleaching, images must be compared and measured before and after the procedure (Figs. 2 and 3). If there is a gradual decrease in the fluorescent signal rather than a sudden disappearance or decrease after dissecting the subcellular structures, then the structure is photobleached rather than dissected by laser nanosurgery.

To make sure that the perturbation observed is specific to the laser ablation, readouts such as cell death indicators or morphological changes of the sample should be used. The readouts

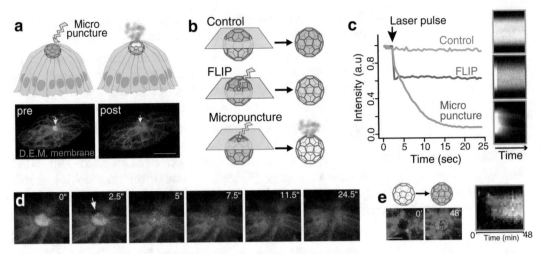

Fig. 3 An example in vivo laser surgery: mechanical disruption of lumen integrity by ablating cell contacts. (**a**) Lumen integrity can be acutely disrupted with two photon laser surgery of cell contacts as monitored by leakage of diffusible extracellular ligands from the luminal space (referred as micro-puncture). *Lower panel* shows ligand filled lumen (*green*) before and after the puncture (*cell membranes in red*). Scale bar, 10 μm. (**b**) Schematics of the micro-puncture experiment. Bleaching during acquisition is controlled by imaging the sample without laser ablation. The specificity of the perturbation and laser pulse induced photo-bleaching are controlled by targeting the lumen center with same laser pulse (called as FLIP, fluorescence loss in photo-bleach). Micropuncture achieved by targeting the lumen lattice is monitored by gradual loss of ligand intensity. (**c**) Plots of mean luminal ligand intensity for each experiment described in (**b**) and kymographs of luminal signal through time (*right panel*). (**d**) Images of a timelapse movie showing ligand leakage upon micropuncture. *Arrow* indicates the time point of puncture and the transient retraction of the membrane (*red*) around the lumen. (**e**) Imaging the microlumen at longer timescale after ablation provides information on the recovery of the system as it refills with ligands. Kymograph (*right*) and single time points of lumen (*left*) show the recovery of the ligand pool. Scale bar, 5 μm

themselves should preferably not be affected by the laser pulses for nanosurgery. This is specifically important for experiments that use fluorescence guided perturbations, which can be misled by photobleaching of the fluorescence signal and hence its readout.

In case of dissecting cytoskeleton the displacement of the newly created ends of the fibers away from each other or recoil due to release of tension is a good indicator of successful nanosurgery (*see* Fig. 2). As shown in Fig. 2, the retraction of the actin fibers can be seen as an increase in the distance between the two cut ends upon laser ablation. And the recoil can be observed as the accumulation of fluorescent intensity at the cut ends. If the aim of nanosurgery is to open membranes or microlumen, leaking of fluorescent reporter can be used as an indicator [27].

One important parameter for successfully monitoring the nanosurgery in the post-cutting period is the frequency of image acquisition. The frame rate of imaging should be adjusted depending on the scope of the experiment. For events occurring at a faster rate the frequency of imaging after the ablation should also be faster and vice versa. For instance, to measure membrane tension, imaging as fast as possible is required whereas monitoring cell ablations may only require imaging every minute. In case of subcellular structures like actin fibers, the imaging can be done every few seconds.

References

1. Amy RL, Storb R (1965) Selective mitochondrial damage by a ruby laser microbeam: an electron microscopic study. Science 150(3697): 756–758

2. Berns W, Strahs R (1979) Laser microirradiation of stress fibers and intermediate filaments in non-muscle cells from cultured rat heart. Exp Cell Res 119(2)

3. Ronchi P, Terjung S, Pepperkok R (2012) At the cutting edge: applications and perspectives of laser nanosurgery in cell biology. Biol Chem 393(April):235–248

4. Colombelli J, Besser A, Kress H, Reynaud EG, Girard P, Caussinus E et al (2009) Mechanosensing in actin stress fibers revealed by a close correlation between force and protein localization. J Cell Sci 122(11):1928–1928

5. Rauzi M, Verant P, Lecuit T, Lenne P-F (2008) Nature and anisotropy of cortical forces orienting Drosophila tissue morphogenesis. Nat Cell Biol 10(12):1401–1410

6. Tängemo C, Ronchi P, Colombelli J, Haselmann U, Simpson JC, Antony C et al (2011) A novel laser nanosurgery approach supports de novo Golgi biogenesis in mammalian cells. J Cell Sci 124(Pt 6):978–987

7. Ronchi P, Tischer C, Acehan D, Pepperkok R (2014) Positive feedback between golgi membranes, microtubules and ER-exit sites directs golgi de novo biogenesis. J Cell Sci 4:4620–4633

8. Yanik MF, Cinar H, Cinar HN, Chisholm AD, Jin Y, Ben-Yakar A (2004) Neurosurgery: functional regeneration after laser axotomy. Nature 432(7019):822

9. Hammarlund M, Jorgensen EM, Bastiani MJ (2007) Axons break in animals lacking beta-spectrin. J Cell Biol 176(3):269–275

10. Timinszky G, Till S, Hassa PO, Hothorn M, Kustatscher G, Nijmeijer B et al (2009) A macrodomain-containing histone rearranges chromatin upon sensing PARP1 activation. Nat Struct Mol Biol 16(9):923–929

11. Chown MG, Kumar S (2007) Imaging and manipulating the structural machinery of living cells on the micro- and nanoscale. Int J Nanomedicine 2(3):333–344

12. Khodjakov A, La Terra S, Chang F (2004) Laser microsurgery in fission yeast; role of the mitotic spindle midzone in anaphase B. Curr Biol 14(15):1330–1340

13. Shimada T, Watanabe W, Matsunaga S, Higashi T, Ishii H, Fukui K et al (2005) Intracellular disruption of mitochondria in a living HeLa cell with a 76-MHz femtosecond laser oscillator. Opt Express 13(24):9869–9880

14. Tirlapur UK, König K (2002) Femtosecond near-infrared laser pulses as a versatile non-invasive tool for intra-tissue nanoprocessing in plants without compromising viability. Plant J 31(3):365–374

15. Austin J, Kimble J (1987) glp-1 is required in the germ line for regulation of the decision between mitosis and meiosis in C. elegans. Cell 51(4):589–599

16. Bargmann CI, Horvitz HR (1991) Control of larval development by chemosensory neurons in Caenorhabditis elegans. Science 251(4998): 1243–1246

17. Ferguson EL, Horvitz HR (1985) Identification and characterization of 22 genes that affect the vulval cell lineages of the nematode Caenorhabditis elegans. Genetics 110(1):17–72

18. McIntire SL, Jorgensen E, Kaplan J, Horvitz HR (1993) The GABAergic nervous system of Caenorhabditis elegans. Nature 364(6435): 337–341

19. Avery L, Horvitz HR (1989) Pharyngeal pumping continues after laser killing of the pharyngeal nervous system of C. elegans. Neuron 3(4):473–485

20. Bargmann CI, Hartwieg E, Horvitz HR (1993) Odorant-selective genes and neurons mediate olfaction in C. elegans. Cell 74(3):515–527

21. Chalfie M, Sulston JE, White JG, Southgate E, Thomson JN, Brenner S (1985) The neural circuit for touch sensitivity in Caenorhabditis elegans. J Neurosci 5(4):956–964

22. Gabel CV, Gabel H, Pavlichin D, Kao A, Clark DA, Samuel ADT (2007) Neural circuits mediate electrosensory behavior in Caenorhabditis elegans. J Neurosci 27(28):7586–7596

23. Gray JM, Hill JJ, Bargmann CI (2005) A circuit for navigation in Caenorhabditis elegans. Proc Natl Acad Sci U S A 102(9):3184–3191

24. Li W, Feng Z, Sternberg PW, Xu XZS (2006) A C. elegans stretch receptor neuron revealed by a mechanosensitive TRP channel homologue. Nature 440(7084):684–687

25. Tsalik EL, Hobert O (2003) Functional mapping of neurons that control locomotory

behavior in *Caenorhabditis elegans*. J Neurobiol 56(2):178–197

26. Ward A, Liu J, Feng Z, Xu XZS (2008) Light-sensitive neurons and channels mediate phototaxis in *C. elegans*. Nat Neurosci 11(8):916–922

27. Durdu S, Iskar M, Revenu C, Schieber N, Kunze A, Bork P et al (2014) Luminal signalling links cell communication to tissue architecture during organogenesis. Nature 515(7525):120–124

28. Bedzhov I, Zernicka-Goetz M (2014) Self-organizing properties of mouse pluripotent cells initiate morphogenesis upon implantation. Cell 156(5):1032–1044

29. Harding MJ, McGraw HF, Nechiporuk A (2014) The roles and regulation of multicellular rosette structures during morphogenesis. Development 141(13):2549–2558

30. Koehler KR, Mikosz AM, Molosh AI, Patel D, Hashino E (2013) Generation of inner ear sensory epithelia from pluripotent stem cells in 3D culture. Nature 500(7461):217–221

31. Bishop D, Nikić I, Brinkoetter M, Knecht S, Potz S, Kerschensteiner M et al (2011) Near-infrared branding efficiently correlates light and electron microscopy. Nat Methods 8(7):568–570

32. Karreman MA, Mercier L, Schieber NL, Shibue T, Schwab Y, Goetz JG (2014) Correlating intravital multi-photon microscopy to 3D electron microscopy of invading tumor cells using anatomical reference points. PLoS One 9(12):e114448

33. Colombelli J, Tängemo C, Haselman U, Antony C, Stelzer EHK, Pepperkok R et al (2008) A correlative light and electron microscopy method based on laser micropatterning and etching. Methods Mol Biol 457:203–213

34. Ronchi P, Pepperkok R (2013) Golgi depletion from living cells with laser nanosurgery. Methods Cell Biol 118: 311–324. 1st edn

35. Kolotuev I, Bumbarger DJ, Labouesse M, Schwab Y (2012) Targeted ultramicrotomy: a valuable tool for correlated light and electron microscopy of small model organisms. Methods Cell Biol 111:203–222

36. Horneffer V, Linz N, Vogel A (2007) Principles of laser-induced separation and transport of living cells. J Biomed Opt 12(5):54016

37. Solon J, Kaya-Çopur A, Colombelli J, Brunner D (2009) Pulsed forces timed by a ratchet-like mechanism drive directed tissue movement during dorsal closure. Cell 137(7):1331–1342

38. Caussinus E, Colombelli J, Affolter M (2008) Tip-cell migration controls stalk-cell intercalation during Drosophila tracheal tube elongation. Curr Biol 18(22):1727–1734

39. Sauteur L, Krudewig A, Herwig L, Ehrenfeuchter N, Lenard A, Affolter M et al (2014) Cdh5/VE-cadherin promotes endothelial cell interface elongation via cortical actin polymerization during angiogenic sprouting. Cell Rep 9(2):504–513

40. Raabe I, Vogel SK, Peychl J, Tolić-Nørrelykke IM (2009) Intracellular nanosurgery and cell enucleation usinga picosecond laser. J Microsc 234:1–8

41. Scheffer LL, Sreetama SC, Sharma N, Medikayala S, Brown KJ, Defour A et al (2014) Mechanism of Ca(2)(+)-triggered ESCRT assembly and regulation of cell membrane repair. Nat Commun 5:5646

42. Jimenez AJ, Maiuri P, Lafaurie-Janvore J, Perez F, Piel M (2015) Laser induced wounding of the plasma membrane and methods to study the repair process. Methods Cell Biol 125:391–408

43. Fink J, Carpi N, Betz T, Betard A, Chebah M, Azioune A et al (2011) External forces control mitotic spindle positioning. Nat Cell Biol 13(7):771–778

44. Rauzi M, Lenne P-F, Lecuit T (2010) Planar polarized actomyosin contractile flows control epithelial junction remodelling. Nature 468(7327):1110–1114

45. Colombelli J, Solon J (2013) Force communication in multicellular tissues addressed by laser nanosurgery. Cell Tissue Res 352(1):133–147

46. Smutny M, Behrndt M, Campinho P, Ruprecht V, Heisenberg CP (2015) UV laser ablation to measure cell and tissue-generated forces in the zebrafish embryo in vivo and ex vivo. Methods Mol Biol 1189:219–235

47. Engelbrecht CJ, Greger K, Reynaud EG, Krzic U, Colombelli J, Stelzer EH (2007) Three-dimensional laser microsurgery in light-sheet based microscopy (SPIM). Opt Express 15(10):6420–6430

48. Rauzi M, Krzic U, Saunders TE, Krajnc M, Ziherl P, Hufnagel L et al (2015) Embryo-scale tissue mechanics during Drosophila gastrulation movements. Nat Commun 6:8677

49. Vogel A, Noack J, Hüttman G, Paltauf G (2005) Mechanisms of femtosecond laser nanosurgery of cells and tissues. Appl Phys B 81:1015–1047

50. Sacconi L, Tolić-Nørrelykke IM, Antolini R, Pavone FS (2005) Combined intracellular three-dimensional imaging and selective nanosurgery by a nonlinear microscope. J Biomed Opt 10(1):14002

51. Rauzi M, Verant P, Lecuit T, Lenne P-F (2008) Nature and anisotropy of cortical forces orienting Drosophila tissue morphogenesis. Nat Cell Biol 10(12):1401–1410

52. Colombelli J, Reynaud EG, Rietdorf J, Pepperkok R, Stelzer EHK (2005) In vivo selective cytoskeleton dynamics quantification in interphase cells induced by pulsed ultraviolet laser nanosurgery. Traffic 6(12):1093–1102

53. Colombelli J, Solon J (2013) Force communication in multicellular tissues addressed by laser nanosurgery. Cell Tissue Res 352(1): 133–147

54. Jiang K, Hua S, Mohan R, Grigoriev I, Yau KW, Liu Q et al (2014) Microtubule minus-end stabilization by polymerization-driven CAMSAP deposition. Dev Cell 28(3):295–309

55. Travers RJ, Shenoi RA, Kalathottukaren MT, Kizhakkedathu JN, Morrissey JH (2014) Nontoxic polyphosphate inhibitors reduce thrombosis while sparing hemostasis. Blood 124(22):3183–3190

56. Sumida GM, Tomita TM, Shih W, Yamada S (2011) Myosin II activity dependent and independent vinculin recruitment to the sites of E-cadherin-mediated cell-cell adhesion. BMC Cell Biol 12(1):48

57. Vogel A, Horneffer V, Lorenz K, Linz N, Huttmann G, Gebert A (2007) Principles of laser microdissection and catapulting of histologic specimens and live cells. Methods Cell Biol 82:153–205

58. Vogel A, Noack J (2001) Numerical simulations of optical breakdown for cellular surgery at nanosecond to femtosecond time scales. In: Proc. SPIE 4260, Optical Diagnostics of Living Cells IV, p 83–93. Accessed from http://proceedings.spiedigitallibrary.org/proceeding.aspx?articleid=900637. doi:10.1117/12.426762

59. Kuetemeyer K, Rezgui R, Lubatschowski H, Heisterkamp A (2010) Influence of laser parameters and staining on femtosecond laser-based intracellular nanosurgery. Biomed Opt Express 1(2):587–597

60. Botvinick EL, Venugopalan V, Shah JV, Liaw LH, Berns MW (2004) Controlled ablation of microtubules using a picosecond laser. Biochem J 87:4203–4212

61. Aist JR, Liang H, Berns MW (1993) Astral and spindle forces in PtK2 cells during anaphase B: a laser microbeam study. J Cell Sci 104(4):1207–1216

62. Heisterkamp A, Maxwell IZ, Mazur E, Underwood JM, Nickerson JA, Kumar S et al (2005) Pulse energy dependence of subcellular dissection by femtosecond laser pulses. Opt Express 13:3690–3696

Part II

Super and High-Resolution Optical Imaging

Chapter 9

Sample Preparation and Choice of Fluorophores for Single and Dual Color Photo-Activated Localization Microscopy (PALM) with Bacterial Cells

Juri N. Bach, Giacomo Giacomelli, and Marc Bramkamp

Abstract

Photo-activated localization microscopy (PALM) is one of the light microscopy techniques providing highest resolution. Single photo-activatable or photo-switchable fluorescent molecules are stochastically excited. The point spread function of this event is recorded and the exact fluorophore position is calculated. This chapter describes how bacterial samples can be prepared for PALM to achieve routinely a resolution of ≤30 nm using fluorophores such as mNeonGreen, Dendra2, and PAmCherry. It is also explained how to perform multicolor PALM and combine it with total internal reflection (TIRF) microscopy to increase resolution.

Key words Localization, Microscopy, PALM, STORM, Dendra2, PAmCherry, mNeonGreen, Super resolution, Dual color PALM

1 Introduction

The resolution of conventional light microscopy is restricted by the diffraction limit of light. Two objects in closer proximity than the diffraction limit of light cannot be separated optically by conventional light microscopy. This effect can be described by the Abbe's criterion (I) $r = \dfrac{0.5\lambda}{NA}$ or by the Rayleigh criterion (II) $r = \dfrac{0.61\lambda}{NA}$ [1, 2]. In both cases, the distance between two points (r) is a function of the wavelength of light λ and the physical properties of the objective, here simplified as NA = numerical aperture. The only difference between the two formulas is in the coefficient used for the calculation, which is the result of the different definition of distinct objects used by Abbe and Rayleigh. The emission of a fluorescent event is generally imaged as a point spread function (PSF).

[\$]Author contributed equally with all other contributors.

Yolanda Markaki and Hartmann Harz (eds.), *Light Microscopy: Methods and Protocols*, Methods in Molecular Biology, vol. 1563, DOI 10.1007/978-1-4939-6810-7_9, © Springer Science+Business Media LLC 2017

If multiple localizations are in closer proximity than the Abbe criterion, the PSFs of these localizations overlap, resulting in a single bright PSF. As a result, exact fluorophore localizations cannot be discriminated. Therefore, the resolution is limited practically to ~250 nm in the x/y direction in conventional light microscopic analyses. Bacteria are small cells, often not bigger than a few micrometers, making cell biological analysis of these cells challenging. Even though, bacterial cells show a remarkably high degree of subcellular compartmentalization the molecular biology tools are limited to investigate these phenomena [3, 4]. Localization microscopy is one of the most powerful techniques to investigate cellular processes at nanometre scale. Generally, three localization microscopy techniques are available that circumvent the resolution limit of light. These are stochastic optical reconstruction microscopy (STORM) [5], photo-activated localization microscopy (PALM) [6], and fluorescence photo-activated localization microscopy (fPALM) [7]. With these super-resolution techniques, single fluorescence events are monitored over a time series, under conditions where only few fluorophores at each given time are stochastically excited. As a result, only a single fluorophore is excited inside a diffraction limited area and it is therefore possible to use the PSF of the molecule to calculate its position with improved resolution. This can be achieved by utilization of synthetic fluorophores (STORM) or fluorescent proteins (fPALM and PALM). The difference between PALM and fPALM is that PALM (similar as STORM) was originally implemented using total internal reflection fluorescence (TIRF) microscopy. In contrast, fPALM was based on a widefield microscope that does not limit the focal plane to the proximity of the coverslip. In PALM, the stochastic activation of single molecules is normally achieved by utilizing photo-activatable (PA), photo-convertible (PC), or photo-switchable (PS) fluorophores. All these fluorophores change their fluorescence spectrum after illumination with light of a certain wavelength. Exemplary, a PC fluorescent protein such as Dendra2 is green fluorescent (Ex. 490/Em. 507); though after illumination with light at 405 nm it switches excitation and emission to red fluorescence (Ex. 553/Em. 573) [8]. These characteristics can be utilized to only convert a single fluorophore per frame. If only single fluorophore is recorded, the center of this localization can be calculated using the formula (III):

$$\sigma\mu_i = \sqrt{\left(\frac{s_i^2}{N}\right) + \left(\frac{a^2}{12N}\right) + \left(\frac{8\pi s_i^4 b^2}{a^2 N^2}\right)}$$, where si is the width of the

distribution (standard deviation in direction I; $\left(\frac{s_i^2}{N}\right)$ is the photon noise), N is the number of photons imaged, a is the pixel size of the imaging (EM) CCD detector ($\left(\frac{a^2}{12N}\right)$ is the finite pixel size of the detector), and b is the standard deviation of the background ($\left(\dfrac{8\pi s_i^4 b^2}{a^2 N^2}\right)$ is the influence of the background on image quality). If hardware and preparation parameters are optimized to a theoretic optimum, the formula (III) may be simplified as (IV) $= \dfrac{1}{\sqrt{N}} * \dfrac{\lambda}{2NA}$. Hence, resolution of PALM is theoretically only limited by the number of photons gathered. Assuming that a theoretic fluorescent molecule would emit 20,000 photons at a wavelength of 600 nm and is imaged using an objective with a NA of 1.4, the resolution would be ~2 nm. However, practically, the hardware setup of the imaging system can hardly be changed and optimization is physically limited. As a consequence, individual image quality is mainly dependent on the number of photons gathered and the background characteristics. The following chapter will focus on the requirements that need to be taken into consideration to increase the number of photons gathered (in single- and multi-color imaging) and on the steps necessary during sample preparation to reduce background. With the protocol described here routinely a resolution of ≤30 nm for PALM with bacterial cells can be obtained. Successful imaging is exemplified here by a soluble, DNA-binding protein, ParB from *Corynebacterium glutamiucm* and membrane micro-domain associated proteins, FloT and FloA, from *Bacillus subtilis*. For both proteins conventional, diffraction-limited wide- filed images have been published before and their subcellular localization is well investigated [9–13].

2 Materials

All aqueous solutions are prepared using ultrapure water (Conductivity at 24 °C: 0.055 μS/cm). Analytical or HPLC grade reagents are used.

2.1 Before Imaging

When planning PALM experiments the choice of an appropriate fluorophore is crucial. Fluorophores may differ in their life time, blinking rate, and quantum yield [14]. Furthermore, only a minority of the fluorophore may be folded properly and fluorophores may have different activation/switching, emission, excitation, and bleaching properties. These characteristics may be altered due to the nature of the experiment itself. This is mainly dependent on the surrounding pH, potential fixation conditions, and tissue thickness. Further differences may occur in 2D or 3D imaging, multicolor experiments, sample density, and potential auto-fluorescence overlap.

Hence, not every fluorescent molecule is suitable for every experiment, and the degree of information that can be collected varies between specific fluorophores. Exemplary, it is not possible to quantitatively count single molecules with a fluorophore with undefined photo-characteristics, though it may be possible to determine cluster size and structures [15].

If the aim of the experiment is to identify structures neglecting the number of proteins inside these structures, a reversible switchable fluorescent molecule may be used, since it allows repeated sampling and, therefore, a better resolution of the structure. If the protein of interest is highly abundant and only its oligomeric form should be studied, split fluorescent proteins can be a good choice [16].

Generally, a fluorophore should not dimerize/cluster, have a good on/off switching ratio, a short maturation time, have a high percentage of correctly folded molecules, emit high number of photons and spectrally not overlap with potential cell auto-fluorescence. Currently, some of the fluorophores most often used for PALM in bacteria are Dendra2, mEOS3.2, PAmCherry [17–19]. Fluorophores for localization microscopy are a strongly emerging research area and, hence, newly developed fluorophores with superior characteristics are described regularly. New, improved fluorophores include mMaple3 and mNeonGreen [20, 21]. An excellent review discussing the most recent developments in fluorophores was recently published by Shcherbakova et al. [22].

The presence of auto-fluorescence can be easily verified by imaging a wild-type strain with the identical imaging parameters that would be used for the fluorophore of choice and by subsequent calculation of the PALM image (Fig. 1a–d). Standard settings for each fluorophore are found in the literature. Although standard settings may not be optimal for each setting and system, it gives a good starting point to evaluate if a particular fluorophore is suited for the planned experiment. If auto-fluorescence is detected (Fig. 1d), it may still be possible to distinguish between auto-fluorescence and the fluorophore by comparing their parameters and filtering accordingly (the most important characteristics in this case are PSF width and photon counts (Fig. 1e–g)). If the filtering parameters chosen manage to separate the events coming from different sources, the PALM image resulting from the WT should be almost empty (Fig. 1c) while the one resulting from the actual sample should maintain its structures (Fig. 1a). If, after filtering, spectral overlap still persists, localization data are not usable and a different fluorophore should be used. Ectopic expression of fluorescent fusion genes is sufficient to test for potential auto-fluorescent overlap of the sample and the fluorophore.

Another problem that can be encountered while acquiring PALM images, especially when the protein of interest is highly abundant or forms dense clusters, is the overlap of multiple events at a certain time in a close spatial proximity. The system will usually not be able to distinguish between the single events and, therefore, register a single event with PSF width and photon number higher

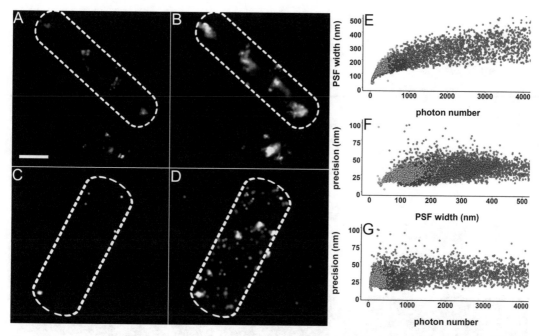

Fig. 1 Application of appropriate filters for PALM image processing: *C. glutamicum* RES 167 cells expressing the partitioning protein ParB C-terminally tagged with mNeongreen are shown after filtering (**a**) and before filtering (**b**). Filtering results in the elimination of both auto-fluorescence events and signals resulting from the co-occurrence of multiple events in the same spot at the same time. When filtering *C. glutamicum* RES 167 cells with the same parameters (before filtering (**d**) and after filtering (**c**)), the number of events drops drastically. The plots (**e–g**) show the different parameter distributions that characterize auto-fluorescence (in *gray*) and ParB-mNeongreen (in *red*). The *blue dots* represent the ParB-mNeongreen events that reside within the chosen filter parameters (PSF width (100–200 nm), precision (1–50 nm), and photon number (400–920)). The plots show that auto-fluorescence is not the only source of noise. Many events show too high PSF width, precision, or photon numbers. This phenomenon is caused by the co-localization of two or more events at a given time. Scale bar 0.5 μm

than the average (Fig. 2). A way to decrease the chance for this to happen is to activate the PA/PC fluorescent protein in a triggered way; by turning on the activating laser (usually a 405 nm laser) only while the signal is transferring to the camera, the number of molecules active at a certain time will decrease, and with it, the chance to have overlapping events. These techniques also prevent photo-activation of a molecule when already acquiring a frame. If the activation laser is not triggered it may be possible to image a molecule only for the last half of one frame and the second half of a following frame. Logically, this would result in an altered number of photons (Fig. 2a, b) and PSF profile (Fig. 2d, e) and hence in decreased resolution. This phenomenon can easily be analyzed by plotting the PSF width of every individual event against the number of photons gathered for this event. To identify optimal imaging settings analyses of the respective fluorophore in vitro may be required (Fig. 2c, f, i), though data for most fluorophores can be found in the original

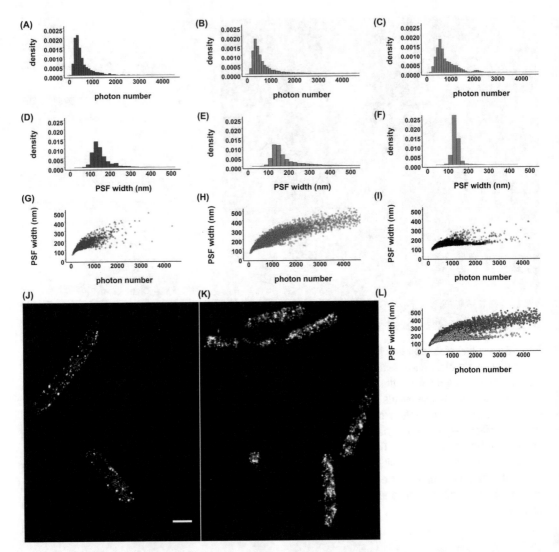

Fig. 2 Effects of laser settings on PALM data. Comparison of the PSF width and photon number distribution with different approaches concerning protein photo-conversion. Activation/conversion of a PA/PC fluorescent protein can be triggered by a 405 nm laser in a continuous way (**b**, **e**, **h**, **k**) or in a triggered way (**a**, **d**, **g**, **j**). In the triggered activation, the 405 nm laser is active only while the signal is transferred to the camera. Characteristics of purified PAmCherry activated by a triggered 405 nm laser are plotted in (**c**, **f**, **i**). (**a–c**) is density of photon numbers of all recorded events; (**d–f**) is the density of the PSF width of all recorded events. (**g–i**) is the PSF width plotted against the photon number of every individual recorded event: (**j**, **k**) are the plotted images of the recorded events. Constant illumination with the activating 405 nm laser causes the distribution of the PSF width and the number of photons to be more scattered compared to triggered laser illumination. Hence, the probability that multiple molecules may be merged in one localization or one event may be split in multiple localizations is higher. When using triggered illumination, 63 % of the events have a PSF width between 100 and 160 nm and a photon number between 100 and 1000 while, when the 405 nm laser is constantly on, the percentage decreases to 52 %. (**l**) Shown is an overlay of events recorded with triggered laser illumination (*blue*), events with constant laser illumination (*red*), and the events detected using purified PAmCherry [26]. Scale bar 1 μm

research paper. However, these data can easily be compared with acquired PALM data (Fig. 2l). Plots of triggered and untriggered PALM experiments can be found in figure (Fig. 2j, k).

Since fluorescence properties of fluorophores are sensitive to environmental changes, it is advisable to test different imaging buffer combinations to gain more localizations or a better photon count and, hence, a higher precision (e.g., it has been shown that the use of heavy water increases the photon count in several fluorophores) [23].

To avoid putative overexpression or labeling artifacts, especially when the objective is the analysis of the structure of protein clusters, it is strongly recommended to express the tagged protein variant as a single copy from the native locus to ensure natural regulation and copy number. This kind of approach can be more time consuming, especially in organisms lacking suitable genetic tools, but allows for an analysis of the protein of interest in the most unbiased and robust possible way.

If multicolor imaging is required, two different approaches are principally available. Channel separation can either be achieved by different activation or emission wavelength. Naturally, either possibilities can be performed using synthetic fluorophores or by protein fusions, though the following part will focus only on combinations of different fluorescent proteins that may be used for PALM. The advantage for activation wavelength is that the channels are naturally aligned and, hence, cross-talk from nonspecific activation does not occur. Combinations of fluorophores that are often used for this approach are the PS proteins Padron and Dronpa [24]. Both emit in an activated state at the same wavelength, thereby avoiding chromatic aberrations. In this case, Dronpa is switched on via ultra violet (UV) light whereat Padron is switched on via blue light and switched off by UV light. Clearly, tight control of switching (On- and Off-state) is absolutely crucial for these experiments.

The most common method is separation by emission wavelength, due to larger choice of different fluorescence proteins. This method has a relatively low crosstalk, but multicolor alignment of raw images is essential after imaging. Established two color PALM fluorophore combinations are PAmCherry combined with PAGFP or mNeonGreen. When PAmCherry and PAGFP are used in combination, both fluorophores are activated by UV laser illumination. Hence, to have a low number of activated molecules at the same time, fluorescence of PAmCherry and PAGFP have to be recorded in an alternating pattern. Easier to handle is the combination of PAmCherry and mNeonGreen (Fig. 3). Since mNeonGreen has to be bleached with blue light (488 nm) prior to imaging, no crosstalk with respect to fluorophore activation or emission occurs.

It is also possible to use PC fluorophores for multicolor imaging. For instance, Dendra2 might be used in combination with mNeonGreen. Though it has to be guaranteed that all Dendra2 molecules are converted to red prior to imaging of mNeonGreen, since the

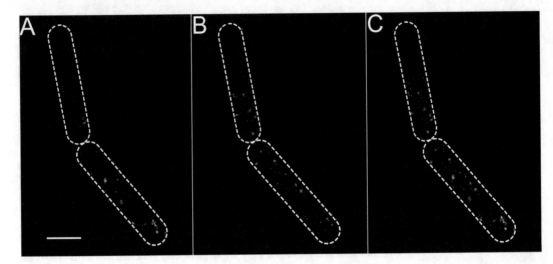

Fig. 3 Dual color PALM: Reconstructed TIRF-PALM image of *B. subtilis* cells expressing two flotillin proteins (FloA and FloT) fused to mNeonGreen (**a**) and PAmCherry (**b**) after drift correction and channel alignment. Overlay of both channels is shown in (**c**). Precision for mNeonGreen ≤35 nm; precision for PAmCherry ≤25 nm. Cells are outlined by *broken white lines*. Scale bar 1 μm

green fluorescence of Dendra2 in its native state may create cross-talk with mNeonGreen fluorescence.

Importantly, when performing multicolor imaging, addition of multicolor beads is essential. The beads allow for drift correction, channel alignment, and adjustment of potential z-axis drift. These corrections are absolutely essential for multicolor imaging. This approach can also be applied to multicolor TIRF-PALM, in which case the beads can also be used for TIRF angle adjustment. Likely, the development of new fluorophores will multiply the possibilities and the combinations available for multicolor PALM. Examples for these are the recently developed fluorophores PSmOrange2 (orange-to-far red) [25] and PS-CFP2 (cyan-to-green; Evrogen).

2.2 Solutions for Sample Preparation

There is not a single solution that can be used for all organisms: fixing agent concentration, medium and buffer used may change significantly and need to be determined empirically.

All solutions are sterile filtered before use!

PBS pH 7.4, 1.78 g/L $Na_2HPO_4 \cdot 2H_2O$, 1.42 g/L Na_2HPO_4, 8 g/L NaCl, 0.2 g/L KCl, 0.27 2 g/l KH_2PO_4.

PBS-G pH 7.4 (PBS, 10 mM glycine), adjust pH with KOH.

Fixing solution, PBS, 2 % formaldehyde (v/v), 2 % paraformaldehyde (v/v)), prepared fresh.

Low fluorescence medium (examples are):

B. subtilis: MD-Medium, 0.7 mg/ml K_2HPO_4, 6 mg/ml KH_2PO_4, 1 mg/ml Na_3 citrate, 20 mg/ml glucose, 20 mg/ml L-tryptophan, 25 mg/ml L-aspartate, mg/ml ferric ammonium citrate, 0.36 mg/ml $MgSO_4$ and mg/ml casamino acids

E. *coli*: M9 medium, MEM amino acids, proline, MEM vitamins, 0.2 % glycerol.

1.1 % (w/v) Poly-L-lysine.

0.02 % (w/v) Na-azide.

2.3 Cleaning Solutions

1.1 M HCl (v/v).

60 % Ethanol (v/v).

2.4 Equipment

Fluorescent beads for drift correction and channel alignment (100 nm diameter).

Sterile filter (pore size of 0.2 μm).

Plasma cleaner (Cressington 208 carbon High Vacuum Carbon Coater).

Water bath sonicator (freq.: 35 kHz).

Immersion Oil (*see* **Note 1**) (e.g., Zeiss Immersol 518 N).

Imaging chamber (*see* **Note 2**) (e.g., Nunc™ Lab-Tek™ II Chamber Slide™ System).

Imaging microscope (e.g., Zeiss ElyraP1) incl. appropriate Imaging Software (e.g., Zeiss ZenBlack) (*see* **Note 3**).
Aluminium foil covered flask (*see* **Note 4**).

3 Methods

3.1 Cleaning of Imaging Chamber

1. Sonicate the imaging chamber for 20 min in 0.1 M HCl.
2. Sonicate the imaging chamber for 20 min in water.
3. Sonicate the imaging chamber for 20 min in 60 % Ethanol.
4. Sonicate the imaging chamber for 20 min in water.
5. Dry under a stream of nitrogen or air (*see* **Note 5**).
6. Plasma clean (15 mA for 30 s) (*see* **Note 6**).
7. The imaging chamber can directly be used or stored in water containing 0.02 % Na-azide for some weeks. Before usage sonicate in water for 20 min and dry under a stream of nitrogen or air.

3.2 Preparation of Beads

1. Dilute beads to appropriate density, e.g., 1:1000 in water containing 0.02 % Na-azide for TetraSpeck beads, sonicate in a water bath for 10 min.
2. Diluted beads can be stored for several weeks in the dark at 4 °C.

3.3 Sample Preparation

1. Grow strain/cells (*see* **Note 4**) in an aluminum foil covered flask (for *Bacillus subtilis* MD—medium may be used) (*see* **Note 7**).
2. When cells reach the cell cycle phase of interest, measure optical density (OD_{600}) and centrifuge cells at $5000 \times g$ for 1 min at

room temperature. The resulting pellet is resuspended in the same volume of fixing solution (*see* **Note 8**).

3. Incubate 15 min at growth temperature in the dark; in parallel continue with **step 7** during incubation.

4. Wash with PBS-G (volume is dependent on imaging dish; for 8-well Nunc™ Lab-Tek™ II Chamber Slide™ System 200 μl should be sufficient).

5. Incubate 10 min at growth temperature in the dark.

6. Wash twice with PBS-G/continue with **step 12.**

7. Wash your imaging dish with water.

8. Remove all liquid and add poly-lysine until the whole cover glass is covered and incubate at RT for 20–60 min.

9. Wash twice with PBS-G and remove all liquid.

10. Add 1.5 μl of diluted beads; homogeneously distribute carefully with a pipette tip. The amount of beads added finally to the imaging chamber should be high enough to ensure that always three to five beads appear in the field of view.

11. Fill chamber with PBS-G.

12. When the last washing step was performed (**step 6**) add cells according to the formula: 15 μl of cells with an OD_{600} of 1 per cm^2 of the imaging dish (*see* **Note 9**).

13. Centrifuge imaging dish in a spin out rotor for ~5 min at $1258 \times g$ to tether cells to the cover glass (*see* **Note 10** and **11**).

14. Place your imaging device on the microscope. Wait till the device reaches the thermal equilibrium (shifts in temperature will dramatically increase drift).

15. Image PALM picture series. The loaded beads can be utilized for channel alignment and drift correction. The beads may also be used to set *z*-axis and angle for TIRF calibration. When performing multicolor imaging, it is necessary to readjust the TIRF angle and *z*-axis before imaging each individual channel. The difference in results with cleaned image chambers can be seen in Fig. 4.

4   Notes

1. Use an immersion oil that fits the refraction index of your sample, objective, and temperature. Using the wrong immersion oil may result in reduced light sensitivity and, in consequence reduced resolution.

2. Generally, high precision glass ware should be used. The usage of imaging chambers is recommenced due to the easier handling during cleaning procedure. However, also high precision

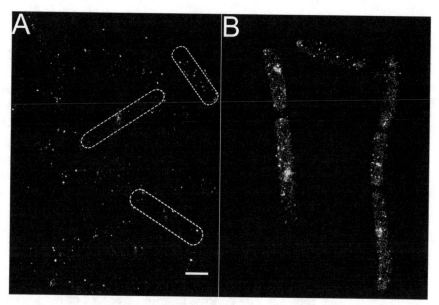

Fig. 4 Effect of efficient imaging chamber cleaning. *B. subtilis* cells expressing a flotillin protein fused to PAmCherry imaged in TIRF-PALM. In (**a**) the used imaging chamber was not cleaned and used as delivered by the manufacturer. The imaging dish used in (**b**) was cleaned as described in this protocol. For plotting of the PALM image a relative intensity scale was used with respect to every individual experiment. Exemplary, few cells are outlined by *broken white lines* (**a**). Precision is ≤25 nm. Scale bar 1 μm

cover glasses may be used with subsequent cleaning (objective slide and cover glass) and sealing.

3. Microscope setup:

   Microscope System ELYRA P.1

   Lasers: 405 nm Diode-Laser 50 mW, 488 nm Laser 200 mW, 561 nm Laser 200 mW, 640 nm Laser 150 mW

   Objectives: alpha Plan-Apochromat 100×/1,46 Oil DIC M27 and Plan-Apochromat 63×/1.4 Oil DIC M27 from Zeiss

   Filter sets: 77 HE GFP + mRFP + Alexa 633 shift free (EX TBP 483 + 564 + 642, BS TFT 506 + 582 + 659, EM TBP 526 + 601 + 688), 49 DAPI shift free (EX G 365, BS FT 395, EM BP 445/50), BP 420–480/LP 750, BP 495–550/LP 750, LP 570 and LP 655

   Camera: Andor EM-CCD camera iXon DU 897

   Optovar: 1.6×

   Hardware focus: Definite Focus

   Table: Piezo table

4. Cells have to be grown in the dark, since light may preactivate/convert PA/PS-fluorophores.

5. Air drying is crucial. Use high air pressure to blow away most liquid. Even ultrapure water may contain some trace elements that may be auto-fluorescent if dried on the imaging dish.

6. Plasma cleaning makes the glass surface hydrophilic, hence remaining dust particles can be removed easier. Generally, cleaning of the imaging dish is absolutely crucial to get rid of auto-fluorescent material sticking to the glass surface (Fig. 4).

7. Even though growth medium will be washed out in later sample preparation steps it is recommended to use a medium with lowest auto-fluorescence. Some organisms even may produce auto-fluorescence only in certain growth media.

8. Fixing conditions may be modified if the used fluorescent protein is less resistant to formaldehyde (compare life cells and fixed cells under an epi-fluorescence microscope; PA proteins can often be activated by simple illumination with DAPI light). It just has to be assured that proteins are no longer dynamic.

9. The volume of cells loaded should be sufficient to image an appropriate amount of cells per spot, though overlapping of cells due to too high cell density should be avoided. (In case of too high cell density, multiple layers of cells will stack at the bottom of the imaging chamber; to decrease background fluorescence coming from cells belonging to other layers, it is good practice to avoid illumination of those cells by using a suitable-TIRF angle. Note that the angle will change between different filter settings).

10. Alternatively, cells can be incubated at RT for ~2 h until cells are properly sedimented. However, cells have to tightly attach to the cover glass prior to imaging. Imaging itself may take ≥30 min. Also any media between the imagining object and the objective decreases resolution due to decreased photon counts, increased background, and increased width of photon distribution. Tethering of the cells to the glass surface is also absolutely crucial if TIRF microscopy is performed since the evanescent wave is restricted to the first ~100 nm of the specimen.

11. Centrifugation of imaging chambers before imaging can result in artifacts due to trapping of molecules between the cells and the glass or due to cell damages caused by the g force. In order to minimize the damages it is mandatory to use a g force as lowas possible.

References

1. Abbe E (1883) XV.—The relation of aperture and power in the microscope (continued)*. J R Microsc Soc 3(6):790–812

2. Rayleigh L (1879) XXXI. Investigations in optics, with special reference to the spectroscope. Philos Mag 8(49):261–274. Series 5

3. Rudner DZ, Losick R (2010) Protein subcellular localization in bacteria. Cold Spring Harb Perspect Biol 2(4):a000307

4. Shapiro L, McAdams HH, Losick R (2009) Why and how bacteria localize proteins. Science 326(5957):1225–1228

5. Rust MJ, Bates M, Zhuang X (2006) Sub-diffraction-limit imaging by stochastic optical reconstruction microscopy (STORM). Nat Methods 3(10):793–795

6. Betzig E et al (2006) Imaging intracellular fluorescent proteins at nanometer resolution. Science 313(5793):1642–1645

7. Hess ST, Girirajan TP, Mason MD (2006) Ultra-high resolution imaging by fluorescence photoactivation localization microscopy. Biophys J 91(11):4258–4272

8. Adam V, Nienhaus K, Bourgeois D, Nienhaus GU (2009) Structural basis of enhanced photoconversion yield in green fluorescent protein-like protein Dendra2. Biochemistry 48(22): 4905–4915

9. Bach JN, Bramkamp M (2013) Flotillins functionally organize the bacterial membrane. Mol Microbiol 88(6):1205–1217

10. Bach JN, Bramkamp M (2015) Dissecting the molecular properties of prokaryotic flotillins. PLoS One 10(1):e0116750

11. Bramkamp M, Lopez D (2015) Exploring the existence of lipid rafts in bacteria. Microbiol Mol Biol Rev 79(1):81–100

12. Donovan C, Schwaiger A, Kramer R, Bramkamp M (2010) Subcellular localization and characterization of the ParAB system from Corynebacterium glutamicum. J Bacteriol 192(13):3441–3451

13. Donovan C, Sieger B, Kramer R, Bramkamp M (2012) A synthetic Escherichia coli system identifies a conserved origin tethering factor in Actinobacteria. Mol Microbiol 84(1):105–116

14. Chozinski TJ, Gagnon LA, Vaughan JC (2014) Twinkle, twinkle little star: photoswitchable fluorophores for super-resolution imaging. FEBS Lett 588(19):3603–3612

15. Annibale P, Vanni S, Scarselli M, Rothlisberger U, Radenovic A (2011) Quantitative photo activated localization microscopy: unraveling the effects of photoblinking. PLoS One 6(7):e22678

16. Jacq M et al (2015) Remodeling of the Z-ring nanostructure during the Streptococcus pneumoniae cell cycle revealed by photoactivated localization microscopy. MBio 6(4)

17. Buss J et al (2013) In vivo organization of the FtsZ-ring by ZapA and ZapB revealed by quantitative super-resolution microscopy. Mol Microbiol 89(6):1099–1120

18. Haas BL, Matson JS, DiRita VJ, Biteen JS (2014) Imaging live cells at the nanometer-scale with single-molecule microscopy: obstacles and achievements in experiment optimization for microbiology. Molecules 19(8):12116–12149

19. Lee SH, Shin JY, Lee A, Bustamante C (2012) Counting single photoactivatable fluorescent molecules by photoactivated localization microscopy (PALM). Proc Natl Acad Sci U S A 109(43):17436–17441

20. Shaner NC et al (2013) A bright monomeric green fluorescent protein derived from Branchiostoma lanceolatum. Nat Methods 10(5):407–409

21. Wang S, Moffitt JR, Dempsey GT, Xie XS, Zhuang X (2014) Characterization and development of photoactivatable fluorescent proteins for single-molecule-based superresolution imaging. Proc Natl Acad Sci U S A 111(23):8452–8457

22. Shcherbakova DM, Sengupta P, Lippincott-Schwartz J, Verkhusha VV (2014) Photocontrollable fluorescent proteins for superresolution imaging. Annu Rev Biophys 43:303–329

23. Ong WQ, Citron YR, Schnitzbauer J, Kamiyama D, Huang B (2015) Heavy water: a simple solution to increasing the brightness of fluorescent proteins in super-resolution imaging. Chem Commun 51(70):13451–13453

24. Andresen M et al (2008) Photoswitchable fluorescent proteins enable monochromatic multi-label imaging and dual color fluorescence nanoscopy. Nat Biotechnol 26(9):1035–1040

25. Subach OM, Entenberg D, Condeelis JS, Verkhusha VV (2012) A FRET-facilitated photoswitching using an orange fluorescent protein with the fast photoconversion kinetics. J Am Chem Soc 134(36):14789–14799

26. Subach FV et al (2009) Photoactivatable mCherry for high-resolution two-color fluorescence microscopy. Nat Methods 6(2):153–159

Chapter 10

STED Imaging in *Drosophila* Brain Slices

Sandra Fendl*, Jesús Pujol-Martí*, Joel Ryan, Alexander Borst, and Robert Kasper

Abstract

Super-resolution microscopy is a very powerful tool to investigate fine cellular structures and molecular arrangements in biological systems. For instance, stimulated emission depletion (STED) microscopy has been successfully used in recent years to investigate the arrangement and colocalization of different protein species in cells in culture and on the surface of specimens. However, because of its extreme sensitivity to light scattering, super-resolution imaging deep inside tissues remains a challenge. Here, we describe the preparation of thin slices from the fruit fly (*Drosophila melanogaster*) brain, subsequent immunolabeling and imaging with STED microscopy. This protocol allowed us to image small dendritic branches from neurons located deep in the fly brain with improved resolution compared with conventional light microscopy.

Key words STED, *Drosophila melanogaster*, Immunofluorescence, Cryostat sectioning, Brain slice

1 Introduction

When imaging biological samples with conventional light microscopy many ultrastructural details kept hidden due to the diffraction barrier. The diffraction barrier was first described by Ernst Abbe in 1873 and is known as the Abbe criterion $d = \lambda/2\,NA$ with the wavelength of light λ and the numerical aperture of the lens NA [1]. The Abbe criterion results in a resolution for standard confocal microscopy of ~250 nm in both the X and Y axes. Fine structures of cells and intracellular compartments are usually much smaller, often occurring very close to each other in the range of tenth of nm, and thus cannot be resolved with conventional light microscopy. Therefore, many efforts have been made to overcome this fundamental limit resulting in super-resolution microscopy methods namely stimulated emission depletion microscopy (STED) and stochastic optical reconstruction microscopy

---

*Author contributed equally with other authors.

Yolanda Markaki and Hartmann Harz (eds.), *Light Microscopy: Methods and Protocols*, Methods in Molecular Biology, vol. 1563, DOI 10.1007/978-1-4939-6810-7_10, © Springer Science+Business Media LLC 2017

(STORM) or photo-activated localization microscopy (PALM) [2–5]. STORM and PALM rely on repetitive nanometer precise localization of single fluorophores which is achieved either by blinking or photo-activation of fluorophores. STED microscopy utilizes the physical concept of stimulated depletion by precise overlay of the excitation beam with the so called STED beam. The donut shape of the STED beam results in fluorescence only from the very center of the two beams.

Even though STED microscopy is a well-established and widely used tool in today's molecular and cell biology research, STED imaging in deep tissue remains challenging. This is mostly due to the fact that light gets scattered in tissue. Consequently, STED microscopy has been mostly used in cells in culture and in the most outer layers of living tissues [6, 7]. Researchers, especially in the molecular, cellular, and circuit neurosciences, have tried to overcome this limitation in recent years. In this direction, optical clearing methods that reduce light scattering while preserving cell morphology and fluorophore brightness have been developed [8]. Such methodology allows for super-resolution imaging of relatively large brain volumes, opening the possibility of large-scale connectome studies based on light-microscopy. Alternatively, super-resolution microscopy applied to thin brain sections has been successfully used to map synaptic inputs onto individual dendrites [9] and to investigate the molecular architecture of synapses in the mouse brain [10]. This methodology, however, has been little explored for imaging in the adult brain of *Drosophila melanogaster* [11].

Here, we present a protocol for super-resolution imaging of subcellular structures of individual neurons located deep in the adult *Drosophila* brain. First, we took advantage of the *Drosophila* genetic toolbox to generate flies with brains expressing a membrane-bound fluorescent protein in a few genetically defined neurons [12–15] (Fig. 1a). Second, we prepared twelve micrometers thin sections from these brains to assure that neurons of interest are closest to coverslip and thus reduce light scattering. We next performed immunostaining and imaged the dendrites of the labeled neurons with STED microscopy (Fig. 1b). After imaging and analysis we found that the overall neuronal morphology seems to be preserved when compared with our results from confocal light-microscopy of whole-mount *Drosophila* brains (compare Fig. 1a, b). Moreover, the

Fig. 1 (continued) the two T4 neurons shown in *top panel*. Thin dendritic branches cannot be resolved. Scale bars = 5 μm. (**b**) Detailed views of individual T4/T5 dendritic arbors labeled after immunostaining and confocal/STED imaging on brain slices. Thin brain slices were prepared as described in this protocol from optic lobes with a few T4/T5 neurons labeled, like the one shown in (**a**). Secondary antibodies used to label the neurons shown here were conjugated with either Atto 647N or Abberior STAR 635P dyes. In both cases, a resolution enhancement from confocal to STED microscopy can be observed, allowing the visualization of small dendritic branches. Scaler bars = 2.5 μm. All images are shown as RAW data and are maximal projections from several confocal planes. Brightness was adjusted for display purposes

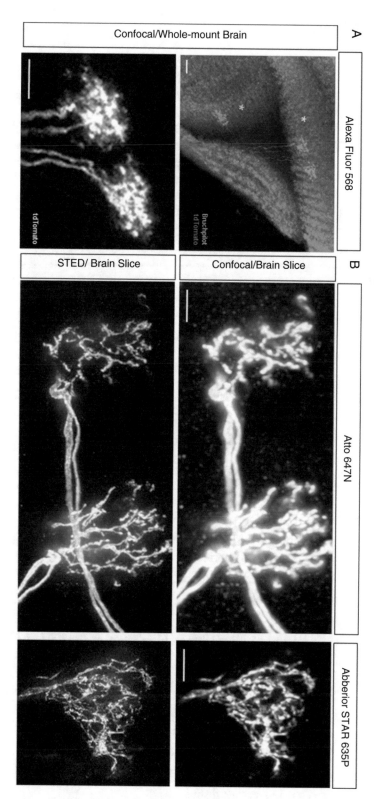

Fig. 1 (a) *Top*: Region of a *Drosophila* optic lobe with two T4 neurons (*white asterisk*) and one T5 neuron (*yellow asterisk*) labeled after immunostaining and confocal imaging of the whole mount adult brain [18]. The optic lobe neuropil was immunolabeled with anti-bruchpilot [19]. The T4/T5 neurons shown express a membrane-bound tdTomato fluorescent protein and were immunolabeled with anti-DsRed. Secondary antibody used to label the neurons was conjugated with Alexa Fluor 568 dye. *Bottom*: Detailed view of the dendritic arbors from

resolution of the STED images improved when compared to conventional light microscopy in brain sections (Fig. 1b). We tested two different secondary antibodies conjugated to either Atto 647N or Abberior STAR 635P dyes. In both cases, a resolution enhancement from confocal to STED microscopy could be observed, allowing a better visualization of small dendritic branches (Fig. 1b). This protocol, when combined with genetic and immunohistochemistry tools, provides a promising starting point to examine the presence and distribution of proteins at the nanoscale level in neurons of *Drosophila*, an extensively used model in current neuroscience research [16, 17].

2 Materials

2.1 Reagents

1. PBS: Phosphate-buffered Saline (pH 7.2).
2. PBST: Phosphate-buffered Saline (pH 7.2) with 0.3 % Triton X-100.
3. Sucrose Buffer: 30 % sucrose in PBST (store at 4 °C).
4. Blocking Buffer: 4 % Bovine Serum Albumin (BSA, Sigma-Aldrich), 5 % Normal Goat Serum (NGS, Sigma-Aldrich) in PBST.
5. Fixation Buffer: 4 % paraformaldehyde (PFA, Electron Microscopy Sciences) in PBST (store at 4 °C).
6. Primary antibody: DsRed Polyclonal Antibody (Source: Rabbit, Clonetech).
7. Secondary antibodies: Anti-Rabbit Atto647N (Source: Goat, Sigma-Aldrich) or Anti-Rabbit Abberior® STAR 635P (Source: Goat, Abberior).
8. TDE mounting medium O (Abberior).
9. Cryostat mounting medium (Richard-Allan Scientific™ Neg-50™ Gefrierschnittmedium, Thermo Fisher Scientific).
10. Adult *Drosophila* of the desired genotype (*see* **Note 1**).

2.2 General Laboratory Equipment

1. 0.2 mL tubes (Thermo Fisher Scientific).
2. Microscope Slides: Superfrost Ultra Plus Adhesion Slides (Thermo Fisher Scientific).
3. Cover glasses: 22 × 40 mm, #1.5 (Thermo Fisher Scientific).
4. Dissecting Microscope.
5. Forceps (#55, Dumont).
6. Dissecting dishes.
7. Kimwipes tissues (Kimberly-Clark).

8. Razor Blades (VWR).

9. Nail Polish (transparent).

10. Lab Rocker (Custom-built).

11. Shandon Coverplate Holder (Thermo Fisher Scientific).

12. Cryostat Leica CM3050 S.

2.3 STED Microscope   Abberior Instruments STED system equipped with a 775 nm pulsed STED laser, 594 nm and 640 nm pulsed excitation laser, UPlan APO 100× 1.4 oil objective (Olympus), 2 APD detectors (Excelitas) for gated detection and a spatial light modulator (Hamamatsu) for generating the donut shape.

Typical gating time was 234 ps between excitation pulse and start of the fluorescence detection.

3   Methods

3.1 Dissection and Fixation of Fly Heads

1. Collect adult flies of the desired genotype and anesthetize them on ice. Transfer them to dissecting dish filled with PBST, use forceps to detach fly heads from body, pull out proboscis, and remove trachea with forceps (*see* **Note 2**).

2. Fix fly heads for 30 min in Fixation Buffer in a 0.2 mL tube at room temperature on a lab rocker (*see* **Note 3**).

3. Remove fixative and wash heads three times for 15 min in PBST.

4. Infiltrate heads with Sucrose Buffer for at least 3 h (up to 24 h) at 4 °C (*see* **Note 4**).

3.2 Cryosectioning of Fly Heads

1. Settings Cryostat: Set chamber temperature to −21 °C and object temperature to −18 °C. Set section thickness to 12–16 μm.

2. Add Cryostat mounting medium to the sample holder and freeze it inside the cryostat until hardened.

3. Trim the block in a square form with a conventional razor blade.

4. Under the dissection microscope transfer the heads to the sample holder with frozen mounting medium block and cover the brains with cryostat mounting medium.

5. Let the block freeze at least 10 min inside the cryostat until hardened.

6. Pick up sections with microscope slides and let them dry at room temperature for at least 10 min. Keep the slides at 4 °C for storage or continue with immunolabeling.

3.3 Immunolabeling of Sections in "Shandon Coverplate Holder"

1. Assemble the microscope slides with head sections in the Shandon Coverplate Holder.
2. Block the slices for 1 h in Blocking Buffer at room temperature.
3. Add primary antibody diluted in PBST (1:300) and incubate the samples overnight at 4 °C.
4. Wash three times with PBST for 15 min each.
5. Add secondary antibody diluted in PBST (1:200 for anti-Rabbit Atto 647 N and 1:500 for anti-Rabbit Abberior ®STAR 635P (*see* **Note 9**)) and incubate the samples overnight at 4 °C (*see* **Note 8**).
6. Wash three times in PBST for 15 min each.

3.4 Mounting

1. Keep microscope slides with head sections in the Shandon Coverplate Holder.
2. Mount slides in TDE Mounting Medium O (for use with oil immersion objectives) (*see* **Note 5**).
3. Add three to five drops TDE Solution A to the slides in the holder. Incubate for 20 min.
4. Repeat **step 7** with TDE Solution B, C, and D.
5. Remove the slides from the Shandon Coverplate Holder. Clean the area around the brain sections with Kimwipes tissues (*see* **Note 6**).
6. Add one drop of TDE Solution D to the brain sections and cover it with a clean cover glass (22 × 40 mm).
7. Seal the edges of the cover glass with clear nail polish and store the samples at 4 °C in the dark (*see* **Note 7**).

3.5 Imaging

1. Find area of interest with 10x objective then switch to 100× oil objective (apply immersion oil).
2. Check quality of labeling and colors in confocal mode (*see* **Note 10**).
3. Apply STED laser and check for best STED power to achieve sufficient depletion. STED power depends on the label and can vary from sample to sample. Gating settings should be adjusted as well.
4. As a general rule we increased excitation power from confocal to STED imaging 3-fold and accumulated 3-5 frames per image.
5. For 3D STED add second donut and adjust STED power accordingly.

4   Notes

1. For sparse labeling of neurons [14, 15], we combined in single flies the following transgenes: R57C10-Flp2::PEST, VT50384-lexA, and LexAop-frt-stop-frt-CD4::tdTomato. The weak flippase FLP2::PEST is expressed pan-neurally and stochastically removes the FRT-flanked stop cassette, allowing LexA-driven expression of a membrane-tagged red fluorescent protein (CD4::tdTomato).

2. The dissection procedure should take ~10–25 min per experiment. It is critical to minimize dissection time to avoid tissue degradation.

3. Add up to ten heads into one tube for proper fixation.

4. Leave heads in Sucrose Buffer until they sink to the bottom. Thereby, the tissue is cryo-protected.

5. TDE Mounting Medium is matching the refractive index of the embedding medium to that of the oil immersion by subsequent steps of incubation in different TDE solutions. Thus, optical aberrations and scattering are minimized. As a result, light penetrates more deeply into the specimen and the imaging contrast is enhanced.

6. It is essential to remove all excess mounting medium around the sections to enable a proper sealing of the cover glass with nail polish.

7. The cover glass should be as clean as possible for STED microscopy. Clean the glass with ethanol if necessary.

8. We tested several dye combinations for simultaneous dual-color STED imaging experiments. We found that Anti-Rabbit Atto594 (Sigma-Aldrich) can be used together with either Atto 647N or Abberior® STAR 635P. In terms of brightness and photo stability all three dyes could be used in our experiments.

9. For dual-color STED imaging, the expression levels of the two proteins to be immunolabeled are critical to avoid bleed-through in the emission channels if not matched properly.

10. This protocol can be used to apply STORM with *Drosophila* brain slices as well. We did some preliminary tests and used Alexa647 and Atto532 as two color dye combinations. For STROM the results would greatly benefit from even thinner brain slices and the structure of interest as close to the cover slide as possible. In addition the mounting medium needs to be changed to a switching buffer containing glucose oxidase and mercaptoethanol or other thiol containing reagents.

Acknowledgments

We are indebted to H. Leonhardt and the BioImaging Network Munich for generous support. We thank Marianne Braun and Ursula Weber for excellent help with technical procedures, and Aljoscha Nern, Gerald M. Rubin, and Barry Dickson for providing transgenic flies.

References

1. Abbe E (1973) Beiträge zur Theorie des Mikroskops und der mikroskopischenWahrnehmung. Archiv für mikroskopische Anatomie 9:413–418

2. Klar TA, Jacobs S, Dyba M, Egner A, Hell SW (2000) Fluorescence microscopy with diffraction resolution barrier broken by stimulated emission. Proc Natl Acad Sci U S A 97:8206–8210

3. Betzig E, Patterson GH, Sougrat R, Lindwasser OW, Olenych S, Bonifacino JS, Davidson MW, Lippincott-Schwartz J, Hess HF (2006) Imaging intracellular fluorescent proteins at nanometer resolution. Science 313(5793):1642–1645

4. Rust MJ, Bates M, Zhuang X (2006) Sub-diffraction-limit imaging by stochastic optical reconstruction microscopy (STORM). Nat Methods 3(10):793–795

5. Hess ST, Girirajan TP, Mason MD (2006) Ultra-high resolution imaging by fluorescence photoactivation localization microscopy. Biophys J 91(11):4258–4272

6. Lau L, Lee YL, Matis M, Axelrod J, Stearns T, Moerner WE (2011) STED super-resolution microscopy inDrosophilatissue and in mammalian cells. Proc SPIE Int Soc Opt Eng 7910:79101N

7. Berning S, Willig KI, Steffens H, Dibaj P, Hell SW (2012) Nanoscopy in a living mouse brain. Science 335(6068):551

8. Ke MT, Nakai Y, Fujimoto S, Takayama R, Yoshida S, Kitajima TS, Sato M, Imai T (2016) Super-resolution mapping of neuronal circuitry with an index-optimized clearing agent. Cell Reports 14(11):2718–2732

9. Sigal YM, Speer CM, Babcock HP, Zhuang X (2015) Mapping synaptic input fields of neurons with super-resolution imaging. Cell 163(2):493–505

10. Dani A, Huang B, Bergan J, Dulac C, Zhuang X (2010) Superresolution imaging of chemical synapses in the brain. Neuron 68:843–856

11. Spühler IA, Conley GM, Scheffold F, Sprecher SG (2016) Super resolution imaging of genetically labelled synapses in Drosophila brain tissue. Front Cell Neurosci 10:142

12. Rodríguez AdV, Didiano D, Desplan, C (2011) Power tools for gene expression and clonal analysis in Drosophila. NatureMethods 9(1):47–55

13. Venken KJT, Simpson JH, Bellen HJ (2011) Genetic manipulation of genes and cells in the nervous system of the fruit fly. Neuron 72:202–230

14. Nern A, Pfeiffer BD, Svoboda K, Rubin GM (2011) Multiple new site-specific recombinases for use in manipulating animal genomes. Proceedings of the National Academy of Sciences of the United States of America 108(34):14198–14203

15. Nern A, Pfeiffer BD, Rubin GM (2015) Optimized tools for multicolor stochastic labeling reveal diverse stereotyped cell arrangements in the fly visual system. Proceedings of the National Academy of Sciences of the United States of America 112(22):E2967–E2976

16. Bellen HJ, Tong C, Tsuda H (2010) 100 years of Drosophila research and its impact on vertebrate neuroscience: a history lesson for the future. Nat. Rev. Neurosci. 11:514–522

17. Kazama H (2015) Systems neuroscience in Drosophila: conceptual and technical advantages. Neuroscience 296:3–14

18. Maisak MS, Haag J, Ammer G, Serbe E, Meier M, Leonhardt M, Schilling T, Bahl A, Rubin GM, Nern A, Dickson BJ, Reiff DF, Hopp E, Borst A (2013) A directional tuning map of Drosophila elementary motion detectors. Nature 500:212–216

19. Wagh DA, Rasse TM, Asan E, Hofbauer A, Schwenkert I, Duerrbeck H, Bucher S, Dabauvalle MC, Schmidt M, Qin G, Wichmann C, Kittel R, Sigrist SJ, Bucher E (2006) Bruchpilot, a Protein with Homology to ELKS/CAST, Is Required for Structural Integrity and Function of Synaptic Active Zones in Drosophila. Neuron 49(6):833–844

Chapter 11

Two-Color Total Internal Reflection Fluorescence Microscopy of Exocytosis in Endocrine Cells

Adam J. Trexler and Justin W. Taraska

Abstract

We describe a comprehensive method for imaging and analysis of local protein dynamics at single sites of exocytosis in living cultured endocrine cells. This method is well suited to quantitatively map the complex dynamics of individual molecules at single sites of vesicle fusion in live cells.

Key words TIRF, Exocytosis, Live-cell imaging, Vesicle fusion, Image analysis, Endocrine cells

1 Introduction

Exocytosis, the regulated secretion of molecules from cells, is critical to many aspects of eukaryotic physiology [1]. During exocytosis, materials packaged into the lumen of secretory vesicles are released into the external environment when the vesicle membrane and plasma membrane fuse. Examples of well-studied exocytic systems are neurotransmitter release at neuronal synapses [2, 3], adrenaline and insulin release from neuroendocrine and endocrine cells [4–7], acrosome and cortical granule fusion during fertilization [8, 9], acetylcholine stimulation of muscle [10], and many more physiological processes.

The process of exocytosis is driven by a molecular complex that includes the proteins Syntaxin1a, SNAP-25, and VAMP [11]. These three SNARE proteins are thought to assemble between the vesicle and plasma membrane, forming a four helix bundle that zippers together and pulls both membranes close to one another. Additional factors including complexin, munc18, munc13, CAPS, tomosyn, and others are thought to regulate SNARE complex assembly in distinct cellular systems [11–17]. Physiologically, membrane fusion is triggered by increases in cytoplasmic calcium concentrations, which is sensed by the protein synaptotagmin [18, 19]. Additional proteins including Rab GTPases and their effectors

Yolanda Markaki and Hartmann Harz (eds.), *Light Microscopy: Methods and Protocols*, Methods in Molecular Biology, vol. 1563, DOI 10.1007/978-1-4939-6810-7_11, © Springer Science+Business Media LLC 2017

help direct vesicles to the plasma membrane and tether them close to sites of fusion [20–22]. While we understand a great deal about the genetics, biochemistry, structures, and mechanisms of many of these factors and their possible roles in exocytosis, it is still unclear which of these molecules are present at sites of fusion before, during, and after exocytosis. To address this central question, we visualize exocytic events using fluorescent proteins to directly interrogate the temporal dynamics of individual molecules at single sites of exocytosis in living cells.

Here, we present detailed methods for two-color through-the-objective total internal reflection fluorescence (TIRF) microscopy (also known as evanescent field microscopy) to visualize exocytosis in living cells [23, 24]. TIRF illumination provides an exponentially decaying fluorescence excitation field around one hundred nanometers above the coverslip/liquid interface [4]. This illumination depth is ideally suited to visualize with high contrast fluorescently labeled 50–300 nm diameter vesicles arriving at, and fusing with, the plasma membrane at the bottom surface of an adherent cell [4]. In objective-based TIRF, adherent cells can be maintained in a bath solution and locally perfused to acutely stimulate exocytosis (Fig. 1).

By visualizing exocytosis in two colors using TIRF, we identify the individual and average behavior of molecules at single sites of exocytosis before, during, and after fusion [5, 25]. This approach is valuable because it provides direct dynamic information about the local behavior of individual molecules, which in turn helps to interpret biochemical data and build mechanistic models to describe the regulation of the exocytic fusion machinery in mammalian cells [26, 27].

2 Materials

2.1 General Cell Culture and Imaging

1. 30 % hydrogen peroxide solution.
2. 27–30 % ammonium hydroxide solution.
3. 25 mm #1.5 glass coverslips.
4. Ceramic or Teflon coverslip holder (Thomas Scientific).
5. Sharp tweezers for coverslip handling, long-handled tweezers, or tongs for handling coverslip holders.
6. Two 2 L glass beakers.
7. 100 % ethanol.
8. Hotplate.
9. Fume hood.
10. Poly-L-lysine solution (0.01 %).

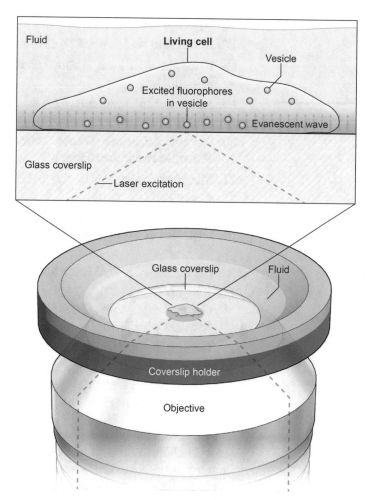

Fig. 1 Diagram of imaging geometry and a cell under TIRF illumination. A coverslip with living cells grown on it is mounted into a coverslip holder with fluid bathing the cells. From below, the excitation laser is directed through the imaging objective and its angle of incidence with the glass coverslip adjusted to achieve total internal reflection. This produces an evanescent illumination field, which decays exponentially, at the glass-water interface to illuminate fluorophores inside vesicles in the cell. With a low-profile coverslip holder, a perfusion pipette can be positioned above the cell using a micromanipulator to locally superfuse cells with stimulation solution

11. RPMI media without phenol red: 10 % FBS, 1 % pen/strep, 11.1 mM glucose, 2 mM glutamine, 1 mM pyruvate, 10 mM HEPES, 50 μM beta-mercaptoethanol.

12. Dulbecco's phosphate buffered saline.

13. 0.25 % trypsin-EDTA solution.

14. 6-well tissue culture plates.

15. T25 or T75 tissue culture flasks.

16. Lipofectamine 2000.

17. Immersion oil (NA: 1.518).

18. FluoSphere0.1 μm yellow-green beads (Thermo Fisher Scientific).

19. Micro-perfusion system (ALA Scientific μFLow-8 with 100 μm diameter tip Quartz manifold).

20. Coverslip chamber (Warner Instruments Series 40 or Thermo Fisher Scientific AttoFluor).

21. Micromanipulator platform (ALA Scientific MT-75 series or similar).

22. Coarse micromanipulator (ALA Scientific MM-3 series or similar) with small manipulator mounted on end (ALA Scientific YOU-2 or similar).

23. Aspirating system (ALA Scientific VWK or similar).

24. Imaging Buffer (IB): 130 mM NaCl, 2.8 mM KCl, 5 mM $CaCl_2$, 1 mM $MgCl_2$, 10 mM HEPES, 10 mM glucose, pH 7.4 (titrated with NaOH).

25. Ionomycin Buffer: IB with 10 μM ionomycin added.

26. Stimulation Buffer: 50 mM NaCl, 105 mM KCl, 5 mM $CaCl_2$, 1 mM $MgCl_2$, 10 mM HEPES, 1 mM NaH_2PO_4, pH 7.4 (titrated with KOH).

2.2 TIRF Microscope Setup

The microscope setup described here is specifically designed for two-color TIRF microscopy optimized for visualizing GFP and mCherry fluorescent proteins. Our system is built around an inverted microscope configured for through-the-objective TIRF. Fluorescence is excited by lasers at 488 nm and 561 nm, and lasers are combined and controlled with an acousto-optic tunable filter (AOTF) and directed into the back port of the microscope via optics for changing TIRF angle, size, and collimation. This microscope uses the Olympus ZDC2 drift correction system which is based on far-red light reflection from the glass/liquid interface on the coverslip. Optical filters and dichroics for excitation light control are bright-line full multi-band LF405/488/561/635 filters (Semrock).

TIRF is achieved through an Olympus 100X 1.45 NA oil immersion objective. The resulting emission is divided by an image splitter's dichroic (565DCXR) and projected side-by-side through 525Q/50 and 605Q/55 emission filters onto the chip of a back-illuminated EMCCD camera. Images are acquired using AndorIQ2 software.

1. Inverted microscope equipped with ZDC correction system (Olympus IX-81).

2. Sapphire 488 nm (Coherent) and 561 nm (Melles Griot LD-561-20A) lasers.

3. Laser-combiner system and AOTF (Andor, 400 Series).

4. 100× 1.45 NA oil-immersion PlanApo objective (Olympus).

5. DualView image splitter (Photometrics DV2).

6. iXon Ultra 897 EM-CCD (Andor DU 897).

7. Software (Andor iQ2).

3 Methods

3.1 Coverslip Preparation

Coverslips must be thoroughly cleaned and sterilized with ethanol prior to use. Our cleaning protocol is adapted from the first step of the classic RCA etch protocol [28]. This protocol removes organic contaminants, substantially reduces background fluorescence on the glass, and imparts partial charge to the glass to help surface-additives adhere.

1. Add coverslips to a ceramic or Teflon coverslip holder.

2. Place coverslip holders in the bottom of a 2 L glass beaker and add 300 mL water (*see* **Note 1**).

3. Add 60 mL of 30 % hydrogen peroxide to the beaker and move into a fume hood.

4. Add 60 mL of 27 % ammonium hydroxide to the beaker. Move the beaker to a hotplate and turn to high. Wait for 5 min and check for gentle bubbling in the beaker (approximately 50 °C). After gentle bubbling begins, incubate the coverslips for 15 min. At the end of the incubation, the solution should be vigorously bubbling at 80–90 °C. CAUTION: the fumes from the beaker are caustic and must not be inhaled.

5. Remaining in the hood, remove the beaker from the hotplate. Using long handled tweezers or wire tongs transfer the coverslip holders to a 2 L beaker filled with 1 L of water. Next transfer coverslip holders to smaller containers of 100 % ethanol for long-term storage.

6. Depending on the cell type, coverslips may need to be coated so that cells will adhere properly. Common surface additives are poly-L-lysine (PLL), poly-D-lysine (PDL), collagen, fibronectin, and others. For INS-1 cells, we briefly coat the coverslips with PLL immediately prior to adding cells. Remove the coverslips from ethanol inside a biological safety cabinet under sterile conditions. Allow the coverslips to air-dry entirely and transfer one coverslip to each well of a six-well plate. Add approximately 100–200 μL of PLL solution to each coverslip. It is not necessary to completely cover the coverslip.

7. Incubate 10 min at room temperature and then aspirate the PLL solution from the coverslip. Wash coverslips twice with

2 mL media and then cover with 2 mL media in preparation for cell addition. It is important to rinse away all of the unbound PLL.

8. Precoated coverslips are also available from several companies. We have used Neuvitro brand (# GG-25-1.5) coverslips with a variety of coatings (poly-D-lysine, poly-L-lysine, fibronection, collagen).

3.2 Cell Culture and Transfection

We study the exocytosis of dense-core vesicles from INS-1/832-13 cells, derived from a rat insulinoma of the pancreas [29]. Other cells that can be used with slight modification to this protocol are rat pheochromocytoma PC12 cells originally derived from the adrenal gland [5]. Cells are passaged using routine tissue culture methods in T-75 plastic tissue culture flasks until approximately passage number 80, after which the culture is discarded.

1. After rinsing cells in DPBS, trypsinizing, and pelleting, cells are resuspended in media and added dropwise to coverslips in six-well plates. Ideally, cells should be plated densely enough to be healthy (INS-1 cells, for example, do not thrive at low density) but not so dense that it will be difficult later to identify single cells in the microscopic field-of-view.

2. After plating, allow cells to rest overnight in a tissue-culture incubator.

3. Transfect the cells using your transfection method of choice one day post-plating. For many transfection methods, maximum transfection efficiency is achieved with freshly plated cells. We routinely obtain ~10–20 % transfection efficiency using Lipofectamine 2000 with INS-1 cells. Nucleofection with Lonza Kit V and protocol T-020 produces much higher transfection efficiency (>50 %).

4. Cells must be transfected with a vesicle cargo marker. For INS-1 cells in our system, we transfect with NPY-GFP using 1 µg of DNA per coverslip (Addgene plasmid #74629).

   (a) Choice of cargo marker will be dependent on the cell line and experiment. In general, useful cargoes are specifically packaged into or associated with secretory vesicles. More general markers of vesicles, such as Rab proteins or VAMPs, often have high levels of diffuse background.

   (b) Other common cargo markers used to visualize dense-core vesicles are tissue plasminogen activator (tPA), phogrin, and chromogranin. TPA can be experimentally useful because after fusion it is released from the vesicle lumen very slowly, allowing for visualization of much longer timescale exocytic events and mechanisms (control of cargo release, for example).

5. Vesicles can be labeled in any convenient color, though probes must be sensitive to the pH changes that vesicles experience during fusion to robustly detect exocytic events. The lumen of most secretory vesicles is acidic (~5.5 pH) and will quench GFP, pH luorin, and other pH-sensitive fluorophores. Upon membrane fusion, the acidic lumen of the vesicle is neutralized by exposure to the extracellular buffer, leading to a sudden and dramatic brightening in the fluorescent signal from the vesicle followed by its loss as the cargo exits the vesicle. This fluorescence behavior is a hallmark of vesicle fusion (Fig. 2b, c). In the absence of pH-sensitivity, exocytosis will manifest as merely a loss of vesicle signal, which could also be caused by vesicle diffusion out of the TIRF field or photobleaching. Probes tagged with mCherry or ECFP which have lower pKa values exhibit this behavior. In most experiments, we co-transfect cells with a second protein-of-interest tagged with a red fluorescent protein such as mCherry or mRFP. Thus if desired, perform co-transfection by adding 1 μg of DNA of a second construct in addition to NPY-GFP to each coverslip.

6. After transfection, allow cells to rest overnight. Cells can be imaged 1–2 days post-transfection. At short timescales post transfection (~6 h), low expression levels of the transgenic protein can be visualized if overexpression is a concern.

3.3 Microscope and Sample Preparation

The following protocol is for an imaging experiment to visualize NPY-GFP labeled vesicles and a mCherry-tagged protein-of-interest using a two-color TIRF microscope, as described in the Materials section. The protocol is broadly applicable to imaging in any other one or two-color modes with different fluorophores, with necessary changes in filters and imaging settings.

Before each round of imaging experiments, the microscope imaging channels must be aligned and the TIRF field calibrated and evaluated for uniformity. Alignment is performed by imaging 100 nm fluorescent beads with 488 nm illumination in TIRF such that the beads are visible in both the green (direct emission) and red (bleed-through signal) channels. These alignment images are essential for processing the data and must be collected prior to each experimental session. We collect these images before each set of experiments to ensure that no mechanical drift in the imaging system is changing the channel alignment.

1. Place a 25 mm coverslip in a coverslip chamber (*see* **Note 2**). The coverslip need not be cleaned. After securing the coverslip, before adding buffer, briefly rub the coverslip with a forefinger, which helps beads stick to the glass. Add 500 μL IB to the coverslip followed by 5 μL diluted fluorescent beads (diluted 1:1000). Transfer bead-coated coverslip to the microscope.

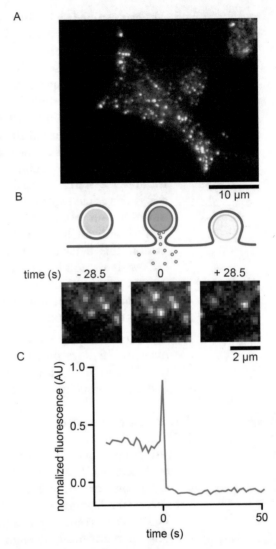

Fig. 2 Representative images of labeled dense-core vesicles in INS-1 cells visualized with TIRF microscopy. (**a**) A TIRF micrograph of an INS-1 cells transfected with NPY-GFP. Diffraction limited spots are vesicles resting near the bottom cell membrane within the evanescent illumination field. The contrast of the image has intentionally been adjusted much higher than normal for print clarity which causes the diffuse background within the cell body. (**b**) A cartoon of exocytosis, shown as a side view of a vesicle resting near the membrane. Upon exocytosis the vesicular and plasma membranes fuse to release cargo. After exocytosis, vesicle fluorescence has been lost. Below the cartoon are representative images of a single dense-core vesicle undergoing exocytosis. The vesicle is present prior to fusion (*left frame*, vesicle at center), its intensity increases dramatically upon fusion (*middle frame*), and is then lost rapidly (*right frame*). (**d**) Fluorescence intensity trajectory extracted from the image sequence in (**b**). The intensity is background subtracted and normalized as described in the text

2. Using the 488 nm laser, focus on the beads stuck to the coverslip. For longer timescale imaging experiments (more than a few minutes) it is useful to employ an auto-focus or drift-correction device. Autofocus devices can usually be calibrated using a bead sample, disengaged to replace the bead sample with a cell sample, and re-engaged to quickly find and keep focus.

3. Adjust the TIRF angle as necessary to produce shallow evanescent illumination. In epi-illumination unbound beads will be visible diffusing freely and briefly contacting the coverslip, while in TIRF illumination, only beads stuck to the coverslip will be visible as immobile spots. Adjust imaging parameters such that the emission in the green channel is in the dynamic range of the camera.

4. Acquire at least three bead images from different fields-of-view using 488 nm illumination. Ideally, the field-of-view should contain at least 20–30 beads but not be so dense that picking out individual beads is difficult.

5. The bead sample is also useful to verify even TIRF illumination over the entire field-of-view, which will be conspicuous in areas of high bead density.

6. Prepare the perfusion apparatus (*see* **Note 3**). Load at least one channel of the perfusion system with IB and one channel with stimulation solution (ionomycin or stimulation buffer, as desired). Check nitrogen pressure and ensure the perfusion apparatus is not clogged by verifying solution flow from the tip of the perfusion manifold from both the IB and stimulation channels.

3.4 Imaging and Stimulation

Exocytosis can be triggered with a variety of stimuli depending on the cell type and secretion process of interest. We trigger secretion by brief (5 s) local superfusion of cells in the field-of-view, which applies a very small volume of stimulation solution. Local superfusion prevents bulk depolarization of the coverslip and allows for multiple rounds of stimulation and imaging in different fields-of-view over the same coverslip.

1. Rinse coverslip with cells three times in IB before placing in coverslip chamber. Rinsing can be easily accomplished by moving the coverslip sequentially through three small dishes filled with IB. Load the coverslip into a coverslip chamber and cover cells with 500 µL IB and place on microscope. Engage the auto-focus device and verify the cells are in focus with bright-field illumination.

2. Using the microscope eyepieces and the micromanipulator controlling the perfusion pipette, position the perfusion tip as near as possible to the focal plane of the cells and to the side of

the field-of-view (*see* **Note 4**). After positioning the perfusion tip, perfuse with IB briefly to ensure no air was trapped in the tip of the perfusion pipette and blow any debris off. Move the stage in the *x-y* plane in all directions to ensure that the tip is not touching cells or the coverslip.

3. If necessary, add an aspirating pipette to the microscope stage insert, positioning the tip just over the desired buffer level in the coverslip (*see* **Note 5**). The aspirating pipette setup is used to maintain constant buffer level in the coverslip chamber after addition of IB for sample rinsing.

4. Switch to fluorescent illumination and scan the coverslip for a cell suitable for imaging. High framerate of 10/s enables easy screening for cells. Ideal cells expressing the vesicle marker show well-defined, diffraction-limited vesicles in the TIRF illumination field (Fig. 2a).

5. If the sample has been co-transfected for two-color imaging, verify that the cell is expressing the second construct.

6. Adjust imaging parameters (laser power, most commonly, or EM gain and exposure time as well) to ensure that the maximum intensity from both the green and red channels is within the dynamic range of the camera.

7. Begin acquiring images, alternating between the green and red channels, for at least 20 frames before perfusing the cells with a stimulation solution. To visualize DCV exocytosis in INS-1 cells using NPY-GFP, we typically use a camera exposure time of 500 ms in both green and red channels, followed by a 500 ms wait, for a total framerate in both channels of 0.67/s. Lower exposure times are, however, possible.

  (a) At lower framerates of 0.67/s, longer movies and more events can be captured at the expense of time resolution. Conversely, high framerates of 10/s or more offer improved time resolution but typically yield fewer events and less total observation time due to photobleaching.

8. Trigger perfusion for 5 s. Perfusion can be triggered manually or automatically via software control. The exact timing of perfusion does not matter greatly as exocytic events will be time aligned later to the moment of exocytosis.

9. After the images have been acquired, rinse the coverslip with 3–5 mL of IB to remove residual stimulation solution. Rinsing can be performed by manually adding IB to the coverslip or with larger volume perfusion systems.

10. After the experiment, save movies as TIFF stacks for further processing.

3.5 Image Analysis   Our analysis pipeline uses custom-written MATLAB scripts to handle TIFF stacks and process image data. The same analysis can be performed in a variety of programming languages or manually with image processing software such as Metamorph or ImageJ. This analysis pipeline assumes a camera-face of 512×512 pixels with DualView setup, as described in Subheading 2.

1. *Split*: Split the raw TIFF stacks into green and red channels by extracting the appropriate frames from the movie and rewriting new TIFF stacks for each channel. These new movies will be half the length of the original acquisition.

2. *Transform*: Using an image of beads acquired before the experiment, map the coordinates of at least six beads from their fluorescence in the green and red channels. Use these coordinates to spatially transform the red channel images onto the same coordinate plane as the green image. This processing step should yield a new red channel movie that can be superimposed on the green channel movie to provide perfect spatial overlap between the two channels (*see* **Note 6**). Bead images are used as fiducials to account for alignment differences between the green and red illumination paths and DualView image splitting.

3. *Identify*: Next exocytic events should be identified by visual inspection of the green channel movies. The rubric for identifying exocytic events will vary depending on the vesicle cargo marker that is used, generally however, events should come from single diffraction limited spots of fluorescence that were stably present at the plasma membrane prior to fusion. Most cargo markers useful to detect vesicle fusion will increase in fluorescence intensity upon membrane fusion, and this dramatic brightening of the fluorescence spot is the marker of an exocytic event (Fig. 2b).

4. *Extract*: Extract the average pixel intensity of a 3×3 pixel region centered at the exocytic event coordinates (F_{center}) over a suitable time interval from the green and red channels. Again the time interval will depend on a variety of factors: the vesicle luminal marker used, the process of interest in the experiment (for example pre-fusion states, the moment of fusion itself, cargo release kinetic post-fusion). The fluorescence intensity should be background subtracted using local cellular background fluorescence (*see* **Note 7**).

5. *Normalize*: Normalize trajectories before averaging to account for differences in brightness from cell-to-cell due to biological or experimental variability. Again there are a variety of methods available, but we normalize each trajectory from 0 to 1 according to:

$$\text{Normalized fluor} = \frac{\left(\left(F_{\text{center}} - F_{\text{surround}}\right) - F_{\text{min}}\right)}{F_{\text{max}} - F_{\text{min}}}$$

where F_{min} is the minimum fluorescence intensity over the F_{center} background-subtracted trace and F_{max} is the maximum. F_{surround} is the background subtraction method used here, where F_{surround} is simply the mean pixel intensity in a 25 pixel box around F_{center}. An example is shown in Fig. 2c.

6. *Time-align*: Time-align fluorescence intensity trajectories to generate average trajectories. Trajectories should be aligned to a moment near fusion, and the fluorescence signal corresponding to this will depend on the vesicle marker. For NPY-GFP, which is our probe of choice for measuring INS-1 dense-core vesicle fusion, the marker is reasonably fluorescent in the vesicle lumen and decays sharply after fusion. We align to the timeframe of maximum intensity decrease, usually occurring in one step at our framerate, as this is the most robust feature of all intensity trajectories independent of how bright the vesicle might be prior to fusion. Probes that are dim in the unfused vesicle lumen (tPA-GFP in INS-1 cells, or pHluorin constructs) can be aligned to the timeframe corresponding to the maximum intensity increase, which should be close in time to when the vesicle fuses. Our analysis pipeline employs a script that detects the maximum intensity decrease or increase in a window around an estimated time of fusion provided by the user when selecting the exocytic events. After time-alignment, trajectories can be averaged and plotted.

4   Notes

1. A round 2 L glass beaker can accommodate four or five of the Thomson ceramic coverslip holders. If more or less coverslips are to be cleaned in one batch, or a different sized beaker used, adjust the total volume of cleaning solution to ensure coverage of the coverslips. Maintain a ratio of water: hydrogen peroxide:ammonium hydroxide at 5:1:1.

2. For imaging stimulated exocytosis, we recommend coverslip chambers from Warner Instruments. These low-profile coverslip chambers occlude a minimal amount of the coverslip and allow for easy access for perfusion, rinsing, and aspirating pipettes. We add custom-cut Parafilm o-rings, approximately the same size as the polycarbonate component of the chamber, which we place over the coverslip after seating it in the aluminum lower component of the chamber. The upper polycarbonate component is then pressed down over the Parafilm ring, which helps to ensure a tight seal and prevent liquid leakage.

We have also used stainless-steel Attofluor chambers from Thermo Scientific, which have great leak protection but occlude more of the coverslip and have a higher profile.

3. The quartz perfusion manifolds from ALA Scientific are much more forgiving and reproducible than glass perfusion pipettes. Care should be taken to clean the perfusion system after each use. Channels used for perfusion must be thoroughly rinsed with water after each experiment or they will clog. Long-term storage in 20 % ethanol is recommended.

4. Proper positioning of the perfusion pipette tip is tricky. The tip must be "found" in the field-of-view by looking for the shadow that it casts in the brightfield illumination light. Begin by using the micromanipulator to position the shaft of the perfusion pipette generally over the objective lens. Using the eyepieces and micromanipulator, move the perfusion tip back-and-forth in the y-plane (where the y-plane is parallel to the direction of the microscope eyepieces) and look for a dark shadow moving through the field-of-view. If no shadow can be found, move the perfusion pipette further away from the objective lens and try again. Once the shadow of the tip is located, center it in the field of view and begin using the micromanipulator controls to slowly step the tip down. After each movement downward, re-center the shadow in the field-of-view. Eventually, the shadow will resolve into the perfusion pipette and the tip will become sharply focused. The ALA quartz perfusion manifold appears somewhat transparent when in the focal plane, which is a good sign the tip is close enough to the coverslip.

5. We use a vacuum pump-driven aspirating system from ALA Scientific. Attached to the aspirating line is a large gauge blunt needle bent downward with a magnet glued to the needle base. The bend of the needle can be changed to suit any particular stage insert or coverslip chamber. The magnet is used to clamp the pipette to our microscope stage insert to position the pipette tip over the coverslip.

6. A good method for validating a transformation method is to acquire a movie of stationary beads, which can then be split and transformed to verify complete overlap of bead fluorescence from each channel.

7. There are a variety of ways to implement a background subtraction and we recommend experimenting with several to identify what is most relevant to the particular experiment and imaging probes being used. For example, high background levels that change in response to fusion, as happens with membrane-bound vesicle lumen markers such as VAMP, can critically confound analysis.

References

1. Jahn R, Lang T, Sudhof TC (2003) Membrane fusion. Cell 112(4):519–533

2. Sudhof TC (2013) Neurotransmitter release: the last millisecond in the life of a synaptic vesicle. Neuron 80(3):675–690. doi:10.1016/j.neuron.2013.10.022

3. Zenisek D, Steyer JA, Almers W (2000) Transport, capture and exocytosis of single synaptic vesicles at active zones. Nature 406(6798):849–854. doi:10.1038/35022500

4. Steyer JA, Almers W (1999) Tracking single secretory granules in live chromaffin cells by evanescent-field fluorescence microscopy. Biophys J 76(4):2262–2271. doi:10.1016/S0006-3495(99)77382-0

5. Taraska JW, Perrais D, Ohara-Imaizumi M, Nagamatsu S, Almers W (2003) Secretory granules are recaptured largely intact after stimulated exocytosis in cultured endocrine cells. Proc Natl Acad Sci U S A 100(4):2070–2075. doi:10.1073/pnas.0337526100

6. Tsuboi T, Rutter GA (2003) Insulin secretion by 'kiss-and-run' exocytosis in clonal pancreatic islet beta-cells. Biochem Soc Trans 31(Pt 4):833–836. doi:10.1042/

7. Gandasi NR, Barg S (2014) Contact-induced clustering of syntaxin and munc18 docks secretory granules at the exocytosis site. Nat Commun 5:3914. doi:10.1038/ncomms4914

8. Tomes CN, Michaut M, De Blas G, Visconti P, Matti U, Mayorga LS (2002) SNARE complex assembly is required for human sperm acrosome reaction. Dev Biol 243(2):326–338. doi:10.1006/dbio.2002.0567

9. Ramalho-Santos J, Schatten G, Moreno RD (2002) Control of membrane fusion during spermiogenesis and the acrosome reaction. Biol Reprod 67(4):1043–1051

10. Heuser JE, Reese TS (1973) Evidence for recycling of synaptic vesicle membrane during transmitter release at the frog neuromuscular junction. J Cell Biol 57(2):315–344

11. Jahn R, Fasshauer D (2012) Molecular machines governing exocytosis of synaptic vesicles. Nature 490(7419):201–207. doi:10.1038/nature11320

12. Brose N, Hofmann K, Hata Y, Sudhof TC (1995) Mammalian homologues of Caenorhabditis elegans unc-13 gene define novel family of C2-domain proteins. J Biol Chem 270(42):25273–25280

13. Fujita Y, Shirataki H, Sakisaka T, Asakura T, Ohya T, Kotani H, Yokoyama S, Nishioka H, Matsuura Y, Mizoguchi A, Scheller RH, Takai Y (1998) Tomosyn: a syntaxin-1-binding protein that forms a novel complex in the neurotransmitter release process. Neuron 20(5):905–915

14. Hata Y, Slaughter CA, Sudhof TC (1993) Synaptic vesicle fusion complex contains unc-18 homologue bound to syntaxin. Nature 366(6453):347–351. doi:10.1038/366347a0

15. Hatsuzawa K, Lang T, Fasshauer D, Bruns D, Jahn R (2003) The R-SNARE motif of tomosyn forms SNARE core complexes with syntaxin 1 and SNAP-25 and down-regulates exocytosis. J Biol Chem 278(33):31159–31166. doi:10.1074/jbc.M305500200

16. Loyet KM, Kowalchyk JA, Chaudhary A, Chen J, Prestwich GD, Martin TF (1998) Specific binding of phosphatidylinositol 4,5-bisphosphate to calcium-dependent activator protein for secretion (CAPS), a potential phosphoinositide effector protein for regulated exocytosis. J Biol Chem 273(14):8337–8343

17. Voets T, Toonen RF, Brian EC, de Wit H, Moser T, Rettig J, Sudhof TC, Neher E, Verhage M (2001) Munc18-1 promotes large dense-core vesicle docking. Neuron 31(4):581–591

18. Chapman ER (2008) How does synaptotagmin trigger neurotransmitter release? Annu Rev Biochem 77:615–641. doi:10.1146/annurev.biochem.77.062005.101135

19. Wang CT, Grishanin R, Earles CA, Chang PY, Martin TF, Chapman ER, Jackson MB (2001) Synaptotagmin modulation of fusion pore kinetics in regulated exocytosis of dense-core vesicles. Science 294(5544):1111–1115. doi:10.1126/science.1064002

20. Fukuda M (2008) Regulation of secretory vesicle traffic by Rab small GTPases. Cell Mol Life Sci 65(18):2801–2813. doi:10.1007/s00018-008-8351-4

21. Geppert M, Goda Y, Stevens CF, Sudhof TC (1997) The small GTP-binding protein Rab3A regulates a late step in synaptic vesicle fusion. Nature 387(6635):810–814. doi:10.1038/42954

22. Wada K, Mizoguchi A, Kaibuchi K, Shirataki H, Ide C, Takai Y (1994) Localization of rabphilin-3A, a putative target protein for Rab3A, at the sites of Ca(2+)-dependent exocytosis in PC12 cells. Biochem Biophys Res Commun 198(1):158–165. doi:10.1006/bbrc.1994.1023

23. Axelrod D (1981) Cell-substrate contacts illuminated by total internal reflection fluorescence. J Cell Biol 89(1):141–145

24. Axelrod D, Burghardt TP, Thompson NL (1984) Total internal reflection fluorescence. Annu Rev Biophys Bioeng 13:247–268. doi:10.1146/annurev.bb.13.060184.001335

25. Sochacki KA, Larson BT, Sengupta DC, Daniels MP, Shtengel G, Hess HF, Taraska JW (2012) Imaging the post-fusion release and capture of a vesicle membrane protein. Nat Commun 3:1154. doi:10.1038/ncomms2158

26. Merrifield CJ, Feldman ME, Wan L, Almers W (2002) Imaging actin and dynamin recruitment during invagination of single clathrin-coated pits. Nat Cell Biol 4(9):691–698. doi:10.1038/ncb837

27. Taylor MJ, Perrais D, Merrifield CJ (2011) A high precision survey of the molecular dynamics of mammalian clathrin-mediated endocytosis. PLoS Biol 9(3):e1000604. doi:10.1371/journal.pbio.1000604

28. Kern W (1990) The evolution of silicon-wafer cleaning technology. J Electrochem Soc 137(6):1887–1892

29. Hohmeier HE, Mulder H, Chen G, Henkel-Rieger R, Prentki M, Newgard CB (2000) Isolation of INS-1-derived cell lines with robust ATP-sensitive K+ channel-dependent and -independent glucose-stimulated insulin secretion. Diabetes 49(3):424–430

Chapter 12

Optical Coherence Microscopy

Rainer A. Leitgeb

Abstract

The present chapter aims at demonstrating the capabilities of optical coherence microscopy (OCM) for applications in biomedical imaging. We furthermore review the functional imaging capabilities of OCM focusing on lable-free optical angiography. We conclude with a section on digital wavefront control and a short outlook on future developments, in particular for contrast enhancement techniques.

Key words Optical coherence tomography, Optical coherence microscopy, OCT angiography, Functional imaging, Bessel beam, Digital aberration correction, Digital wavefront sensing, Beam engineering

1 Introduction

Optical coherence tomography (OCT) can be seen as the missing link in medical imaging between high-resolution microscopy techniques on the one hand, and the full body imaging methods such as magnetic resonance imaging, computed tomography, or ultrasound imaging, on the other hand [1, 2]. As an optical technique it has excellent lateral resolution in the order of micrometers, with still decent penetration depth of some millimeters. The higher penetration into scattering tissue as compared to confocal microscopy is due to the additional coherence gating leading to a strong rejection of light from out of focus and from out of the coherence gate. In addition, the coherent amplification of the light from the sample allows for shot-noise limited detection even at high imaging speeds. Many pathologic changes start from superficial layers of skin or internal organs within the first 100 μm. Hence, OCT has been seen as the most promising candidate for performing in-situ virtual biopsy without the need of tissue extraction, and thereby overcoming the randomness and invasiveness of conventional tissue biopsies and histopathology [3]. Still, for true histopathologic tissue assessment, cellular resolution is required. Optical coherence microscopy (OCM) shares with OCT the distinct advantages of

Yolanda Markaki and Hartmann Harz (eds.), *Light Microscopy: Methods and Protocols*, Methods in Molecular Biology, vol. 1563, DOI 10.1007/978-1-4939-6810-7_12, © Springer Science+Business Media LLC 2017

potentially millimeter deep tissue imaging at high speed and sensitivity due to the coherence gating, but exhibits on the other hand high lateral resolution of 1 µm and less. The axial resolution in OCT and OCM is decoupled from the lateral resolution, and is given by the coherence gate width, which in turn is defined by the coherence length of the employed light source. The axial resolution is related to the spectral properties of the light source as $\delta z \propto \lambda_c^2 / \Delta\lambda$, with λ_c the central wavelength of the light source, and $\Delta\lambda$ the optical bandwidth. The choice of the optimal center wavelength is determined by light scattering on the one hand, and water absorption on the other hand. In the shorter wavelength region scattering is dominant whereas water absorption dominates in the near infrared region. Typical OCT imaging wavelengths are centered at 800 nm, or at 1300 nm, for strongly scattering tissue such as skin. Water absorption has also a minimum at 1060 nm, which is an interesting alternative to 800 nm for retinal imaging. Given the strong dependence of the axial resolution on the center wavelength, 800 nm is a good candidate for OCM with still better penetration into tissue as for example 400 nm light. In order to achieve axial resolution in the order of 1 µm at 800 nm, large optical bandwidths of 200 nm and more are needed. First implementations of ultrahigh resolution OCT employed femtosecond Ti:Sapph lasers [4]. The main challenge was the dispersion management to avoid loss of axial resolution due to chromatically unbalanced optical path lengths between the interferometer arms. Other light sources capable of delivering such large bandwidths are supercontinuum sources, which intrinsically suffer from higher random intensity noise due to the nature of the light generation itself [5, 6]. Alternatively, one could employ thermal sources, which however deliver only small optical power into a coherent single mode channel. An advantage of those sources is their spatial incoherence, which leads to increased contrast and improved image quality, as speckle noise is suppressed [7]. They are employed for full field OCT of static tissue samples, with sufficient time for signal integration using a 2D sensor. Each pixel of the 2D sensor records the full sample structure in depth, during a piezo-modulated reference arm scan. The reference arm scan displaces the coherence gate axially within the sample. In order to keep the confocal gate and thus the optimum lateral resolution within the coherence gate, the focus plane is at the same time axially displaced within the sample. Whereas the axial resolution is only dependent on the spectral light source properties, the lateral resolution is still dependent on the numerical aperture (NA) of the detection optics. Dynamic focusing in OCM has been first described by Schmitt et al. [8], and accounts for the different scaling of the depth position of confocal gate and coherence gate by a factor of n^2, with n being the sample refractive index.

The complexity of dynamic focusing outlines already the challenge to improve lateral resolution in OCM. Time domain OCT is ideally suited for high-resolution imaging as the scanned reference arm position selects specific depth layers sequentially. En-face OCT is a variant of TD OCT, where the fast scanning priority is in the transverse plane allowing to obtain in-focus en-face cross-sections with high frame rates [9, 10]. The first en-face OCM system has been demonstrated already in 1994 [11, 12]. However, TD OCT is nowadays largely replaced by FDOCT, which enables for impressive high-speed imaging due to its intrinsic higher sensitivity. Since in FDOCT, the reference arm is kept fixed, and the full depth structure is recorded in parallel, dynamic focusing cannot directly be applied. Alternatively, one can stitch several in-focus volumes, recorded with different focus position settings [13]. A naturally extended focus configuration can be achieved by employing Bessel beams [14]. Bessel-like beams have the attractive property of propagating over significant distance without apparent diffraction. It consists of a central lobe, surrounded by a large number of concentric side-lobes that roughly carry the same amount of energy as the central lobe. Hence, although the central lobe stands out in intensity, the energy is distributed over a relatively large area. Bessel beams are easily obtained by employing conical lenses, called axicons. Ding et al. were the first to replace the conventional objective lens in front of the sample with an axicon lens [15] there by illuminating the sample with a Bessel pattern and defining an identical detection mode. However, the back-coupling on the detection path through the axicon is highly inefficient and leads to a sensitivity penalty of 20 dB and more. Such signal loss can hardly be compensated by employing higher illumination power, given further the strict exposure limits for in-vivo imaging. Another disadvantage of such straightforward implementation is the inherently strong side lobes, which are only slightly reduced by virtue of the large bandwidth employed in OCM. Those limitations have been shared also by implementations of micro-axicon lens, or conically etched fiber tips for enhanced depth of field (DOF) OCT endoscopy [16, 17]. In case only moderate DOF extension is required, phase or intensity masks offer an attractive compact solution [18, 19]. The performance in scattering media of symmetric Bessel beam configurations has recently been well described both mathematically and experimentally and demonstrated the limitations in comparison to Gaussian beams.

Decoupling the illumination from detection and engineering both individually for enhanced depth ranging, on the one hand, and sufficient detection sensitivity, on the other hand, allows avoiding the critical sensitivity loss due to the axicon double pass [20]. As a result, the asymmetric configuration gave excellent results for Fourier domain OCM even in highly scattering tissue. Illumination with a high NA Bessel beam and enhanced focus depth and detection in a Gaussian mode with a lower NA provides an interesting compromise between axial imaging range, lateral resolution, and sensitivity. Such an extended focus scheme benefits from the FDOCM intrinsic parallel signal acquisition along depth without the time consuming need to readjust the focus position. The gained flexibility enables in addition to include beam steering and scanning units with appropriate relay optics. Fast galvo-scanners or MEMS scanners are indispensable to exploit the full speed advantage of OCM to dynamically acquire tissue volumes and to overcome respiratory or heart-beat-induced artifacts during in-vivo applications.

Despite its extraordinary sensitivity, OCM still has the drawback of low tissue-specific contrast. This certainly limits its attractiveness for applications in biology and medicine. Functional extensions such as polarization contrast [21, 22], angiography and blood flow quantification [23], and recently elastography [24] help to partially mitigate the missing specificity [25]. They make use of the fact that OCM provides not only the backscattered light intensity but the full complex light field. This allows for quantitative displacement measurements in the order of the light wavelength, which can be used for highly sensitive tissue deformation sensing under external stress yielding the local tissue biomechanical properties, as well as for determining blood flow speed. The unique availability of phase information opens furthermore the ability to measure the wavefront of the backscattered field. Recent research showed promising results for digitally refocusing the scattered field distribution, measured by the complex valued OCT signal, to recover an extended DOF [20, 26–28].

The present chapter aims at demonstrating the capabilities of extended focus Fourier domain OCM for applications in biomedical imaging. We furthermore review the functional imaging capabilities of OCM focusing on label free optical angiography. We conclude with a section on digital wavefront control and a short outlook on future developments, in particular for contrast enhancement techniques.

2   Methods

2.1   Extended Focus Fourier Domain OCM Configurations

In the following, we would like to focus on the practical implementation of extended focus OCM. For those not familiar with OCT or OCM we shortly review the signal characteristics. More detailed analysis of the OCM signal generation can be found in [29]. The method is based on short coherence interferometry, and senses the differential optical path length delays between different axial sample reflectors and a reference reflector. In the simplified case of discrete axially distributed reflectors at positions z_i with associated intensity reflectivities R_i the structure can be described by the function $g(z) = \sum_i \sqrt{R_i}\delta(z - (z_0 - z_i)) + R_r\delta(z - (z_0 - z_r))$, where R_r is the reference reflectivity at axial optical distance z_r, and $\delta(z)$ is the delta functional, and z_0 is a common reference position. The backscattered signal from the sample at the common reference position z_0, which can be assumed as the detector position, can be written as $ED(z_0, t, k) = \int g(z - z_0)E_0(k) \exp(i\omega t - 2ikz)dz$, where $I_0(k) = E_0(k)E_0^*(k)$ is the total spectral intensity of the light source, and k is the wavenumber. The expression for the field can be rewritten as $ED(z_0, t, k) = E_0(k) \exp(i\omega t)Fk\{g(z - z_0)\}$, where the operator $F\{\}$ stands for the Fourier transform. The detected intensity becomes then $ID(k) = E_0(k)E_0^*(k)|Fk\{g(z)\}|^2$. This relation is central to the Fourier domain OCT signal reconstruction. The structure is retrieved by calculating the inverse Fourier transform of the recorded spectral intensity. In fact, it yields the autocorrelation function of the structure function $g(z)$ convoluted with the Fourier transform of the spectral field intensity as

$$\mathcal{F}\{I_D(k)\} = \mathcal{F}\{I_0(k)\} \otimes ACF\{g(z)\} = I_0\gamma(\tau = z / c) \otimes ACF\{g(z)\}, \quad (1)$$

where the operator ACF{} stands for the autocorrelation function, and $\gamma(\tau)$ is the complex degree of temporal coherence. The latter is related to the power spectral density via Fourier transform according to the Wiener-Khintchin theorem. The width of the coherence function $\gamma(\tau)$, which serves as axial PSF, depends inversely proportional on the optical bandwidth and scales with the square of the central wavelength as has been already mentioned in the introduction. The fact that not the actual structure function $g(z)$ but its autocorrelation function is retrieved has several implications on the Fourier domain OCM signal, which we do not want to discuss in detail. The interested reader is referred to [30]. What is important to note is the in general complex valued result of the Fourier transform of the spectral interference pattern $I_D(k)$. The argument of the Fourier transform is directly related to the phase of the backscattered field. Calculating changes in the phase between successive recordings allows assessing axial structural displacements in the order of fractions of the center wavelength in a fully quantitative manner.

Let us now return to the actual optical configuration of OCM. As already mentioned in the introduction, the central idea is the decoupling of illumination and detection path. Figure 2 shows the respective configuration of high NA Bessel beam illumination and lower NA Gaussian detection mode. The Bessel beam is generated by an axicon lens, and relayed via scanning system finally to the sample space. The first realization achieved isotropic resolution of 1.3 μm laterally and 2 μm axially, over an axial range of 200 μm. This corresponds to a tenfold extended DOF when compared to a Gaussian mode with the same lateral resolution. The light source was a broad bandwidth Ti:Sapph laser centered at 800 nm. The spectral interference pattern was recorded by a fiber coupled spectrometer equipped with a fast line sensor at the exit if the interferometer. Further details are found in [20, 29]. As mentioned earlier, the efficient and rapid scanning of this extended focus beam over the sample is crucial to benefit from the advantage of the extended focus scheme and necessary for in vivo imaging to overcome motion artifacts. As seen from Fig. 1, the Bessel beam illumination has another advantageous feature: it is effectively a dark field illumination. The dark field effect is efficiently enhanced by using the masks in the illumination and detection path denoted by M1 and M2 respectively in Fig. 1. The masks suppress spurious backscattering light and light from the tip of the axicon, which otherwise degrade the contrast. Alternatively, one can decouple illumination and detection by using a central mirror within the ring-shaped Fourier plane of the Bessel beam the position of M1 in Fig. 1 as demonstrated in [32].

First application of the introduced xf-OCM scheme in life sciences was in diabetes research to image the islets of Langerhans in mice [31, 33]. The islets, which are scattered throughout the pancreas, are agglomerations of beta cells that produce insulin. They exhibit an excellent backscattering contrast in OCM which is dominantly caused by the zinc-insulin crystals in the pancreatic beta cells. They are strongly vascularized releasing insulin to contribute to the glucose homeostasis. Using a mouse model of type I diabetes, islets down to a size corresponding to a cluster of only a few beta cells could be visualized and quantitatively assessed (Fig. 2) [31]. The strength of OCM is the ability to assess the beta cells in their natural volumetric environment in a fully lable-free manner; a perfect situation for longitudinal studies for example on drug and treatment efficacy.

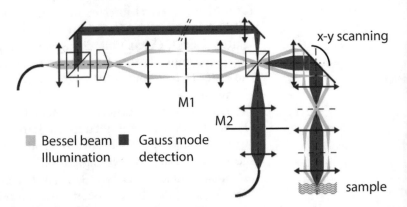

Fig. 1 Schematic layout of xf OCM, depicting the decoupling of the illumination and the detection paths. The masks M1 and M2 help to exhibit the full dark field properties of this configuration

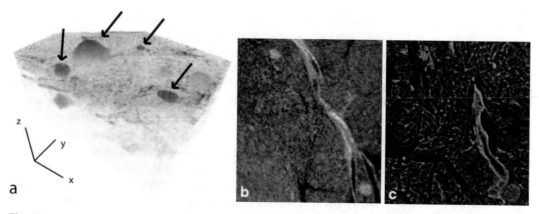

Fig. 2 Imaging of Langerhans islets: (**a**) 3D rendering of murine pancreas exhibiting strong contrast for Langerhans islets (*arrows*) (**b**) En-face view of pancreas with islets and duct-like structure. (**c**) Corresponding histological section with immune-labeling for insulin (*red*), PECAM (*green*), and DBA lectin (*blue*) [31]

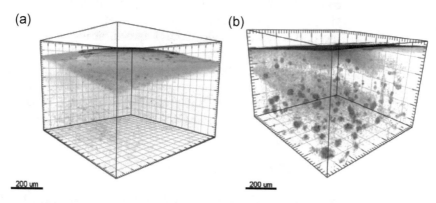

Fig. 3 Imaging of Alzheimer plaques: Three-dimensional rendering of an ex vivo xfOCM image of the parietal cortex of the transgenic mouse brain. (**a**) 1 month-old predepositing brain sample. (**b**) 3 month-old brain sample showing amyloid plaque deposits (courtesy T. Lasser, EPFL, Switzerland) [34]

xf-OCM yields not only high contrast for beta cells, but has recently been shown to provide excellent contrast for amyloid-β (Aβ) peptide accumulations in cerebral plaques [34, 35]. Those plaques are characteristic for the pathology of Alzheimer's disease (AD) and can be studied on an APPPS1 mouse model of AD. Figure 3 shows volume rendered xf-OCM images of the AD brain structure clearly revealing Aβ plaques without exogenous contrast agents. Again, the minimal invasive assessment through a cranial window allows for longitudinal studies of plaque formation and drug responses.

2.2 Extended Focus Microcirculation Imaging

The missing molecular specific contrast is a strong limitation of OCM. Functional extensions of OCM on the other hand provide intrinsic contrast, yielding unique insight into tissue physiology. In particular OCT angiography holds great promise, as it yields microangiographic tissue details down to the level of individual capillaries without the need of contrast agents [23, 36, 37]. Blood flow and vascular structure is key information for understanding tissue health condition, as well as for effective treatment monitoring. Insight into capillary structure, its integrity, and perfusion, would create new diagnostic capabilities in clinical practice and research. The advancement of high-speed Fourier domain OCT technology was of particular benefit for the development of highly sensitive optical angiography techniques. The method of OCT angiography (OCTA) itself is simple, as it detects differences in the OCT signal between successive tomograms taken at the same position. Those differences are only due to dynamic structural changes induced by moving red blood cells, whereas the surrounding tissue remains static. The signal fluctuations can be contrasted on the level of speckle changes [38], or on the level of signal phase changes [39], or of the full complex signal [40, 41]. Sufficiently large motion will cause loss of speckle or phase correlation, which can be visualized using correlation or decorrelation analysis. The simplest method is based on calculating logarithmically scaled intensity differences between successive tomograms. Using the intensity information instead of the phase is easily implemented and better suited to high-speed swept source laser sources. An angiographic image volume P, contrasting flow against static tissue, is obtained by calculating the squared intensity difference between successive tomograms [42]:

$$P(x, y_i, z) = (I(x, y_i, z) - I(x, y_{i+1}, z))^2 \tag{2}$$

where $I(x, y, z) = 20 \cdot \log[|FFT\{I(x, y, k)\}|]$ are the spatial pixel coordinates corresponding to fast and slow scanning, and depth coordinate, respectively, and k is the wavenumber. Averaging over several difference tomograms helps to enhance the motion contrast and to reduce speckle noise. For visualization, the maximum intensity projection within the motion contrast volume is calculated over a selected depth range, yielding en-face projection views. Figure 4 shows the vascular structure for healthy skin, demonstrating impressively the performance even in strongly scattering media [42].

In the previous section, we demonstrated the capabilities of xf-OCM to image the Langerhans islets $ that exhibit extraordinary backscattering contrast. Still, important metabolic information is missing. Performing the angiography yields completely new insights into the health state of those islets. This is of importance when trying to assess the function of implanted islets and for studying the autoimmune response, which leads to beta-cell loss in diabetes I. Figure 4 shows an example of visualizing beta cell loss with functional OCM over time of human islets, which are implanted into the iris of a mouse [43]. The effect is perfectly seen

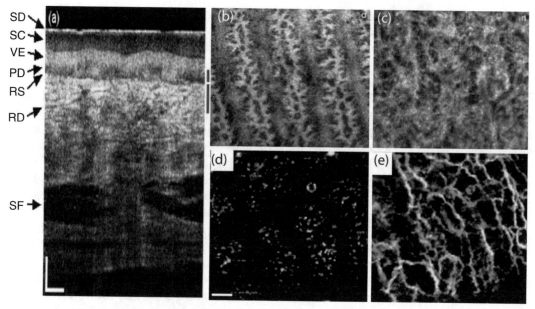

SD
SC
VE
PD
RS
RD

SF

Fig. 4 OCTA of healthy skin of the palm. (**a**) OCT tomogram. Side bars indicate depth ranges for calculating the intensity projection views in (**b**) and (**c**), as well as the angiograms in (**d**) and (**e**) respectively. *SD* stratum disjunctum, *SC* stratum corneum, *VE* viable epidermis, *PD* Papillary dermis, *RS* Rete subpapillare, *RD* reticular dermis, *SF* subcutaneous fat. Scale bars indicate 250 μm in each picture (reproduced from Blatter et al. [42])

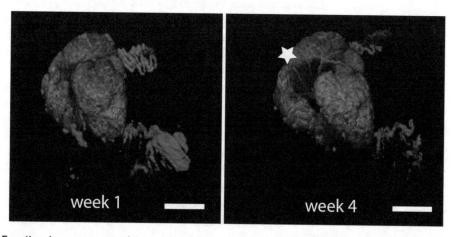

Fig. 5 Functional assessment of Langerhans islet: assessed longitudinally with xf-OCM over 4 weeks. Structural xf-OCM data are displayed in *green*, microvascular structure obtained with OCTA is displayed in *red*. Beta cell loss is visible over time at the location indicated by the star at week 4 (courtesy T. Lasser, EPFL, Switzerland) [43]

both on the structural and on the microvascular level as loss of beta cell mass is accompanied by loss of vascular structure. Other research demonstrated impressively the capability of OCT angiography to study neovascular growth in tumor environments and the response to anti-VEGF drugs [44]. Furthermore, the combination of angiography and quantitative assessment of flow promises to be a powerful tool in neuroscience to study physiologic responses and get further insight into neuronal function [45, 46].

2.3 Digital Focus and Aberration Correction

The goal of OCM is to image microscopic cellular structural details in their natural volumetric environment without the need of cumbersome tissue preparation. We have seen how Bessel beams help to improve penetration depth beyond the standard Gaussian mode FOV. Still, the improvement came at the expense of loss of sensitivity and contrast as well as higher system complexity. Bessel beam illumination can be seen as one example of wavefront engineering.

Having in OCM the full complex field information available opens another exciting possibility of manipulating the wavefront. It has been shown by several authors that this information can be used to fully refocus the recorded OCM images far beyond the nominal DOF, depending on the scattering properties of the sample. For correcting higher order aberrations apart from defocus, iterative methods have been employed. Kumar et al. showed a different approach for focus correction and aberration correction based on pupil splitting, which works noniteratively, and does not require any knowledge about system parameters. In the following, the algorithm will be reviewed with a few examples of the performance.

The most efficient implementation of digital wavefront correction is based on full field OCM. This variant of OCM images an area of the sample onto a 2D sensor, and uses then either depth scanning in time domain OCM [7] or spectral scanning in swept source OCM for recording the depth structure [47–49]. The advantage is the intrinsic extraordinary lateral phase stability, which is indispensable for efficient wavefront reconstruction and correction. A disadvantage of full field swept source OCM is the missing confocal gating, which leads to strong scattering artifacts and critical loss of contrast. Line field OCM scans the structure by a line, thereby keeping confocal gating at least in one dimension. In general, a scanning OCM system needs to be fast enough to keep appropriate lateral phase correlation. For in-vivo imaging of the retina, for example, tomogram rates of more than 2000 per second are required.

The pupil splitting algorithm is graphically explained in Fig. 6. It operates on en-face slices taken from a recorded 3D volume of complex valued image data. The availability of phase information is crucial for the algorithm to work correctly. In FD OCM the phase is readily available after the signal reconstruction as argument of the spectral Fourier transform according to Eq. 1. In a first step the 2D spatial Fourier transform of the complex-valued image data is calculated. The Fourier or pupil plane is then split into sub-tiles, and the inverse Fourier transform of each sub-tile is calculated. As seen in Fig. 7 this results in low resolution copies of the original

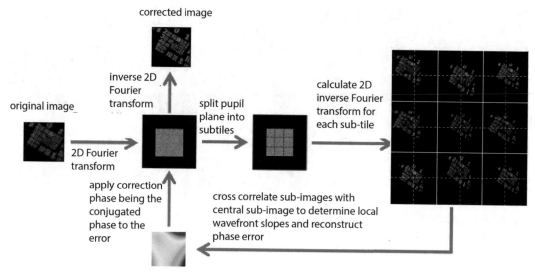

corrected image

inverse 2D
Fourier
transform

original image

2D Fourier
transform

split pupil
plane into
subtiles

calculate 2D
inverse Fourier
transform for
each sub-tile

apply correction
phase being the
conjugated
phase to the
error

cross correlate sub-images with
central sub-image to determine local
wavefront slopes and reconstruct
phase error

Fig. 6 Split aperture method: Graphical explanation [50]

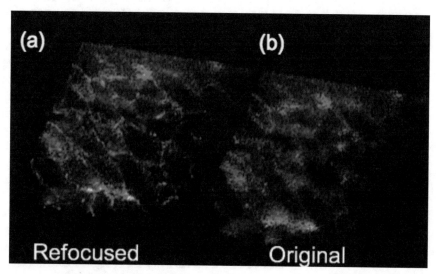

Fig. 7 Result of digital refocusing: En-face slice through a 3D rendered reconstructed volume of an onion at 430 μm distance from the focus plane. (**a**) digitally refocused volume; (**b**) original data

image, with its centers slightly shifted. The shift is in fact proportional to the local slope of the wavefront. The set of obtained slopes over the pupil field of view can then be used to reconstruct the wavefront phase. It can be either represented by polynomials or by Zernike modes. The digital wavefront sensing may be seen as scene-based equivalent of a Hartman-Shack wavefront sensor. The important feature of this reconstruction is that it does not need any iteration and works in a single step. If only defocus error needs to

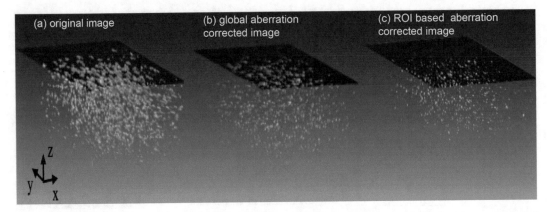

Fig. 8 Anisotropic digital aberration correction: Volume-rendered image of iron oxide test target. (**a**) Original image; (**b**) globally corrected aberrations using the split aperture method for each depth slice; (**c**) ROI-based aberration corrected image (*see* text) [51]

be corrected, simple tiling of the pupil plane into two halves is sufficient. Details on the performance of the split aperture method are found in [50]. The correction has to be applied for each depth slice individually. Since the calculations are independent, the correction can be significantly speeded up by parallel computing using multicore CPUs or on a GPU. Figure 7 shows an image slice from an onion sample, with Fig. 7b being the original image, and Fig. 7a the digitally refocused image. The image was obtained with a full field swept source OCM setup operating at 840 nm center wavelength with a detection NA of 0.14 yielding a lateral resolution of 6.5 μm and a depth of focus of 130 μm. The image slice was taken at 430 μm depth distance from the focus plane demonstrating the effective focus depth enhancement.

In case, high numerical aperture microscope objectives are used, aberrations will become anisotropic across the field of view and in particular outside the isoplanatic patch. The split aperture method can then be applied only for a region of interest, correcting locally for aberrations. Stitching then all ROIs together results in a large FOV aberration corrected image beyond the isoplanatic patch. Figure 8 shows volume-rendered images of a test target with iron oxide nanoparticles suspended in resin. The data was obtained with a point-scanning Fourier domain OCM system, employing a microscope objective of 0.8 NA, with a measured lateral resolution of 0.81 μm and a depth of field of 9 μm. The light source was a Ti:Sapph laser centered at 790 nm with a bandwidth of 290 nm and an axial resolution of 1.6 μm in air. Figure 8a shows the original image, Fig. 8b is the global aberration corrected image, and Fig. 8c is the ROI-based aberration correction. With the latter method a 30× focus depth enhancement has been achieved.

Digital aberration correction holds not only great promise to improve image quality by focus depth enhancement and aberration correction, but also to help characterizing tissue optical properties. Since the split aperture method does not need a-priori knowledge about local tissue refractive index, the latter could be deduced as a free parameter from the algorithm.

3   Notes

The chapter reviewed the capabilities of optical coherence microscopy as in-vivo imaging tool in biomedical applications. Its strength is certainly the high speed, capturing dynamic tissue processes in a volumetric manner, as well the relatively high tissue penetration as compared to confocal microscopy. We further reviewed focus extension strategies, which help to fully exploit the speed advantage of Fourier domain OCM, which records full depth profiles in a parallel manner. In particular, Bessel beam illumination and Gaussian detection helps to efficiently extend the focus and to maintain high detection sensitivity. The missing molecular specificity of OCM can be mitigated by novel contrast mechanism, such as lable-free angiography or optical elastography. We showed results from tissue imaging, as well as from applications in diabetes research, where blood flow and vascular status yields immediate information about organ health.

A more straightforward solution to the missing intrinsic molecular contrast of OCM is to employ multimodal imaging platforms. OCM could be combined with other molecular sensitive microscopy and sensing techniques such as fluorescence microscopy, Raman spectroscopy, or nonlinear microscopy techniques [52]. Such solutions are currently hot candidates for realizing virtual biopsies. Assessing the tissue in-situ using OCM or OCT first as guidance, and then a molecularly specific technique for lesion grading and staging would help avoiding unnecessary tissue excisions. This would ultimately improve patient comfort as well as in general the histopathologic evaluation process. Another candidate for providing spectroscopic information based on absorption contrast is photoacoustics (PA) [53]. It is fully complementary to optical coherence microscopy that shows high endogenous contrast of tissue scattering but lacks absorption sensitivity [54, 55].

The combination of OCM with holographic wavefront detection shows great promise to enhance focus depth and might ultimately be used in combination with spatial light modulators such as deformable mirror to further enhance penetration into scattering media. This would mark another milestone development in the history of optical coherence tomography and microscopy.

Acknowledgments

Acknowledged are the contributions of Abhishek Kumar, Laurin Ginner, Daniel Fechtig, Cedric Blatter, Branislav Grajciar, and Wolfgang Drexler, from the Medical University Vienna (Austria), Theo Lasser, Martin Villiger, Adrian Bachmann from the Ecole Polytechnique Fédérale de Lausanne (Switzerland), Robert Huber from the Ludwig Maximillian University in Munich (Germany) as well as the following financial support: European Commission FP7-HEALTH (grant 201880, FUN OCT), Austrian Christian Doppler Association, and Swiss National Fonds (SNF grant 205321-10974).

References

1. Fercher AF, Drexler W, Hitzenberger CK, Lasser T (2003) Optical coherence tomography—principles and applications. Rep Prog Phys 66(2):239–303

2. Huang D, Swanson EA, Lin CP, Schuman JS, Stinson WG, Chang W, Hee MR, Flotte T, Gregory K, Puliafito CA, Fujimoto JG (1991) Optical coherence tomography. Science 254(5035):1178–1181

3. Fujimoto JG, Brezinski ME, Tearney GJ, Boppart SA, Bouma B, Hee MR, Southern JF, Swanson EA (1995) Optical biopsy and imaging using optical coherence tomography. Nat Med 1(9):970–972

4. Drexler W, Morgner U, Kartner FX, Pitris C, Boppart SA, Li XD, Ippen EP, Fujimoto JG (1999) In vivo ultrahigh-resolution optical coherence tomography. Opt Lett 24(17):1221–1223

5. Povazay B, Bizheva K, Unterhuber A, Hermann B, Sattmann H, Fercher AF, Drexler W, Apolonski A, Wadsworth WJ, Knight JC, Russell PSJ, Vetterlein M, Scherzer E (2002) Submicrometer axial resolution optical coherence tomography. Opt Lett 27(20):1800–1802

6. Kray S, Spöler F, Fürst M, Kurz H (2009) High-resolution simultaneous dual-band spectral domain optical coherence tomography. Opt Lett 34(13):1970–1972

7. Vabre L, Dubois A, Boccara AC (2002) Thermal-light full-field optical coherence tomography. Opt Lett 27(7):530–532

8. Schmitt JM, Lee SL, Yung KM (1997) An optical coherence microscope with enhanced resolving power in thick tissue. Opt Commun 142(4–6):203–207

9. Podoleanu AG, Dobre GM, Jackson DA (1998) En-face coherence imaging using galvanometer scanner modulation. Opt Lett 23(3):147–149

10. Hitzenberger C, Trost P, Lo P-W, Zhou Q (2003) Three-dimensional imaging of the human retina by high-speed optical coherence tomography. Opt Express 11(21):2753–2761

11. Izatt JA, Hee MR, Owen GM, Swanson EA, Fujimoto JG (1994) Optical coherence microscopy in scattering media. Opt Lett 19(8):590–592

12. Pircher M, Baumann B, Götzinger E, Sattmann H, Hitzenberger CK (2009) Phase contrast coherence microscopy based on transverse scanning. Opt Lett 34(12):1750–1752

13. Huber R, Wojtkowski M, Fujimoto JG, Jiang JY, Cable AE (2005) Three-dimensional and C-mode OCT imaging with a compact, frequency swept laser source at 1300 nm. Opt Express 13(26):10523–10538

14. Herman RM, Wiggins TA (1991) Production and uses of diffractionless beams. J Opt Soc Am A Opt Image Sci Vis 8(6):932–942

15. Ding ZH, Ren HW, Zhao YH, Nelson JS, Chen ZP (2002) High-resolution optical coherence tomography over a large depth range with an axicon lens. Opt Lett 27(4):243–245

16. Lee KS, Rolland LP (2008) Bessel beam spectral-domain high-resolution optical coherence tomography with micro-optic axicon providing extended focusing range. Opt Lett 33(15):1696–1698

17. Tan KM, Mazilu M, Chow TH, Lee WM, Taguchi K, Ng BK, Sibbett W, Herrington CS, Brown CTA, Dholakia K (2009) In-fiber common-path optical coherence tomography using a conical-tip fiber. Opt Express 17(4):2375–2384

18. Liu L, Gardecki JA, Nadkarni SK, Toussaint JD, Yagi Y, Bouma BE, Tearney GJ (2011) Imaging the subcellular structure of human coronary atherosclerosis using micro-optical coherence tomography. Nat Med 17(8):1010–1014. doi:10.1038/nm.2409

19. Lorenser D, Yang X, Sampson DD (2012) Ultrathin fiber probes with extended depth of focus for optical coherence tomography. Opt Lett 37(10):1616–1618

20. Leitgeb RA, Villiger M, Bachmann AH, Steinmann L, Lasser T (2006) Extended focus depth for Fourier domain optical coherence microscopy. Opt Lett 31(16):2450–2452

21. de Boer JF, Milner TE (2002) Review of polarization sensitive optical coherence tomography and Stokes vector determination. J Biomed Opt. 7(3):359–371. doi:10.1117/1.1483879

22. Pircher M, Hitzenberger CK, Schmidt-Erfurth U (2011) Polarization sensitive optical coherence tomography in the human eye. Prog Retin Eye Res 30(6):431–451. doi:10.1016/j.preteyeres.2011.06.003

23. LeitgebRA, WerkmeisterRM, BlatterC, SchmettererL (2014) Doppler optical coherence tomography. Prog Retin Eye Res 41(0):26–43. doi:http://dx.doi.org/10.1016/j.preteyeres.2014.03.004

24. Kennedy BF, McLaughlin RA, Kennedy KM, Chin L, Curatolo A, Tien A, Latham B, Saunders CM, Sampson DD (2014) Optical coherence micro-elastography: mechanical-contrast imaging of tissue microstructure. Biomed Opt Express 5(7):2113–2124. doi:10.1364/BOE.5.002113

25. Leitgeb RA (2011) Current technologies for high-speed and functional imaging with optical coherence tomography. In: Hawkes PW (ed) Advances in imaging and electron physics, Advances in imaging and electron physics, vol 168. Elsevier Academic Press Inc, San Diego, pp 109–192. doi:10.1016/b978-0-12-385983-9.00003-x

26. Ralston TS, Marks DL, Carney PS, Boppart SA (2006) Inverse scattering for optical coherence tomography. J Opt Soc Am A 23(5):1027–1037

27. Ralston TS, Marks DL, Carney PS, Boppart SA (2008) Real-time interferometric synthetic aperture microscopy. Opt Express 16(4):2555–2569

28. Yasuno Y, Sando Y, Sugisaka JI, Endo T, Makita S, Aoki G, Itoh M, Yatagai T (2005) In-focus Fourier-domain optical coherence tomography by complex numerical method. Opt Quantum Electron 37(13–15):1185–1189

29. Villiger M, Lasser T (2010) Image formation and tomogram reconstruction in optical coherence microscopy. J Opt Soc Am A 27(10):2216–2228

30. WojtkowskiM, LeitgebR, KowalczykA, FercherA (2002) Fourier domain OCT imaging of human eye in vivo. In:Coherence domain optical methods in biomedical science and clinical applications vi, vol 3. Proceedings of the society of photo-optical instrumentation engineers (SPIE), pp 230–236

31. Villiger M, Goulley J, Friedrich M, Grapin-Botton A, Meda P, Lasser T, Leitgeb RA (2009) In vivo imaging of murine endocrine islets of Langerhans with extended-focus optical coherence microscopy. Diabetologia 52(8):1599–1607

32. Blatter C, Grajciar B, Eigenwillig CM, Wieser W, Biedermann BR, Huber R, Leitgeb RA (2011) Extended focus high-speed swept source OCT with self-reconstructive illumination. Opt Express 19:12141–12155.

33. Berclaz C, Goulley J, Villiger M, Pache C, Bouwens A, Martin-Williams E, Van de Ville D, Davison AC, Grapin-Botton A, Lasser T (2012) Diabetes imaging-quantitative assessment of islets of Langerhans distribution in murine pancreas using extended-focus optical coherence microscopy. Biomed Opt Express 3(6):1365–1380

34. Bolmont T, Bouwens A, Pache C, Dimitrov M, Berclaz C, Villiger M, Wegenast-Braun BM, Lasser T, Fraering PC (2012) Label-free imaging of cerebral beta-amyloidosis with extended-focus optical coherence microscopy. J Neurosci 32(42):14548–14556. doi:10.1523/Jneurosci.0925-12.2012

35. Radde R, Bolmont T, Sa K, Coomaraswamy J, Lindau D, Stoltze L, Calhoun ME, Jäggi F, Wolburg H, Gengler S, Haass C, Ghetti B, Czech C, Hölscher C, Mathews PM, Jucker M (2006) Abeta42-driven cerebral amyloidosis in transgenic mice reveals early and robust pathology. EMBO Rep 7:940–946

36. Makita S, Hong Y, Yamanari M, Yatagai T, Yasuno Y (2006) Optical coherence angiography. Opt Express 14:7821–7840

37. Spaide RF, Fujimoto JG, Waheed NK (2015) Optical coherence tomography angiography. Retina 35(11):2161–2162. doi:10.1097/iae.0000000000000881

38. Mariampillai A, Standish BA, Moriyama EH, Khurana M, Munce NR, Leung MKK, Jiang J, Cable A, Wilson BC, Vitkin IA, Yang VXD (2008) Speckle variance detection of microvasculature using swept-source optical coherence tomography. Opt Lett 33(13):1530–1532

39. Kim DY, Fingler J, Werner JS, Schwartz DM, Fraser SE, Zawadzki RJ (2011) In vivo volumetric imaging of human retinal circulation with phase-variance optical coherence tomography. Biomed Opt Express 2(6):1504–1513

40. An L, Qin J, Wang RK (2010) Ultrahigh sensitive optical microangiography for in vivo imaging of microcirculations within human skin tissue beds. Opt Express 18(8):8220–8228

41. SchmollT, IvascuIR, SinghASG, BlatterC, LeitgebRA (2015) Intra-and inter-frame differential doppler optical coherence tomography. Sovremennye Tehnologii v Medicine 7 (1):34–42. doi:10.17691/stm2015.7.1.05

42. Blatter C, Weingast J, Alex A, Grajciar B, Wieser W, Drexler W, Huber R, Leitgeb RA (2012) In situ structural and microangiographic assessment of human skin lesions with high-speed OCT. Biomed Opt Express 3(10):2636–2646

43. Berclaz C, Schmidt-Christensen A, Szlag D, Extermann J, Hansen L, Bouwens A, Villiger M, Goulley J, Schuit F, Grapin-Botton A, Lasser T, Holmberg D (2016) Longitudinal three-dimensional visualisation of autoimmune diabetes by functional optical coherence imaging. Diabetologia 59(3):550–559. doi:10.1007/s00125-015-3819-x

44. Vakoc BJ, Lanning RM, Tyrrell JA, Padera TP, Bartlett LA, Stylianopoulos T, Munn LL, Tearney GJ, Fukumura D, Jain RK, Bouma BE (2009) Three-dimensional microscopy of the tumor microenvironment in vivo using optical frequency domain imaging. Nat Med 15(10):1219–U1151. doi:10.1038/nm.1971

45. Bouwens A, Bolmont T, Szlag D, Berclaz C, Lasser T (2014) Quantitative cerebral blood flow imaging with extended-focus optical coherence microscopy. Opt Lett 39(1):37–40. doi:10.1364/OL.39.000037

46. Srinivasan VJ, Sakadi S, Gorczynska I, Ruvinskaya S, Wu W, Fujimoto JG, Boas DA (2010) Quantitative cerebral blood flow with optical coherence tomography. Opt Express 18(3):2477–2494

47. Choma MA, Ellerbee AK, Yang C, Creazzo TL, Izatt JA (2005) Spectral-domain phase microscopy. Opt Lett 30(10):1162–1164

48. Hillmann D, Lührs C, Bonin T, Koch P, Hüttmann G (2011) Holoscopy—holographic optical coherence tomography. Opt Lett 36(13):2390–2392. doi:10.1364/OL.36.002390

49. Povazay B, Unterhuber A, Hermann B, Sattmann H, Arthaber H, Drexler W (2006) Full-field time-encoded frequency-domain optical coherence tomography. Opt Express 14(17):7661–7669. doi:10.1364/OE.14.007661

50. Kumar A, Drexler W, Leitgeb RA (2013) Subaperture correlation based digital adaptive optics for full field optical coherence tomography. Opt Express 21(9):10850–10866. doi:10.1364/OE.21.010850

51. Kumar A, Kamali T, Platzer R, Unterhuber A, Drexler W, Leitgeb RA (2015) Anisotropic aberration correction using region of interest based digital adaptive optics in Fourier domain OCT. Biomed Opt Express 6(4):1124–1134. doi:10.1364/BOE.6.001124

52. Drexler W, Liu M, Kumar A, Kamali T, Unterhuber A, Leitgeb RA (2014) Optical coherence tomography today: speed, contrast, and multimodality. J Biomed Opt 19(7):071412-071412. doi:10.1117/1.JBO.19.7.071412

53. Wang LV (2009) Multiscale photoacoustic microscopy and computed tomography. Nat Photon 3(9):503–509

54. Blatter C, Grajciar B, Zou P, Wieser W, Verhoef AJ, Huber R, Leitgeb RA (2012) Intrasweep phase-sensitive optical coherence tomography for noncontact optical photoacoustic imaging. Opt Lett 37(21):4368–4370

55. Liu M, Chen Z, Zabihian B, Sinz C, Zhang E, Beard PC, Ginner L, Hoover E, Minneman MP, Leitgeb RA, Kittler H, Drexler W (2016) Combined multi-modal photoacoustic tomography, optical coherence tomography (OCT) and OCT angiography system with an articulated probe for in vivo human skin structure and vasculature imaging. Biomed Opt Express 7:3390–3402

Part III

Quantitative and Computational Image Analysis

Chapter 13

Designing Image Analysis Pipelines in Light Microscopy: A Rational Approach

Ignacio Arganda-Carreras and Philippe Andrey

Abstract

With the progress of microscopy techniques and the rapidly growing amounts of acquired imaging data, there is an increased need for automated image processing and analysis solutions in biological studies. Each new application requires the design of a specific image analysis pipeline, by assembling a series of image processing operations. Many commercial or free bioimage analysis software are now available and several textbooks and reviews have presented the mathematical and computational fundamentals of image processing and analysis. Tens, if not hundreds, of algorithms and methods have been developed and integrated into image analysis software, resulting in a combinatorial explosion of possible image processing sequences. This paper presents a general guideline methodology to rationally address the design of image processing and analysis pipelines. The originality of the proposed approach is to follow an iterative, backwards procedure from the target objectives of analysis. The proposed goal-oriented strategy should help biologists to better apprehend image analysis in the context of their research and should allow them to efficiently interact with image processing specialists.

Key words Light microscopy, Image analysis, Image processing, Image segmentation, Watershed transform

1 Introduction

Continuous improvements and innovations in light microscopy techniques result in increasing amounts of image data. In parallel, formal approaches imported from mathematics, statistics, and computer science are progressively penetrating biological sciences. In light microscopy, quantitative image analysis can be used to answer many different questions about biological specimens. Automatizing image analysis by means of a set of consecutive techniques or *pipeline* presents three main advantages: first, it prevents the bias inherent to human vision; second, it grants the extraction of information that is not accessible by eye; and finally, it allows to process very large amounts of image data, otherwise unmanageable. Consequently, there is an increasing need for biologists to

Yolanda Markaki and Hartmann Harz (eds.), *Light Microscopy: Methods and Protocols*, Methods in Molecular Biology, vol. 1563, DOI 10.1007/978-1-4939-6810-7_13, © Springer Science+Business Media LLC 2017

gain fundamental knowledge and practical experience to fully exploit acquired images and extract from these data as much quantitative and relevant information as possible.

However, there are two potential difficulties for biologists to use image analysis. The first one is that, as opposed to wet experiment protocols, there is no such thing as a standard image processing and analysis pipeline. An imaging experiment generally corresponds to a unique combination of biological system, sample preparation, microscopic apparatus, acquisition conditions, etc. It therefore requires the design of a specific image processing and analysis chain. Users are here confronted to the combinatorial explosion that results from the numerous methods available at each step in a typical image processing pipeline. The second difficulty is that image processing textbooks and introductory articles are generally structured according to the mathematical or computational underlying principles and following the chronological order of application of operations. This is not the most appropriate approach for biologists, who focus on end analysis objectives and output measures rather than on the technical means, and their theoretical foundations, to attain these goals.

We present here a general approach to help biologists design specific pipelines suited to their scientific problems. The originality of this methodology is to put the emphasis on the ultimate goals of the analysis and to incrementally introduce the intermediate processing steps according to a binary decision scheme. This shift of focus from the "how" to the "why" of image analysis leads to completely reverse the traditional order of considering image processing steps at the design stage. Though this may sound paradoxical in the first place, several years of teaching and research experience demonstrate that the proposed iterative, goal-oriented approach is both natural and efficient.

2   Materials

2.1   Hardware Equipment

The methods described here can be run on any modern computer with standard configuration. However, applying these methods to large volume images (roughly, from 1 Gb and more) may require above standard RAM equipment. A high performance accelerated graphics card may also be required, especially if demanding 3D rendering is desired. Images can be stored locally on hard disk or on distant server. In the latter case, images can be accessed with remote access protocols such as Samba or NFS.

2.2   Software Equipment

Though most of the methods described in the sequel may be found in several bioimage analysis software, the popular free Fiji platform [1] is recommended unless otherwise needed. Fiji can be installed on the Windows, Mac OS, and Linux platforms. Fiji is written in

Java and will run with preinstalled Java Runtime Environment. If required, a Fiji version with an embedded Java distribution can also be downloaded. Users requiring more than 2 GB RAM usage in Fiji should run on a 64-bit operating system due to limitation in Java memory management on 32-bit systems. The core functionalities of the software can be extended using plugins. Fiji installation bundles a number of preselected plugins, and additional plugins can be added after installation. Fiji and the plugins implementing the methods described below can be found with installation instructions from the imagej.net website.

2.3 File Formats

Acquired images in light microscopy are generally obtained in proprietary formats such as LSM, ZVI, or LIF. Many image analysis software can read these formats. In Fiji, the LOCI BioFormats plugin reads a wide range of file formats used in biological science. Alternative formats not specific to light microscopy can be used as well. File formats supporting lossless compression, such as TIF (from which several proprietary formats such as LSM are derived), are recommended. Formats with lossy compression, such as JPEG, should be avoided for the purpose of scientific image analysis. The adoption of systematic, standardized file naming conventions is strongly recommended.

3 Methods

3.1 Quantifying Biological Information Using Image Analysis

Digital image analysis consists in extracting biologically meaningful information by performing quantitative measurements on acquired images. Of particular interest are the measurements or the so-called *descriptors* with properties that facilitate the reusability and generalization of results. These descriptors are invariant to image transformations (such as translation, rotation, or scaling), robust against noise and image artifacts, and easy to interpret and validate.

The spectrum of quantitative information that can be extracted using image analysis is quite large, ranging from simple measurements such as object numbers to more elaborate ones such as texture descriptors. In this section, we describe the main quantitative measurements and types of analysis that are of special relevance to study biological samples using light microscopy.

Digital images are matrices of pixel (2D) or voxel (3D) values. In acquired images, these values range from 0 to 255 or more, depending on the encoding of intensity signals and image bit-depth. The purpose of image processing is to transform acquired images (Fig. 1a) into images of objects (Fig. 1b), in which values represent labels that typically range from 0 (background) to N (number of objects). Some object measurements can be made using label images only (geometrical parameters); others require to use label images as masks defining where to perform measurements on the original images (photometrical parameters).

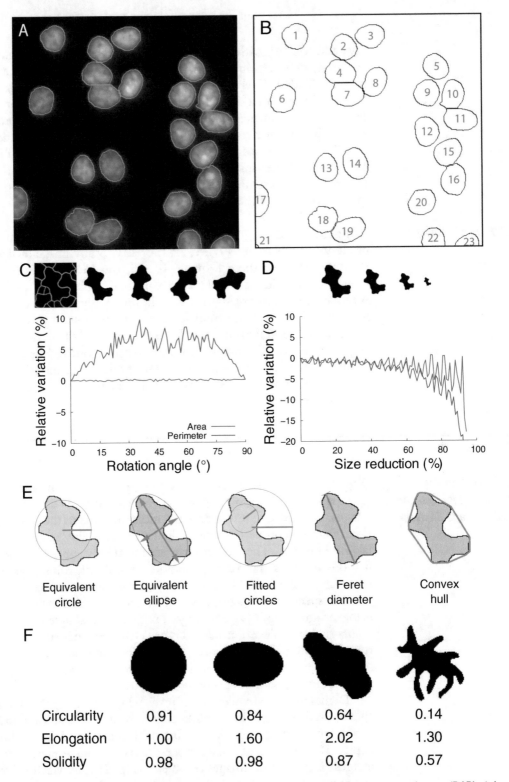

Fig. 1 Morphological and photometric measurements. (**a**) Grayscale light microscopy image (DAPI-stained nuclei). Cell borders are highlighted in *green*. (**b**) Cell boundaries with cell count numbers. (**c**) Influence of rotation on object area and perimeter measurements. (**d**) Influence of scale on object area and perimeter measurements. (**e**) Geometrical features. Many size and shape measurements are derived from the equivalent circle, the equivalent ellipse, the circumscribed and inscribed circles, the Feret diameters, and the convex hull. (**f**) Shape measures for different object shapes

3.1.1 Detecting and Counting Objects

The first information provided by image analysis is the detection and counting of objects of interest (Fig. 1b). This type of information is relatively easy to retrieve, insofar as it does not require a perfect image of object shapes. However, care must be taken when converting object counts to densities if acquired images correspond to sample windows. Corrections for object intersections with image borders must be applied to avoid over- or underestimating densities. Stereology provides methods to compute unbiased estimators from sampled image data [2].

3.1.2 Measuring Sizes and Quantifying Shapes

Other frequently relevant measurements are those related to the size and shape of the objects under study. In image analysis, area is one of the most popular measures of object size. Object area is defined as the product of pixel area by the number of pixels in the object. Pixel area can be computed from the spatial calibration of the images, which gives, in physical distance units, the width and height of a pixel in the real space (*see* **Notes 1** and **2**). Area is a robust size descriptor (Fig. 1c, d). However, at a given spatial calibration, the relative error on area measurement increases when object size decreases (*see* **Note 3**). Image acquisition conditions should be adjusted according to the scale of the smallest objects for which area measurements are desired.

Since it is given in square distance units, area is not easy to interpret. Parameters expressed in distance units may be preferred, such as object perimeter. A straightforward perimeter estimate is obtained from the chain-code representation of object boundary by summing lengths of straight and diagonal moves. This is a biased estimate which in addition is not robust to scale or rotation [3, 4] (Fig. 1c, d). Formulas with statistical corrections terms have been proposed [5]. Unbiased estimates can be obtained using the Crofton formula, which computes the perimeter from the number of intersections between object contour and parallel lines at various orientations [3, 4]. Unfortunately, this perimeter estimation is seldom implemented in bioimaging software [6].

Robust size measurements expressed in distance units can be derived by assimilating objects to ideal shapes (Fig. 1e). The equivalent circular diameter ($\sqrt{4 \times area \div \pi}$) is the diameter of a disk with the same area as the object. Approximating an object with its equivalent inertia ellipsis provides two diameter measures known as major and minor axis lengths. Alternative measures of object extent are provided by the Feret diameters, defined by the spacing at all angles of a virtual caliper rotating around the object. Image analysis software generally report only the largest and the smallest values.

Shape parameters quantify the geometrical information that is independent of absolute size. These measures can be performed even when the spatial calibration of the images is not known (as long as pixels/voxels are square/cubic) because their definitions encompass a scale normalization. Probably the most popular shape parameter (sometimes called *The Shape Factor*) is circularity ($4 \times$ area/perimeter^2). Circularity takes its maximum value 1 for a disk and decreases towards 0 when shape complexity increases. Another useful parameter is solidity (area ÷ area of the convex hull), which decreases when shape concavity increases (Fig. 1e; **Note 4**). Solidity is related to the local behavior of the object silhouette. Other parameters capture global shape traits. The most popular is probably elongation, which is computed from the object's equivalent ellipsis (length of largest axis ÷ length of shortest axis). Circularity depends on both global and local shape properties.

Any of these shape parameters only captures some aspects of the object form. Users should be aware of what specific shape features are quantified by different parameters and should remember that shape is never completely represented by these measurements (Fig. 1f). Alternative shape measures, such as Fourier descriptors [7], provide complete representations. However, they are more complex to interpret and are seldom available in bio-imaging software.

Size and shape parameters derived by an integration over the entire object, such as equivalent radius and elongation, are generally robust. Conversely, parameters relying on extreme values, such as Feret diameters, are less robust. The popularity of the circularity index is paradoxical, given that this is one of the least robust shape parameters due to its dependence on perimeter (*see* **Note 5**). The drawback of integration-based parameters is that they are not always as easy to interpret and to relate to physical reality.

3.1.3 Quantifying
Intensities

Complementary to morphometric parameters, photometric measurements are obtained by quantifying intensity values. They are typically quantiles (minimum, maximum, median) and moments (mean, variance, skewness, kurtosis) of intensity distributions within objects or regions-of-interest. For instance, measuring the total amount of fluorescence on each detected cell in an image can be used to determine cells with high expression of a specific gene. The simplicity of the few measures that are generally made in intensity-based analysis is misleading. It is counterbalanced by the number of issues that can potentially affect measurements [8].

3.1.4 Measuring
Positions and Analyzing
Spatial Distributions

Object position is frequently represented by the centroid, the point of average coordinates in the image plane (*see* **Note 6**), or by the center-of-mass (intensity-weighted barycenter of object pixels). While absolute positions in the image plane are useful on a control environment, relative positions with respect to other structures are generally more relevant. Euclidean distances or angles can be used for this purpose. Various descriptors such as radial analysis measures are also used to quantify the relative positioning of objects included within other structures [9].

One particular and very popular case of spatial analysis is colocalization analysis. It provides a measure of the spatial co-occurrence between two or more types of objects labeled with different fluorophores. There exist two major ways of performing a colocalization analysis, either by a photometric approach (using coefficients to express the intensity correlation between different channels) or by a geometrical approach (using the overlap between the pre-detected objects). Photometric studies should be conducted with caution since the reliability of the correlation coefficients depends on many factors, including a number of different sources of noise [10, 11].

Based on distance measurements, spatial interactions in the relative positioning of objects can be analyzed using spatial statistics. For example, spatial point pattern analysis [12] provides methods for characterizing the spatial distribution of the objects of interest and to test if they are located at random (independently of each other's location), tend to form clusters (indicating a possible attraction) or follow a regular distribution (which suggests a repulsion among the objects). Furthermore, specific spatial models can be statistically tested to find the distribution that fits best the underlying spatial organization. Spatial statistics are not yet popular in bioimage analysis, probably because they have essentially been developed in the context of ecology and forestry applications. Methods for handling issues specific to biological studies, such as replicated data, arbitrarily sized objects and exhaustive sampling within confined domains, have to be developed [13].

3.1.5   Motion Analysis and Tracking

Motion analysis quantifies the apparent object motion between consecutive images on an image sequence. The simplest application consists on detecting the motion, i.e., the points in the image that are moving. More complex analysis can be performed to group moving points belonging to the same object, determine the motion velocity and direction of each point, or follow specific points or objects over time, which is known as tracking [14].

3.2   Finding Objects in Images: The Segmentation Problem

Prior to analysis, objects must be detected and defined according to a representation suitable for quantification by the computer. This is achieved through segmentation, the process of partitioning an image into multiple homogeneous regions or segments (Fig. 2). Segmentation constitutes a major transition in the image analysis pipeline, replacing intensity values (quantitative information) by region labels (qualitative information). In this section we describe some of the most popular methods for segmenting light microscopy data. The reader should keep in mind that there is no universal segmentation method. It is recommended to try different approaches to determine which one works best for his/her specific image data.

3.2.1   Binarization by Grey Level Thresholding

Binarization, the simplest image segmentation method, consists in classifying pixels into two classes: pixels belonging to objects of

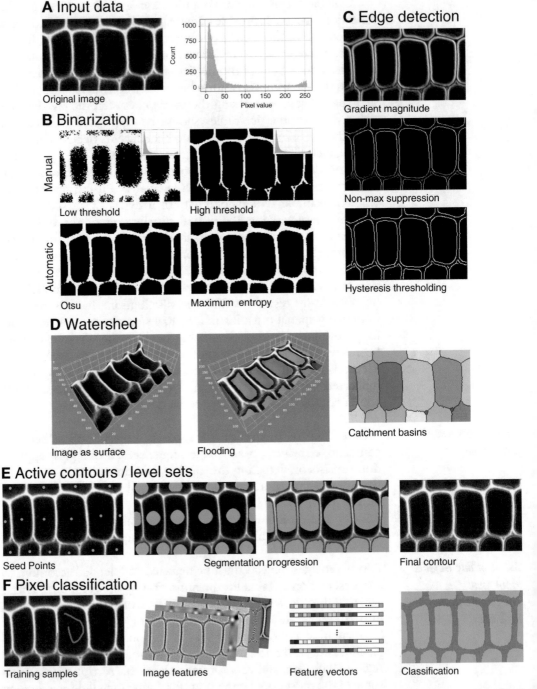

Fig. 2 Segmentation methods. (**a**) Example of input image data and corresponding histogram (crop of confocal *XY* plane of *Arabidopsis* embryo [45]). (**b**) Binarization by thresholding (manual and automatic methods). (**c**) Edge detection by gradient operator, followed by non-maximum suppression and hysteresis thresholding. (**d**) Watershed segmentation by flooding, considering the image as a topographic surface. *Right*: segmentation result. (**e**) Segmentation by active contours/level sets from manually placed seed points. (**f**) Segmentation by pixel classification. A set of pixels is selected for training (*green* and *red markings*), image features are extracted from the original image, the pixels are then represented in the feature space and a classification method is trained and applied to classify all other pixels

interest (*foreground*) and pixels belonging to other parts of the image (*background*). This binary classification is performed by comparing the intensity value of each pixel to a threshold value. All pixels above the threshold are marked as foreground (usually by setting them to white) and the rest of pixels are marked as background (usually black) (Fig. 2b). This approach is very common to segment light microscopy data, especially fluorescence images where the areas of interest are substantially brighter than the rest of the image.

Even under fixed image acquisition conditions, using the same threshold over a collection of images is generally not recommended because of uncontrolled fluctuations in intensity values across images. Hence, a new threshold value should be computed for each image, using an automated threshold selection technique. Some thresholding methods are global and use the same threshold value over the entire image. Local methods adapt the threshold to compensate for regional intensity variations. All automatic thresholding methods consist in optimizing some objective criterion that can be statistical (e.g., maximization of inter-class variance [15] or of entropy [16]), probabilistic (e.g., minimization of pixel classification error [17]) or structural (e.g., circularity of detected objects).

Binarization generates an image where the objects of interest are connected regions of white pixels called connected components. Labeling the different connected components allows distinguishing different objects prior to quantitative analysis (Fig. 1b).

3.2.2 Defining Objects by Their Contours

Sometimes the objects of interest do not have homogeneous intensities but their contours are easily identifiable by their contrast difference with the background. In those cases it might be interesting to use edge detection to segment the images. Edge detection is the process of estimating the boundaries of objects by highlighting places of large intensity variations. This is usually accomplished by calculating the first or second order derivatives of the pixel intensities, followed by thresholding (Fig. 2c). Very frequently additional steps are required to transform those estimations into continuous borders and then close objects.

3.2.3 Watershed Transform

The watershed transform is a popular segmentation method in biological imaging. This method draws an analogy between the image and a topographic surface where bright areas define peaks and dark ones represent valleys. The algorithm simulates the flooding of the surface from water sources placed at its lowest points and builds dams when the water from different sources meet [18]. Each separate region is a *catchment basin* that defines an object, while the separation lines between them are known as *watersheds*.

This approach requires the borders of the regions of interest to be brighter than the background and than the interior of the regions. In light microscopy, it is very frequently applied to data expressing a membrane marker (Fig. 2d). On images where the whole objects are stained rather than just their boundaries, it is necessary to preprocess the image with an edge detector.

3.2.4 Constraining Segmentation Using Geometrical Knowledge

In some cases, the objects of interest are not completely defined by the information in the image. For example, cell membranes might appear with gaps produced by different problems during the image acquisition. In those cases, it is convenient to apply a segmentation method such as active contours, which makes use of prior knowledge on object shape to geometrically constrain the iterative search of the outline (in 2D) or surface (in 3D) that enclose best the objects [19]. The final contours are a compromise between geometric constraints (continuity, elasticity, flexibility) and the location at strong intensity variations. There exist many variants of this strategy. One of the most popular ones makes use of the level set method to efficiently address the curve propagation and topological changes, advancing the contour like a rubber band until it reaches the object boundaries [20] (Fig. 2e).

3.2.5 Classifying Pixels and Learning Segmentation by Example

Image segmentation can be cast as a pixel classification problem, where each pixel has to be labeled as belonging to one class depending on its similarity (in intensity, position, etc.) with other pixels of the same class. The classification can be unsupervised, i.e., without any guidance, or supervised, where the user provides some samples of each class so the classifier learns how to label the rest of pixels in the image. One of the most popular and fastest unsupervised methods is K-means, that groups pixels into K classes or clusters based on how similar they are to the mean of each cluster. Supervised methods are usually a bit slower, because they need a training phase, but more precise since they mimic the classification by an expert.

All these methods can deal with images having n-dimensional pixel values. Grayscale images have $n = 1$, each pixel bearing a single intensity value, and multichannel images have n equal to the number of channels. For example, it is common to use K-means on RGB images ($n = 3$) to separate objects based on color (*see* **Note 7**). Popular tools have emerged recently to segment microscopy images by combining high-dimensional pixel representations (using predefined image features) and supervised classifiers in an interactive way, where the user introduces new training samples and the segmentation results get updated on-the-fly [21, 22] (Fig. 2f). These methods, while slower than classic clustering methods, provide very robust solutions improved by the continuous user feedback (*see* **Note 8**).

3.3 Post-processing Images to Facilitate Analysis

Prior to analysis, it may be needed to improve the segmented images to correct some errors or to transform the object representation to allow the extraction of desired measurements. Typical corrections at this stage include regularizing object shapes, filling holes inside the segmented regions (false negatives), removing artifacts in the background (false positives) and rearranging the topology of segmented regions (splitting or merging). It is often necessary as well to extract the contours or the center-lines of the objects to simplify the analysis of their structure. As they operate downstream of segmentation on object rather than on intensity images, these transformations are referred to as post-processing operations. This section describes the most common techniques used at this step.

3.3.1 Shape Operations Using Binary Mathematical Morphology

Mathematical morphology is a theory and a set of methods that operate on objects based on their size and shape [23, 24]. The basic operators are a set of morphological filters that can be combined to provide a large variety of image transforms. They are local filters, in the sense that they consider the neighborhood of each pixel/voxel according to a structuring element of given size and shape.

The base morphological filters are the dilation (background pixels where the structuring element intersects the object are turned to object pixels) and the dual operation of erosion (Fig. 3a). Dilation and erosion are generally used in combination to preserve object sizes. For example, the morphological closing (dilation followed by an erosion) removes background regions smaller than the structuring element. Symmetrically, the morphological opening (erosion followed by a dilation) removes objects smaller than the structuring element (Fig. 3a).

3.3.2 Separation of Touching Objects

Due to the low image resolution of the microscope being used or the limited accuracy of the chosen segmentation method, it is frequent that neighboring objects end up connected and therefore considered as a single object (for instance, two cells or nuclei with a separation smaller than the spatial resolution). Morphological opening can be used to separate objects if the spatial extent of object connections is at least one order of magnitude smaller than object sizes. A popular alternative when object connections are too large consists in applying the distance transform to the binary segmented image and then running the watershed method on its inverse to recover the boundaries between objects. This strategy works very well on convex (circular or elliptical) objects such as cells or nuclei (Fig. 3b).

3.3.3 Filling Holes and Gaps

Mathematical morphology also provides with tools to fill holes within objects or to close gaps between parts of objects that would have been split during segmentation. Morphological closing can be used when the spatial extent of holes and gaps is small. Otherwise, hole filling based on morphological reconstruction (*see* below Subheading 3.4) is generally preferred. In light microscopy images, these operators offer a simple and very fast way to make sure that objects like nuclei do not present holes or that cell membranes are completely closed (Fig. 3c).

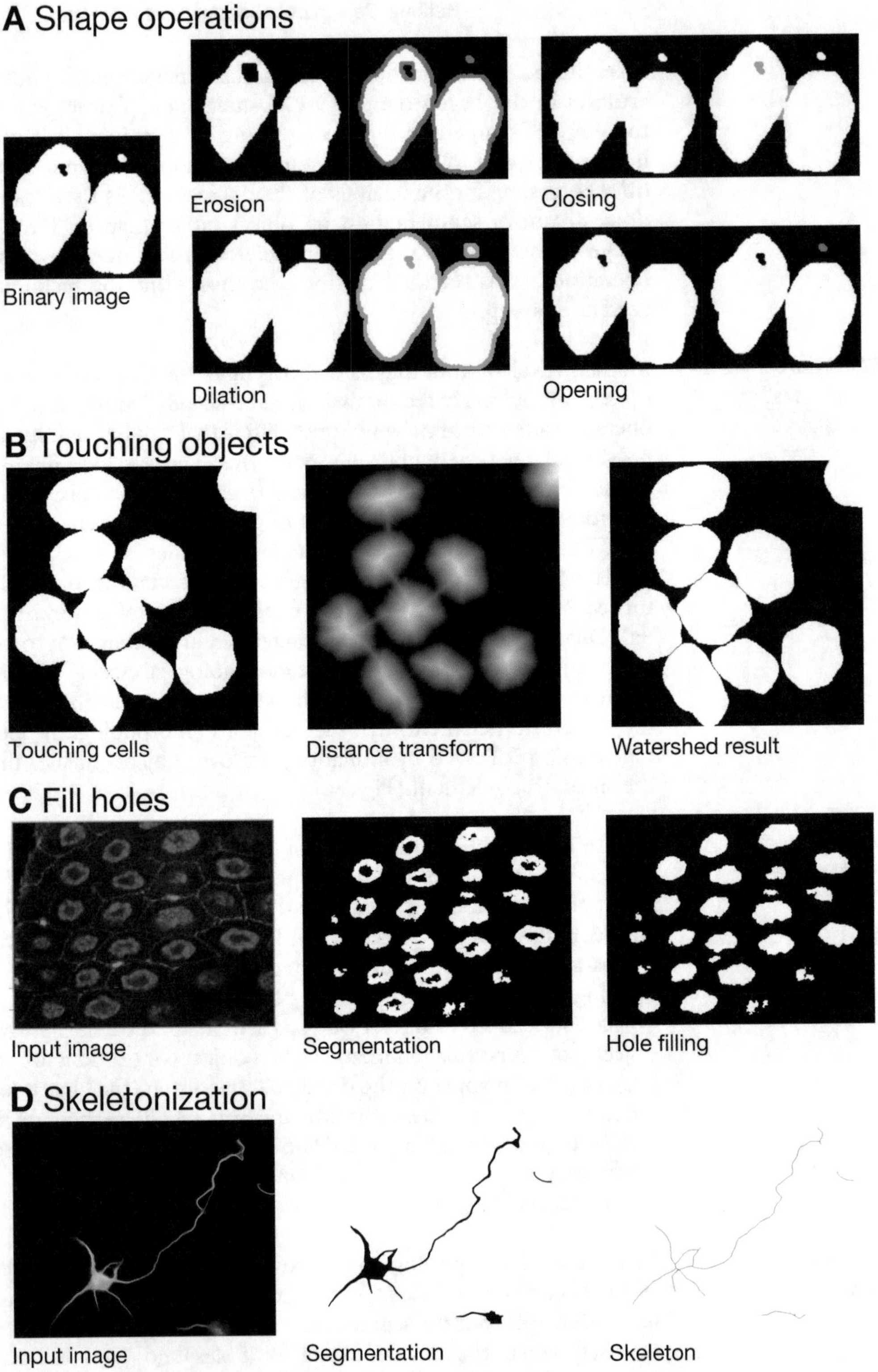

A Shape operations

Binary image

Erosion

Closing

Dilation

Opening

B Touching objects

Touching cells

Distance transform

Watershed result

C Fill holes

Input image

Segmentation

Hole filling

D Skeletonization

Input image

Segmentation

Skeleton

Fig. 3 Post-processing operations. (**a**) Basic morphological operations on a binary image using a 3×3 square structuring element. *Red/Green*: object pixels removed/added during operation. (**b**) Separation of touching objects using watershed and distance transform. Watershed was run on the inverted distance map of the binary input image. (**c**) Hole filling applied on a binary segmentation. (**d**) Skeletonization of the binary image of a neuron. Original fluorescence images (**c, d**) from the Cell Image Library (CIL39686 and CIL8476 respectively)

3.3.4   Simplifying Shapes
Using Skeletonization
and Border Thinning

Finally, reducing the representation of objects to pixel-wide skeletons or to contours through morphological operations is a very common strategy to facilitate the analysis of linear structures such as membranes or of treelike organizations such as neuronal arborescences (Fig. 3d).

3.4   Preprocessing Images to Enable Better Object Segmentation

In many applications, it is difficult, if not impossible, to generate a correct image of segmented objects using segmentation and postprocessing operations only. The acquired images must then be filtered to make them easier to process at the segmentation step and onward (*see* **Note 9**). The common principle underlying all preprocessing operators is to increase the separability between object and background pixels. This is achieved either by increasing homogeneity within each class or by increasing the contrast between the two classes.

3.4.1   Increasing Region
Homogeneity
by Attenuating Noise

Noise is one of the major sources of heterogeneity in input images. Noise can result from the stochastic nature of the sampled physical property (e.g., fluorescence emission) as well as from the acquisition process (thermal, read-out, and quantification noise). Noise induces wide dispersion around histogram peaks and fast fluctuations of intensity values in the spatial domain. At the segmentation step, this potentially hampers the automated detection of correct intensity thresholds and leads to high numbers of background/foreground classification errors.

Standard operators to attenuate noise are spatial linear filters such as the mean and the Gaussian filters (Fig. 4a). These filters replace the value of each pixel by a linear combination of pixel values in its neighborhood. The Gaussian filter is optimal in the case of Gaussian-distributed noise. The degree of smoothing can be tuned by adjusting the size of the neighborhood.

One major drawback of linear filters is that they reduce local contrast by blurring object boundaries. Suboptimal filters that better preserve local contrast may be preferred. The median filter, which replaces each pixel by the median value in its neighborhood, is a popular alternative to linear filters (Fig. 4a). Preserving local contrast can also be achieved by extending neighborhoods from the spatial to the photometric domain. Blurring is then limited by allowing only similar intensities to be combined. Early examples of this approach are the α-trimmed mean and the sigma filters [25]. Adaptive filters such as anisotropic diffusion [26] (Fig. 4a) and bilateral filter [27, 28] were subsequently introduced. Recent developments extended spatial neighborhoods to regions or to the whole image scale, as in the Non-Local Means filter [29], or extended the similarity in the photometric domain from individual values to local patches [30]. The additional cost that comes with most of these adaptive filters compared to classical ones is an increased number of parameters. Identifying the best combination of parameters is therefore more complicated.

3.4.2 Reducing Uncertainty on Object Boundaries by Enhancing Local Contrast

Local contrast corresponds to the slope of an intensity transition at object boundary. A low contrast visually manifests itself by a blurry border. Low contrast is problematic for automatic segmentation because it makes object boundary detection highly sensitive to intensity thresholds. Convolution by the optics of the microscope is the major source of blur in acquired images. Local contrast can be enhanced by subtracting to the image a fraction of its second derivatives, as is classically done using the Laplacian filter or the related unsharp masking operator (Fig. 4b). Deconvolution methods can also be used to remove blur in acquired images [31, 32]. Deconvolution aims at inverting the degradation of the signal that was introduced by the optics of the acquisition system, described by the Point Spread Function (PSF). Theoretical (mathematical model) or empirical (experimentally acquired using fluorescent beads) PSF are used as input in deconvolution methods.

3.4.3 Trade-off Between Preprocessing Operations

Smoothing filters reduce noise but may also reduce local contrast. Conversely, filters enhancing local contrast may increase intensity fluctuations caused by noise. A practical consequence is that a trade-off has to be made between noise reduction and local contrast enhancement and that defects cannot be completely removed from acquired images. It is therefore highly recommended to optimize the conditions of image acquisition to limit as much as possible the need for preprocessing operations (*see* **Note 10**).

3.4.4 Specifically Enhancing Objects of Interest

Noise and contrast filters are applied to reduce defects in images. Preprocessing operations can also be applied to specifically enhance the objects of interest at the expense of other structures. Mathematical morphology on gray level images provides a large spectrum of tools for this purpose [24].

As in the binary case (Subheading 3.3.1), gray level mathematical morphology relies on two basic operations, erosion and dilation, that are applied in tandem in the composite opening and closing operations. In their simplest form, grayscale erosion and dilation consist in replacing each pixel by the minimum (resp. maximum) value over its neighborhood (*see* **Note 11**). Neighborhood size and shape (structuring element) are arbitrary but usually correspond to a discretized version of a disk. Generalizing their binary counterparts, grayscale opening and closing respectively remove bright and dark objects smaller than the structuring element (Fig. 4c).

Small objects such as vesicles are frequently of interest in microscope image analysis. The top-hat transform generates an image where only small bright objects are retained, by subtracting to the original image the result of its opening (dark objects are similarly specifically enhanced by subtracting the original image to the result of its closing) (Fig. 4c). Top-hat is a particular case of background removal techniques, which allow to correct for intensity variations due to uneven illumination over the image (Fig. 4d).

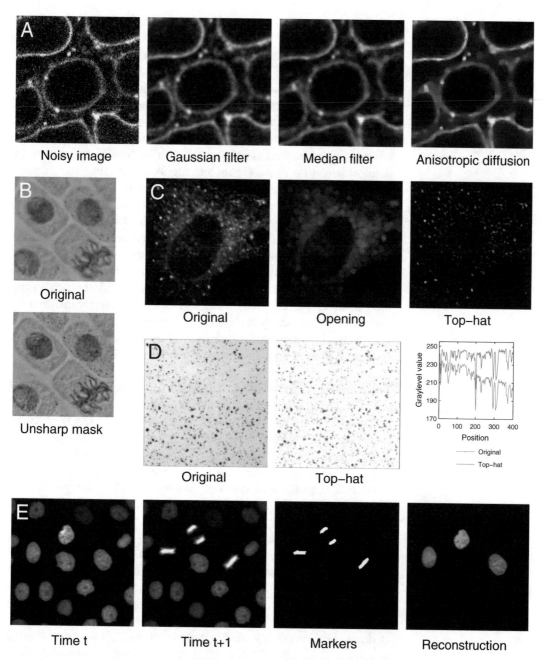

Fig. 4 Preprocessing operations. (**a**) Noise attenuation by spatial filters. Image by S. Vernhettes, INRA Versailles, France. (**b**) Blur removal (local contrast enhancement) using the unsharp mask filter. Original image from the Cell Image Library (CIL43552). (**c**) Size-based object enhancement using the top-hat transform. Small vesicles were enhanced (*right*) by subtracting from the original image (*left*) its morphological opening (*middle*). Original image from the Cell Image Library (CIL13568). (**d**) Background correction using the top-hat transform. The uneven illumination was removed by subtracting the original image from its morphological closing. The graph shows graylevel profiles along the horizontal midline in both images. (**e**) Marker-based object enhancement and selection using gray level morphological reconstruction. Reconstruction was used to find in an image sequence the nuclei at time *t* that have divided at time *t*+1. The markers were obtained by thresholding image at *t*+1 and were used for the reconstruction by dilation of image at *t*. Original image from http://www.codesol-orzano.com/celltrackingchallenge/Cell_Tracking_Challenge/Datasets.html [46]

Geodesic reconstruction is another class of powerful mathematical morphology operators that can be used to filter objects in an image (called the mask) based on markers in another image [33]. Markers in this context refer to sets of pixels that tag the objects of interest. Reconstruction by dilation proceeds by repeatedly dilating the marker image while constraining it to remain below the mask image. When stability is reached, the marker image contains a reconstructed version of the objects in which markers where initially located (Fig. 4e). Many other useful operations are defined based on geodesic reconstruction, including the removal of peaks of height below a threshold (h-maxima transform) or the imposition of minima at specified positions. The latter operation is used as a preprocessing step in the marker-based watershed. It greatly contributes to improve the watershed segmentation results by limiting the amount of over-segmentation. Due to the frequent use of multiple channels corresponding to as many experimental labels, geodesic operations are particularly suited for processing biological images acquired using light microscopy. Unfortunately, they are not frequently available in bioimage analysis software [6]. The same holds for other classes of mathematical morphology operators such as area and other attribute openings [34].

3.5 Validation of Image Analysis Pipeline and Results

Several factors can affect the validity of measurements obtained with an automated image processing and analysis pipeline. The presence of noise can lead to false-positive detection of objects; an incorrect intensity threshold affects size measurements; programming errors (e.g., in user-defined macros) can lead to incorrect values; etc. Results of quantitative analysis should systematically be examined critically and checked through a validation procedure. The validation process can also be applied at intermediate stages in the pipeline, such as the segmentation step.

The most common validation strategy is to compare the results obtained with the image analysis pipeline to a set of reference measurements (*gold-standard*) obtained by manual analysis of sample images by a human expert. How the comparison between automatic and expert results is performed largely depends on the type of measurement and the image processing step at which evaluation is done. Object counts are typically evaluated using a correlation criterion. Evaluation at the segmentation stage is generally performed by quantifying the overlap between automatic and manual segmentation masks, using criteria such as the Jaccard or Dice coefficients [35, 36]. The limit of this evaluation strategy is that human expertise is itself affected by uncertainty due to intra- and inter-operator variability. Another limitation is that it is not always possible in practice to manually generate a dataset of sufficient size, as for example to validate a 3D segmentation.

An alternative validation strategy consists in using image simulation algorithms to generate a gold standard. Given models of object geometries and of the physics of the image formation process (microscope characteristics such as PSF, geometrical and photometrical alterations such as noise, etc.), algorithms can be used to generate artificial images that simulate real images of cells or particles [37, 38]. Model parameters can be set arbitrarily and adjusted by trials-and-errors. Alternatively, they can also be learned from sample images [39]. The usefulness of such image generators of course depends on the ability to model accurately the biological structures and the physical processes that determine image contents.

Lastly, image measurements can be compared and cross-validated with results obtained using alternative experimental methods than image analysis. However, a few numbers of measurements can be validated along this approach (such as concentration of molecules in ratiometric fluorescence imaging), given that many parameters can hardly be obtained using other methods than image analysis (e.g., shape measurements).

When validation based on a gold standard is not feasible, confidence on the obtained results can be quantitatively assessed by evaluating the sensitivity of measurements to the parameter setup in the image analysis pipeline. Due to the possibly large number of parameters and to the resulting combinatorial explosion, this approach is however applicable to a limited number of parameters, such as threshold values at the segmentation step [40].

3.6 The Whole Picture: A Goal-Oriented, Iterative Approach

The previous sections presented the building blocks (ingredients) of a typical image processing and analysis pipeline. This section presents a goal-oriented generic strategy (recipe) to assemble these elements and instantiate them in practice. Designing an image analysis solution is not a one-pass process. It generally proceeds by trial-and-error and involves several rounds before converging to a final solution. Since it is generic, the "algorithm" for pipeline design presented here is of course to some extent idealized. It is intended as a general guideline for rationalizing and optimizing the design of image analysis pipelines. A key point of the proposed methodology is that it does not follow the chronological order of operations in the final pipeline, but instead proceeds backwards from the analysis objective (Fig. 5).

1. Step 1 is to specify formally the analysis objectives by identifying the quantitative measurements to perform. At this stage, the objectives are translated from the biological to the mathematical or computer science terminology. For example, "nucleus position" or "cell shape" are ambiguous terms for image analysis; "centroid" or "solidity," for example, should be used instead. Care should be taken that the chosen parameters actually and faithfully quantify the biological features of interest (*see* comments and notes in Subheading 3.1).

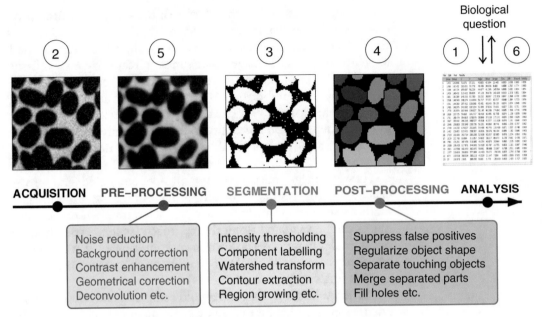

Fig. 5 Main steps in a generic image processing and analysis pipeline. Typical operations performed at each processing step are mentioned in the related *box*. *Circled numbers* refer to the ordering in which the different steps are progressively introduced in the proposed strategy (*see* Subheading 3.6)

2. Step 2 is to perform image acquisition using appropriate conditions given the objectives defined at **step 1**. A first important point to consider at this stage is a sufficient resolution for the desired measurements (*see* Subheading 3.1). Optical resolution primarily depends on the numerical aperture of the objective and on light wavelength. The pixel size should be not set arbitrarily but small enough to preserve the resolution of the microscope image. It can generally be set by microscope software to its optimal value given the imaging conditions, following the Nyquist–Shannon criterion [41] (*see* **Note 12**).

A second important point is to ensure the largest possible range of intensity values in the acquired images while preventing saturation at both ends of the dynamic range (*see* Subheading 3.2). On a confocal microscope, this is obtained by tuning the gain of the photomultiplier (*see* Note 13). When acquiring collections of images, a trade-off has to be found to meet this requirement while at the same time keeping acquisition conditions constant.

A final important point is to improve as much as possible the signal-to-noise ratio to ease the segmentation step (*see* Subheading 3.2) and to limit the needs for preprocessing operations (*see* Subheading 3.4). On a confocal microscope, this can be tuned by adjusting the laser power, the pinhole aperture and the total time spent on each pixel [42]. Trade-offs have to be made, since for example longer exposure times and increased laser power may induce other issues such as photobleaching and photodamage.

3. Step 3 is to perform image segmentation using one of the methods presented in Subheading 3.2. Which method to use depends on the origin of the contrast that defines the objects of interest. However, image thresholding is frequently an appropriate initial choice in light microscopy because of the use of extrinsic labeling. If a correct segmentation is obtained, then go to **step 6**. Otherwise, go to **step 4**.

4. Step 4 is to remove moderate errors in the images of segmented objects, using the post-processing techniques presented in Subheading 3.3. If post-processing is sufficient to generate a correct image of objects, then go to **step 6**. Otherwise, go to **step 5**.

5. Step 5 is to enhance acquired images using the preprocessing techniques presented in Subheading 3.4 to make them easier to process at the subsequent segmentation and post-processing steps. Given that the less image transformations, the better, preprocessing should be considered only when everything else (segmentation and post-processing) fails at producing correct object images.

    There is generally a mix of degradation in acquired images. Diagnosing the most important ones and among them, those that make segmentation difficult, is essential to select the appropriate operators that should be applied at this stage. Simple tools such as variance of local histograms within structurally homogeneous regions and gray level profiles can be used to evaluate noise levels and local contrast.

    Validating preprocessing operations is more difficult than segmentation and post-processing steps, because they involve intensity rather than label images. The validity of a preprocessing operation is therefore evaluated based on the success it confers to the downstream segmentation and post-processing steps.

    Generally, several rounds of **steps 3–5** sequences will be applied before converging to a satisfactory pipeline. In some situations, it will not be possible to generate correct object images from the input images. In such a case, go to **step 2** to reconsider sample preparation and image acquisition conditions.

6. Step 6, the final step, is to run the image analysis proper by performing on the segmented objects the measurements defined at **step 1**. There is no practical recommendation at this stage except the ones already formulated in Subheading 3.1.

4   Notes

1. In biological imaging, the spatial calibration of an image is typically expressed in μm or nm. It is frequently interpreted as the size of the square covered by a pixel in the real space.

Actually, spatial calibration refers to the spacing between consecutive pixels. Pixel width and height are generally identical on modern image acquisition instruments.

2. Pixel calibration is generally stored automatically by acquisition systems in the meta-data section of the image files and can be read by most image analysis software. It is however good practice to check that this is indeed the case. In ImageJ/Fiji, this information appears in *Image → Properties....*

3. In practice, image analysis software will report areas for any object size. It is not recommended to rely on area values for objects smaller than 5–10 pixels in diameter, given the large relative uncertainty that may affect these measures.

4. There is ample room for confusion in the nomenclature of shape parameters. The same definition is frequently referred to under different names (for example, circularity is also known as compactness; elongation may be called aspect ratio). The same name can also refer to different parameter definitions (e.g., the inverse formula is sometimes used for circularity). Lastly, the vocabulary, that mostly originates from material science, may be inappropriate in biology. For example, solidity actually quantifies shape convexity, and would probably be better referred to as such in a biological context. In any case, we advise to systematically check the actual definitions of size and shape parameters reported by image analysis software.

5. We recommend using the solidity parameter rather than circularity everywhere possible. Though it depends on the extreme points of object silhouette, solidity is more robust since it relies on area measurements only (object and convex hull). A robust alternative to the classical circularity measure was proposed in [43].

6. The centroid of an object is not systematically a representative point of this object. The centroid can be located outside an object with a non-convex shape. Alternatives such as the ultimate eroded point may be preferred in such situations.

7. The Ridler and Calvard thresholding technique available as the default method in the ImageJ/Fiji software is a special case of K-means clustering, run with $K=2$ in the 1-dimensional space of grayscale values. It is also an iterative version of Otsu's method [44].

8. The speed of the interactive learning segmentation depends on the number and size of the selected image features and the choice of the classifier method. In the Trainable Weka Segmentation plugin [22] of Fiji [1], these parameters can be tuned in the settings dialog. We recommend to start with the default configuration and to set the maximum sigma to a radius larger than the structures that can be confused with objects at a pixel level (for example the radius of bright spots when the

aim is to segment membranes). The number of features can be reduced to save computer memory and calculation time when the segmentation accuracy does not get affected.

9. We only consider in this section preprocessing operations that enhance the image in the perspective of segmentation. Techniques improving the visual appearance of images for display purposes, such as histogram transforms, are generally not to be applied in an automated image processing and analysis pipeline and are therefore not considered in this chapter.

10. Ideally, all preprocessing would be taken care of at the image acquisition stage. Investing time to optimize sample preparation, mounting, and microscope setup is highly beneficial for the subsequent image processing steps.

11. The general definition of erosion and dilation operations actually involves minimum and maximum after point-wise subtraction or addition to neighboring pixels of intensity values stored in a structuring element. This reduces to mere minimum and maximum operations when these values are constant ("flat" structuring element). Using a non-flat structuring element brings robustness to noise. The use of such elements has become less popular since the introduction of the powerful reconstruction operators, which rely on minimum and maximum operations only.

12. It is generally recommended to set pixel/voxel size 2–3 times smaller than optical resolution. For identical acquisition conditions, optimal values reported by different microscope software can vary due to the different formulas used to compute resolution from numerical aperture and wavelength.

13. The offset parameter is sometimes used to remove background noise, setting the corresponding pixel values to zero. When images are acquired to be digitally processed and analyzed, this is not necessary. This may even be detrimental since background noise may be useful for some preprocessing or segmentation operators (for example, for estimating a noise level).

References

1. Schindelin J, Arganda-Carreras I, Frise E et al (2012) Fiji: an open-source platform for biological-image analysis. Nat Methods 9:676–682

2. Howard CV, Reed MG (1988) Unbiased stereology: three-dimensional measurement in microscopy. BIOS Scientific Publishers, Oxford

3. Pirard E, Dislaire G (2005) Robustness of planar shape descriptors of particles. Proc. Int. Assoc. Math. Geol. Conf. Toronto, CA

4. Lehmann G, Legland D (2012) Efficient N-dimensional surface estimation using Crofton formula and run-length encoding. Insight J. http://hdl.handle.net/10380/3342

5. Dorst L, Smeulders AWM (1987) Length estimators for digitized contours. Comput Vis Graph Image Process 40:311–333. doi: http://dx.doi.org/10.1016/S0734-189X(87)80145-7

6. Legland D, Arganda-Carreras I, Andrey P (2016) MorphoLibJ: mathematical morphol-

ogy library for ImageJ. Release 1(2):2. doi:10.5281/zenodo.51734

7. Pincus Z, Theriot JA (2007) Comparison of quantitative methods for cell-shape analysis. J Microsc 227:140–156. doi:10.1111/j.1365-2818.2007.01799.x

8. Waters JC (2009) Accuracy and precision in quantitative fluorescence microscopy. J Cell Biol 185:1135–1148. doi:10.1083/jcb.200903097

9. Ronneberger O, Baddeley D, Scheipl F et al (2008) Spatial quantitative analysis of fluorescently labeled nuclear structures: problems, methods, pitfalls. Chromosom Res 16:523–562

10. Bolte S, Cordelieres FP (2006) A guided tour into subcellular colocalization analysis in light microscopy. J Microsc 224:213–232

11. Dunn KW, Kamocka MM, McDonald JH (2011) A practical guide to evaluating colocalization in biological microscopy. Am J Physiol Physiol 300:C723–C742

12. Diggle PJ (2014) Statistical analysis of spatial and spatio-temporal point patterns, 3rd edn. Chapman and Hall/CRC Press, Boca Raton

13. Andrey P, Kiêu K, Kress C et al (2010) Statistical analysis of 3D images detects regular spatial distributions of centromeres and chromocenters in animal and plant nuclei. PLoS Comput Biol 6:e1000853

14. Meijering E, Smal I, Danuser G (2006) Tracking in molecular bioimaging. IEEE Signal Process Mag 23:46–53. doi:10.1109/MSP.2006.1628877

15. Otsu N (1979) A threshold selection method from gray-level histograms. IEEE Trans Syst Man Cybern 9:62–66

16. Kapur JN, Sahoo PK, Wong AKC (1985) A new method for gray-level picture thresholding using the entropy of the histogram. Comput Vis Graph Image Process 29:273–285

17. Kittler J, Illingworth J (1986) Minimum error thresholding. Pattern Recognit 19:41–47

18. Vincent L, Soille P (1991) Watersheds in digital spaces: an efficient algorithm based on immersion simulation. IEEE Trans Pattern Anal Mach Intell 13:583–598

19. Kass M, Witkin A, Terzopoulos D (1988) Snakes: active contour models. Int J Comput Vis 1:321–331

20. Sethian JA (1999) Level set methods and fast marching methods: evolving interfaces in computational geometry, fluid mechanics, computer vision, and materials science. Cambridge University Press, Cambridge

21. Sommer C, Straehle C, Koethe U, Hamprecht FA (2011) ilastik: interactive learning and segmentation toolkit. In: 2011 IEEE international symposium on biomedical imaging: from nano to macro, pp 230–233

22. Arganda-Carreras I, Cardona A, Kaynig V, Schindelin J (2011) Trainable weka segmentation. Fiji website

23. Serra J (1982) Image analysis and mathematical morphology. Academic Press, London

24. Soille P (2003) Morphological image analysis: principles and applications, 2nd edn. Springer-Verlag, Berlin, Germany

25. Lee J-S (1983) Digital image smoothing and the sigma filter. Comput Vis Graph Image Process 24:255–269. doi: http://dx.doi.org/10.1016/0734-189X(83)90047-6

26. Perona P, Malik J (1990) Scale-space filtering and edge detection using anisotropic diffusion. IEEE Trans Pattern Anal Mach Intell 12:629–639

27. Tomasi C, Manduchi R (1998) Bilateral filtering for gray and color images. In: Sixth Int. Conf. Comput. Vis. pp 839–846

28. Smith SM, Brady JM (1997) SUSAN—a new approach to low level image processing. Int J Comput Vis 23:45–78

29. Buades A, Coll B, Morel J-M (2005) A review of image denoising algorithms, with a new one. Multiscale Model Simul 4:490–530

30. Kervrann C, Boulanger J (2006) Optimal spatial adaptation for patch-based image denoising. IEEE Trans Image Process 15:2866–2878

31. Wallace W, Schaefer LH, Swedlow JR (2001) A workingperson's guide to deconvolution in light microscopy. Biotechniques 31:1076–1097

32. Cannell MB, McMorland A, Soeller C (2006) Image enhancement by deconvolution. In: Pawley BJ (ed) Handb. Biol. Confocal Microsc. Springer, Boston, MA, pp 488–500

33. Vincent L (1993) Morphological grayscale reconstruction in image analysis: applications and efficient algorithms. IEEE Trans Image Process 2:176–201

34. Breen EJ, Jones R (1996) Attribute openings, thinnings, and granulometries. Comput Vis Image Underst 64:377–389. doi: http://dx.doi.org/10.1006/cviu.1996.0066

35. Jaccard P (1912) The distribution of the flora in the alpine zone. New Phytol 11:37–50

36. Dice LR (1945) Measures of the amount of ecologic association between species. Ecology 26:297–302

37. Lehmussola A, Ruusuvuori P, Selinummi J et al (2007) Computational framework for simulating

fluorescence microscope images with cell populations. IEEE Trans Med Imaging 26:1010–1016. doi:10.1109/TMI.2007.896925

38. Svoboda D, Kozubek M, Stejskal S (2009) Generation of digital phantoms of cell nuclei and simulation of image formation in 3D image cytometry. Cytom A 75:494–509. doi:10.1002/cyto.a.20714

39. Murphy RF (2016) Building cell models and simulations from microscope images. Methods 96:33–39. doi:10.1016/j.ymeth.2015.10.011

40. Eils R, Dietzel S, Bertin E et al (1996) Three-dimensional reconstruction of painted human interphase chromosomes: active and inactive X chromosome territories have similar volumes but differ in shape and surface structure. J Cell Biol 135:1427–1440

41. Pawley JB (2006) Points, pixels, and gray levels: digitizing image data. In: Pawley BJ (ed) Handb. Biol. Confocal Microsc. Springer, Boston, MA, pp 59–79

42. Sheppard CJR, Gan X, Gu M, Roy M (2006) Signal-to-noise ratio in confocal microscopes. In: Pawley BJ (ed) Handb. Biol. Confocal Microsc. Springer, Boston, MA, pp 442–452

43. Žunić J, Hirota K, Rosin PL (2010) A Hu moment invariant as a shape circularity measure. Pattern Recognit 43:47–57. doi: http://dx.doi.org/10.1016/j.patcog.2009.06.017

44. Xue J-H, Zhang Y-J (2012) Ridler and Calvard's, Kittler and Illingworth's and Otsu's methods for image thresholding. Pattern Recognit Lett 33:793–797. doi:10.1016/j.patrec.2012.01.002

45. Bassel GW, Stamm P, Mosca G et al (2014) Mechanical constraints imposed by 3D cellular geometry and arrangement modulate growth patterns in the Arabidopsis embryo. Proc Natl Acad Sci U S A 111:8685–8690

46. Maška M, Ulman V, Svoboda D et al (2014) A benchmark for comparison of cell tracking algorithms. Bioinformatics 30:1609–1617. doi:10.1093/bioinformatics/btu080

Chapter 14

Automated Analysis of Intracellular Dynamic Processes

Yao Yao*, Ihor Smal*, Ilya Grigoriev, Maud Martin, Anna Akhmanova, and Erik Meijering

Abstract

The study of intracellular dynamic processes is of fundamental importance for understanding a wide variety of diseases and developing effective drugs and therapies. Advanced fluorescence microscopy imaging systems nowadays allow the recording of virtually any type of process in space and time with super-resolved detail and with high sensitivity and specificity. The large volume and high information content of the resulting image data, and the desire to obtain objective, quantitative descriptions and biophysical models of the processes of interest, require a high level of automation in data analysis. Two key tasks in extracting biologically meaningful information about intracellular dynamics from image data are particle tracking and particle trajectory analysis. Here we present state-of-the-art software tools for these tasks and describe how to use them.

Key words Intracellular dynamics, Fluorescence microscopy, Image analysis, Particle tracking, Trajectory analysis, Feature extraction, Feature visualization, Software tools

1 Introduction

Living organisms depend on a multitude of interconnected dynamic processes that are of crucial importance for their development, functioning, and maintenance [1]. Examples of such processes within the cell include the growth and shrinkage of microtubules to enable intracellular transport and cell division [2], the formation and regulation of focal adhesions needed for cell migration during development and tissue repair [3], and DNA damage repair mechanisms for genome maintenance [4]. Many of the most devastating diseases such as cancer and dementia originate from malfunctioning intracellular dynamic processes, thus making extensive study of these processes of fundamental importance for developing effective drugs and therapies. A powerful tool in this endeavor is fluorescence microscopy [5]. Widely available

*These authors contributed equally to this work

Yolanda Markaki and Hartmann Harz (eds.), *Light Microscopy: Methods and Protocols*, Methods in Molecular Biology, vol. 1563, DOI 10.1007/978-1-4939-6810-7_14, © Springer Science+Business Media LLC 2017

fluorescent proteins and nanocrystals [6] nowadays allow specific labeling of virtually any type of structure or particle within the cell, which may subsequently be imaged in space and over time by a wide range of advanced time-lapse light microscopy imaging techniques [7], with or without super-resolved localization [8]. However, to come to a deep understanding of the biological processes of interest, merely producing pretty pictures of them is not sufficient. Instead, thorough analyses are required, and the large volume and high information content of the image data produced by state-of-the-art fluorescence microscopy techniques call for a high level of automation in these analyses [9–11].

The first step in converting the raw image data of the studied intracellular dynamic process into biologically useful information is to detect each and every fluorescently labeled particle in each and every time point, and then to optimally link the detections between successive time points, resulting in particle trajectories. In recent years, many image analysis methods and software tools have been developed for detection as well as for linking [12]. For a detailed treatment of these we refer to previous works comparing particle detection methods [13–17], particle linking methods [18], and specific combinations of particle detectors and linkers, collectively called particle tracking methods [19]. While particle tracking is a crucial first step, by itself it does not directly produce biologically meaningful numbers. To this end, as a second step, trajectory analysis is needed, which computes a broad range of dynamics features from the trajectories. For this step, there are as yet few automated methods and tools. In the literature, trajectory analysis is typically limited to computing average velocities, traveled distances, or the mean-squared displacement [20]. However, for both discovery and modeling of dynamic phenomena, it is of crucial importance to fully exploit all available information and thus to consider as many features as possible.

Here we describe software tools we have developed for particle tracking as well as for trajectory analysis to facilitate detailed studies of intracellular dynamic processes. We provide comprehensive step-by-step descriptions of how to use the tools along with brief explanations of the theoretical principles of the underlying methods. The tools work with any two-dimensional time-lapse microscopy image and we are in the process of extending them to work also with three-dimensional and multichannel time-lapse microscopy images based on the same steps. All described tools are freely available for noncommercial use and we give an example of their use in analyzing vesicle dynamics. While the particle tracking and the trajectory analysis tools are used together in these examples, they are in fact separate modules and can be easily combined with other tools.

2   Materials

The software tools presented here are plugins of ImageJ [21–24], the most widely used open-source image processing and analysis platform, originally developed at the National Institutes of Health (Bethesda, Maryland, USA). ImageJ and its plugins are written in the Java programming language, which implies that in principle they run on all major computer platforms, including Microsoft Windows, Mac OS, and Linux, as long as an appropriate Java runtime environment is installed. To simplify finding the tools, we refer to a web page (https://github.com/imagescience/SOS-SAID) corresponding to this article which provides the reader with all relevant links.

2.1   ImageJ Platform

There exist various distributions of ImageJ but we recommend using the Fiji distribution [25] as it facilitates keeping up to date with the latest versions of all relevant ImageJ components (*see* **Note 1**). This includes the components (specifically the MTrackJ plugin and the ImageScience and JAMA libraries) that are required to use the two plugins described hereafter. If the reader prefers to use the plain ImageJ distribution, the relevant components must be installed manually.

1. Go to the Fiji download site (follow the link in the mentioned GitHub page) and download the Fiji version pertaining to your operating system (*see* **Note 2**).

2. Unpack the downloaded file in an appropriate place on your computer (*see* **Note 3**).

3. Launch Fiji by clicking the Fiji application (on Mac OS computers) or the executable file within the Fiji root folder (on Microsoft Windows and Linux computers).

4. Update Fiji by running the menu item **Help > Update Fiji** (if the program does not already do this automatically upon first startup). In the resulting **ImageJ Updater** window, click the button **Manage update sites**, select the **ImageScience** update site from the list, click the **Close** button, and finally click **Apply changes** to download the updates.

5. Install the SOS and SAID plugins (as described next).

6. Restart Fiji to activate all downloaded components.

2.2   SOS Plugin

The plugin for particle tracking is called SOS (short for Smart Optics Systems, the name of one of the projects in which it was developed) and is not part of Fiji by default but must first be installed. This is done simply by downloading the corresponding Java archive (jar) file (click the link in the mentioned web page) into the **plugins** folder within the Fiji root folder (Mac users should drag the downloaded file onto the running Fiji application, confirm to save into the plugins folder, and restart).

2.3 SAID Plugin   The plugin for trajectory analysis is called SAID (short for Supra-Analysis of Intracellular Dynamics) and, similar to SOS, is not part of Fiji by default but must first be installed by the user. Again this is done by downloading the corresponding jar file (click the link in the mentioned web page) into the **plugins** folder within the Fiji root folder (Mac users should drag the downloaded file onto the running Fiji application, confirm to save into the plugins folder, and restart).

3   Methods

Analysis of intracellular dynamic processes is accomplished by first applying particle tracking and then running trajectory analysis on the output of the tracking step. Here we detail how to perform these two steps using, respectively, the SOS and the SAID plugins. To begin, launch Fiji and load a time-lapse microscopy image of interest (*see* **Note 4**) using either the menu item **File > Open...** (if the image is a single file containing all time points) or **File > Import > Image Sequence...** (if the time points are stored as separate image files). Make sure the image properties are correctly set by opening the menu item **Image > Properties...** and modifying the listed parameters where necessary.

3.1 Particle Tracking   Particle tracking is generally implemented as a two-step procedure: particle detection and particle linking. The SOS plugin comprises various modules to perform these steps and related operations. Here we limit ourselves to describing the two basic modules: **SOS > Gaussian Fitting** for particle detection and **SOS > Nearest Neighbor Tracking** for particle linking.

3.1.1 Particle Detection   1. Launch **SOS > Gaussian Fitting** to open the parameters dialog (Fig. 1).

2. Specify in the respective dialog fields **Minimum spot intensity (above the background)** and **Maximum spot intensity (above the background)** the expected minimum and maximum intensity of the particles above the local background (*see* **Note 5**).

3. Specify in the respective dialog fields **Minimum stdev (sigma) of Gaussian PSF** and **Maximum stdev (sigma) of Gaussian PSF** the expected minimum and maximum size (in pixels) of the particles as the standard deviation of the Gaussian PSF model (*see* **Note 6**).

4. Specify in the dialog field **Step in the spot intensity range (for greedy search)** the intensity step size used by the search algorithm to find the optimal Gaussian PSF model fit between the minimum and maximum intensity (*see* **Note 7**).

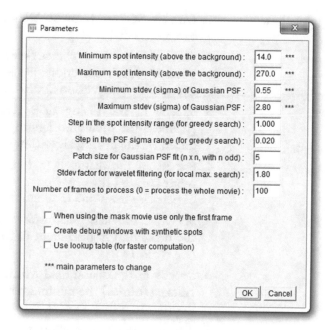

Fig. 1 Parameters dialog of the SOS plugin for particle detection

5. Specify in the dialog field **Step in the PSF sigma range (for greedy search)** the sigma step size (in pixels) used by the search algorithm to find the optimal Gaussian PSF model fit between the minimum and maximum sigma (*see* **Note 8**).

6. Specify in the dialog field **Patch size for Gaussian PSF fit (n × n, with n odd)** the patch size (in pixels) used to sample the Gaussian PSF model (*see* **Note 9**).

7. Specify in the dialog field **Stdev factor for wavelet filtering (for local max. search)** the factor with which the standard deviation of the wavelet coefficients is multiplied in order to determine their threshold (*see* **Note 10**).

8. Specify in the dialog field **Number of frames to process (0 = process the whole movie)** for how many time points (starting from the first) particles should be detected (*see* **Note 11**).

9. The remaining options in the dialog can be left unchecked.

10. Upon clicking the **OK** button of the dialog the specified parameters are stored in a file named **parameters.txt** in the same folder as the image. Then the detection algorithm is automatically started (its progress is shown in the **Log** window) and, after completion, the detection results are stored in a file named **detections.txt** in the same folder as the image. In addition they are stored in the MTrackJ data format, in a file named **detections.mdf**, and MTrackJ is launched for the image to show the detections (Fig. 5). After inspection the Log and MTrackJ windows may be closed.

3.1.2 Particle Linking

1. Launch **SOS > Nearest Neighbor Tracking** to open the parameters dialog (Fig. 2).

2. Specify in the dialog choice **Select file with detections** (at the bottom) which detections file to use in the linking step (by default this is **detections.txt** from the detection step).

3. Specify in the dialog field **Remove tracks shorter than [frames]** the minimum length (in frames) of the tracks produced by the linking algorithm (*see* **Note 12**).

4. Specify in the dialog field **Maximum interframe displacement [pixels]** the expected maximum displacement (in pixels) of particles from one frame to the next (*see* **Note 13**).

5. Specify in the dialog field **Maximum displacement gap factor** the maximum displacement factor for retaining gaps in tracks (*see* **Note 14**).

6. Specify in the dialog field **Minimum time gap for splitting tracks [frames]** the minimum number of time points in a gap in order to split tracks (*see* **Note 15**).

7. The remaining parameters in the dialog (the minimum and maximum spot intensity, the minimum and maximum spot size in terms of Gaussian sigma, and the number of frames to process) have already been described (Subheading 3.1.1) and can be kept as is (*see* **Note 16**).

8. The options at the bottom of the dialog can be left unchecked.

9. Upon clicking the **OK** button of the dialog the specified parameters are stored in a file named **parameters.txt** (the same

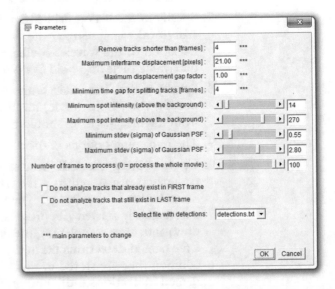

Fig. 2 Parameters dialog of the SOS plugin for particle linking

file as in the detection step). Then the linking algorithm is automatically started (its progress is shown in the **Log** window) and, after completion, the linking results are stored to a file in the same folder as the image, with the same base name as the image file but with extension **.mdf**, and MTrackJ is launched for the image to show the tracks (Fig. 5). After inspection the Log and MTrackJ windows may be closed.

3.2 Trajectory Analysis

Particle trajectory analysis with the SAID plugin can be done in two ways: feature tabulation and feature visualization. In both cases a wide variety of dynamics features (Tables 1–4) can be computed, but in the former case they are presented in tabulated form while in the latter they are visualized in color coding in the image. The corresponding menu items are, respectively, **SAID > Feature Tabulation** and **SAID > Feature Visualization**.

3.2.1 Feature Tabulation

1. Launch **SAID > Feature Tabulation**. If the image for which tracking results are to be analyzed is already open in Fiji, the SAID plugin works with that image (if multiple images are open it takes the one whose window is active), otherwise it opens a file dialog to select an image file. The plugin then automatically loads the tracks file corresponding to the image (*see* **Note 17**), and opens a dialog (Fig. 3) for selecting the features of interest.

2. Select in the left panel, in the tabs named **Particle**, **Trajectory**, **Cluster**, and **Overall** (*see* **Note 18**), which features (Tables 1–4) to compute and tabulate.

3. Select in the **Statistics** panel which statistical measures to compute and tabulate for supra-analysis (*see* **Note 19**) of the selected features. Click option **ALL** to toggle the selection of all other options in the panel.

4. Check in the **Parameters** panel whether the **Sampling time** (frame interval) and **Pixel size** (in X/Y and in Z) are set correctly and make modifications where necessary (*see* **Note 20**). Also set the parameters **Angle ALPHA** (*see* **Note 21**) and **Persistence angle** (*see* **Note 22**).

5. Select in the **Export choices** panel how to export the computed features. Select option **Show tables** to show the results in tabular form in a new window (*see* **Note 23**). Select option **Export to files** to export the results to the specified files (*see* **Note 24**).

6. Upon clicking the **OK** button of the dialog the specified features are computed and exported as indicated by the user (Fig. 5).

3.2.2 Feature Visualization

1. Launch **SAID > Feature Visualization**. If the image for which tracking results are to be analyzed is already open in Fiji, the

Table 1
Particle features computed by the SAID plugin

Feature	Description
Instant displacement	Distance between the particle position in the current frame and in the previous frame (is zero in the first frame)
Distance from origin	Distance between the particle position in the current frame and in its start frame
Displacement from origin	Total distance traversed by the particle from its start frame to the current frame (sum of instantaneous displacements)
Maximum relative displacement from origin	Largest distance of the particle to its position in the start frame within the interval from the start to the current frame
Maximum jump	Largest displacement of the particle between any two frames within the interval from the start to the current frame
Growth or shrinkage length	Difference between the particle displacement from origin in the current frame and in the previous frame
Time point	Frame index
Duration from origin	Time difference between the current frame of the particle and its start frame
Instant speed	Instant displacement of the particle divided by the frame interval
Instant acceleration	Instant speed of the particle divided by the frame interval
Growth or shrinkage rate	Growth or shrinkage length divided by the frame interval
Instant angle	Angular direction (in degrees) the particle moved into from the previous frame to the current frame
Turning angle	Difference between the instant angle in the current frame and in the previous frame
Angular speed	Turning angle divided by the frame interval
Straightness	Mean of the cosine of the turning angle from the start to the current frame
Bending	Mean of the sine of the turning angle from the start to the current frame
Angle with respect to the reference point	Angle (in degrees) of the line connecting the particle position in the current frame with the reference point
Instant intensity	Pixel intensity in the image at the particle position

SAID plugin works with that image (if multiple images are open it takes the one whose window is active), otherwise it opens a file dialog to select an image file. The plugin then automatically loads the tracks file corresponding to the image, and opens a dialog (Fig. 4) for selecting the features of interest.

Table 2
Trajectory features computed by the SAID plugin

Feature	Description
Total distance	Total distance traversed by the particle (spatial length of the track or the sum of instantaneous displacements)
Net displacement	Euclidean distance between the start position and the end position of the particle in the track
Rescue frequency	Frequency of switching back from shrinkage to growth in the track
Maximum relative displacement from origin	Largest distance of the particle to its position in the start frame within the interval from the start to the end frame
Maximum jump	Maximum displacement within the track between any two time points from the start to the end
Confinement ratio	Ratio of the net displacement and the total distance of the track
Displacement ratio	Ratio of the net displacement and the maximum relative displacement from origin of the track
Outreach ratio	Ratio of the maximum relative displacement from origin and the total distance of the track
McCutcheon index	Ratio of the net distance moved in the direction of **Angle ALPHA** (user parameter) and the total distance of the track
Track distance with respect to the reference point	Distance between the center point of the convex hull of the track and the reference point
Total duration	Difference between the end and the start time of the track
Persistence time	Total time for which the angular difference between the net direction of the track and its instant directions is less than the **Persistence angle** (user parameter)
Mean curvilinear speed	Mean of the instant speeds computed over the track (equal to the mean speed if the frame rate is constant)
Mean speed	Ratio of the total distance and the total duration of the track
Mean straight line speed	Ratio of the net displacement and the total duration of the track
Linearity of forward progression	Ratio of the mean straight line speed and the mean curvilinear speed of the track
Straightness of velocity	Ratio of the mean straight line speed and the mean angular speed of the track
Mean acceleration	Mean of the instant acceleration of the particle computed over the track
Mean growth or shrinkage rate	Mean growth or shrinkage rate of the particle computed over the track
Net direction	Angle of the line connecting the start and end positions of the track

(continued)

Table 2
(continued)

Feature	Description
Angular change rate	Mean of the turning angles divided by the total distance
Angular symmetry	Difference between the angle of the line from the start point to the middle point, and the angle of the line from the end point to the middle point of the track
Angular directionality	Ratio of the sum of the turning angles that are centrally located in the turning angles histogram and the total sum of turning angles computed over the track
Straightness	Mean of the cosine of the turning angle from the start to the end of the track
Bending	Mean of the sine of the turning angle from the start to the end of the track
Angle with respect to the reference point	Angle between the line from the start point to the end point of the track, and the line from the reference point to the end point
Perimeter	Total distance plus net displacement of the track
Area	Area of the polygonal shape made up by the track when connecting its start and end points
Area change rate	Area divided by the total duration of the track
Area change rate CV	Area of the convex hull divided by the total duration of the track
Convexity	Ratio of the perimeter of the convex hull of the track and the perimeter of the track
Concavity	Reciprocal of convexity
Solidity	Ratio of the area of the track and the area of the convex hull of the track
Roundness	Area of the track times 4π divided by the square of the perimeter of the convex hull of the track
Compactness	Square of the perimeter divided by 4π times the area of the track
Circularity	Reciprocal of compactness
Rectangularity	Area of the track divided by the area of the minimum bounding rectangle
Eccentricity	Ratio of the lengths of the major and minor axes of the minimum bounding rectangle
Ellipticity	One mines the eccentricity
Elongation	Binary logarithm of the eccentricity
Dispersion	Binary logarithm of the ratio between π times the major axis length times the minor axis length and the convex hull area of the track
Sphericity	Ratio of the areas of the inscribed and the circumscribed circles of the convex hull of the track

Table 3
Cluster features computed by the SAID plugin

Feature	Description
Mean distance between tracks	Mean of the distance between the convex hull centers of two tracks computed over all possible track pairs within the cluster
MSD	Mean squared displacement computed over all tracks in the cluster
Area	Area of the convex hull of all tracks in the cluster
Track area rate	Number of tracks divided by the area of the convex hull of all tracks within the cluster
Rectangularity	Area of the cluster divided by the area of the minimum bounding rectangle of the cluster
Eccentricity	Ratio of the lengths of the major and minor axes of the minimum bounding rectangle of the cluster
Ellipticity	One mines the eccentricity
Elongation	Binary logarithm of the eccentricity
Dispersion	Binary logarithm of the ratio between π times the major axis length times the minor axis length and the convex hull area of the cluster
Sphericity	Ratio of the areas of the inscribed and the circumscribed circles of the convex hull of the cluster

Table 4
Overall features computed by the SAID plugin

Feature	Description
Mean distance between clusters	Mean of the distance between the convex hull centers of two clusters computed over all possible cluster pairs
MSD	Mean squared displacement computed over all tracks
Area	Area of the convex hull of all tracks
Track area rate	Number of tracks divided by the area of the convex hull of all tracks
Rectangularity	Area divided by the area of the minimum bounding rectangle of all tracks
Eccentricity	Ratio of the lengths of the major and minor axes of the minimum bounding rectangle of all tracks
Ellipticity	One mines eccentricity
Elongation	Binary logarithm of eccentricity
Dispersion	Binary logarithm of the ratio between π times the major axis length times the minor axis length and the convex hull area of all tracks
Sphericity	Ratio of the areas of the inscribed and the circumscribed circles of the convex hull of all tracks

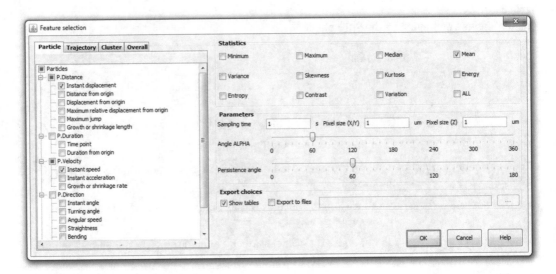

Fig. 3 Parameters dialog of the SAID plugin for feature tabulation

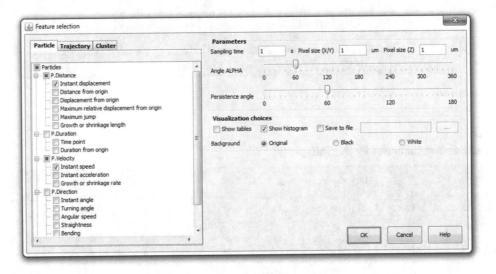

Fig. 4 Parameters dialog of the SAID plugin for feature visualization

2. Select in the left panel, in the tabs named **Particle**, **Trajectory**, and **Cluster**, which features (Tables 1–3) to compute and visualize.

3. Check in the **Parameters** panel whether the **Sampling time** (frame interval) and **Pixel size** (in X/Y and in Z) are set correctly and make modifications where necessary (*see* **Note 20**). Also set the parameters **Angle ALPHA** (*see* **Note 21**) and **Persistence angle** (*see* **Note 22**).

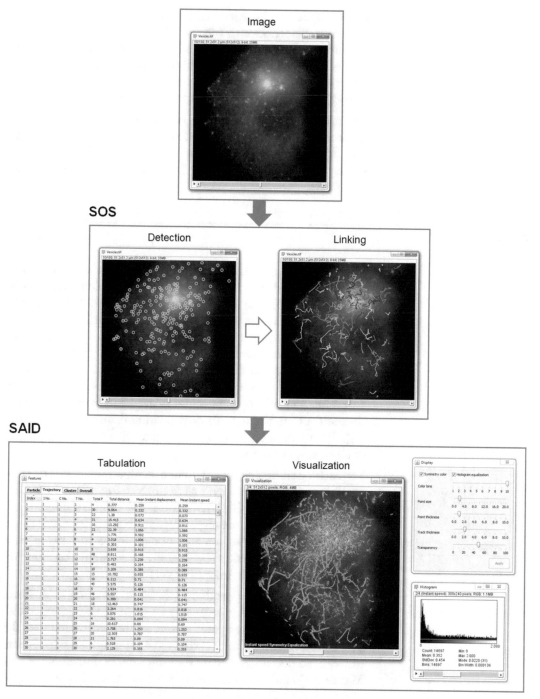

Fig. 5 Example of vesicle tracking using SOS and trajectory analysis using SAID

4. Select in the **Visualization choices** panel how to visualize the computed features. By default the plugin creates a new image stack window, with as many slices as the number of features selected, visualizing the results. The background value in the

slices is specified by selecting **Original** (*see* **Note 25**), **Black**, or **White**. Select **Save to file** to also save the stack to the specified image file. Select option **Show tables** to also show the results in tabular form in a new window (*see* **Note 23**). And select option **Show histogram** to also show for each selected feature the histogram of values.

5. Upon clicking the **OK** button of the dialog the specified features are computed and visualized as indicated by the user (Fig. 5). On the left side of the new image window a dialog is shown that allows to further fine-tune the visualization (*see* **Note 26**).

4 Notes

1. The presented plugins should in principle work with any recent distribution of ImageJ but compatibility problems may occur in the future as the plugins are updated and may become dependent on newer versions of specific ImageJ components. Plain ImageJ requires the user to personally keep track of this and to update the relevant components manually when needed. By contrast, the Fiji distribution of ImageJ has an automated updating system. Every time Fiji is launched it checks whether a new version of any component is available from the update sites and offers the user to download and install it automatically. We recommend staying up to date with the latest versions of all components.

2. For each operating system the Fiji download site offers the latest Fiji version bundled with a specific version of the Java runtime environment (JRE) to ensure full compatibility of all components. Since not every computer has a JRE installed by default, and because in practice not all Fiji components may work with all Java versions by default, we strongly recommend downloading a JRE-bundled Fiji version.

3. Fiji is distributed as a portable application, meaning there is no need to run an installer but only to unpack the downloaded file, after which the program is immediately ready for use. Be sure to unpack into a folder where the program has permission to write, so that it can update its components. For example, on Microsoft Windows, it is strongly recommended to avoid system folders (such as C:\Program Files).

4. It is best to have images in the tagged image file format (TIFF) as it is a widely accepted file format that allows lossless storage of image data along with its metadata. That said, Fiji is able to read a large variety (> 100) of image file formats through the Bio-Formats library [26], including proprietary file formats of many microscope manufacturers.

5. The local background intensity around the spots is automatically estimated by the SOS plugin. This is done by taking the median of the pixels that directly touch the n × n patch defined in **step 6** of Subheading 3.1.1. Thus the user needs to specify only how much the intensity of the particles is expected to rise above the background. Estimates for the minimum and maximum particle intensity above the background can be obtained by studying the intensity profiles of straight lines through various representative spots. This is done by selecting the straight-line drawing tool in the Fiji toolbar, then drawing a line, and running the Fiji menu item **Analyze > Plot Profile**.

6. To discriminate between true particles and noise the SOS plugin uses a weighted least-squares Gaussian fitting algorithm [27]. This is justified by the fact that intracellular particles are typically smaller than the optical resolution limit of the microscope, as a result of which their intensity profiles in the images resemble the microscope's point-spread function (PSF), which in turn can be modeled very accurately by a Gaussian [28]. The expected particle size (sigma) in the images can be computed directly from the Gaussian PSF model corresponding to the type of microscope used [28], in which case the minimum and maximum can be taken to be, e.g., minus or plus 50 % around this value. Alternatively, estimates of the minimum and maximum particle size (sigma) can be obtained by studying the intensity profiles of straight lines through various representative spots (drawn as described in **Note 5**). The standard deviation (sigma) of a Gaussian-like intensity profile is roughly half of the width of the profile halfway between the minimum and maximum intensity.

7. The smaller the intensity step size, the more accurate the fit can be, but also the more time and memory is needed for the computations. A typical step size is 1 intensity unit for 8-bit images and 10 (or up to 100, depending on the particle intensity range) for 16-bit images.

8. The smaller the sigma step size, the more accurate the fit can be, but also the more time and memory is needed for the computations. A typical sigma step size is 1/100th of the range between the minimum and maximum expected particle size (sigma in pixels).

9. Depending on the pixel size of the image, particles may cover more or fewer pixels. In the case of subresolution particles and Nyquist pixel sampling, a patch size of 5 × 5 pixels should theoretically be adequate. Alternatively, the user may visually inspect the particle spots in the image to get a practical estimate of their size in pixels. But in order to ensure symmetry, the patch width and height (n) must always be an odd number.

10. To save computation time, Gaussian fitting in the SOS plugin is not applied to every possible location in the image, but only to the local maxima found by wavelet filtering. Specifically, a three-scale isotropic undecimated wavelet transform [29] is computed, and the wavelet coefficients of the second and third scales below a given threshold are discarded, while the remaining coefficients are summed to yield a reconstructed image with reduced noise and low-frequency background variation. The threshold for each scale is equal to the specified factor times the standard deviation of the wavelet coefficients at that scale. Typical values for this factor are 1.5–2.5 depending on the signal-to-noise ratio (SNR). For images with high SNR (> 5) this factor can be as high as 3.0, but in practice, due to variable fluorescence levels and noise, particles may appear as rather dim spots, and to include these spots the factor should be lowered accordingly. This likely also results in more false-positive detections, but most of these are filtered out in the subsequent particle linking step (Subheading 3.1.2). Local maxima in the reconstructed image after wavelet filtering are taken as the candidate particle positions for the fitting procedure.

11. To save computation time in trying different parameter values for particle detection, it could be handy to process only a few time points at first. Once the user is satisfied with the results, particle detection can be applied to all time points (by setting this parameter to 0).

12. Depending on the (unknown) errors made in the particle detection step and the complexity of the (true) particle motion, shorter tracks may be more suspicious or erroneous than longer tracks. This parameter allows the user to set a threshold on the minimum length of the tracks returned by the linking step (shorter tracks are discarded).

13. For the linking of detections to generate tracks, the SOS plugin uses a gated nearest-neighbor assignment procedure [18]. That is, a detection in one frame is in principle linked to the spatially nearest detection in the next frame, but only if the distance between them is less than the specified maximum interframe displacement (the gate radius).

14. The construction of tracks [18] starts by forming short track fragments consisting solely of detections in successive frames that fall within the gate (*see* **Note 13**). By definition these fragments do not contain gaps. Subsequently, any two track fragments are merged to form a longer track if the distance between the end (the temporally last position) of one fragment and the start (the temporally first position) of another is less than the specified factor times the maximum interframe displacement. This process is repeated to create full tracks, which may contain any number of shorter and longer gaps.

15. If a full track (*see* **Note 14**) contains a gap consisting of the specified number of successive time points or more, the track is split into two parts around that gap. That is, the part up to and including the last detection before the gap, and the part starting from the first detection after the gap, become two separate tracks. This is repeated for all such gaps in a track.

16. These parameters are repeated here so that the user can refine the detections without having to rerun the detection algorithm.

17. A prerequisite for both SAID modules is that there exists a file with tracking results corresponding to the image file for which the analysis is to be performed. This file should have the same base name as the image file but with extension **.mdf** (MTrackJ Data File) or **.xml** (eXtensible Markup Language) for SAID to load it automatically, otherwise a dialog is opened for the user to select a file. The former file format is produced by the SOS plugin (and can be loaded by MTrackJ) while the latter is produced by various alternative tracking tools. In addition to the MDF format the SAID plugin is able to read tracking results in XML format from the Particle Tracking Challenge [19], TrackMate [24], and Icy [30]. If a track in the loaded file contains gaps (particle coordinates are missing for some time points between the start and end of the track), they are automatically filled using linear interpolation from the time points before and after the gap for which particle positions are available.

18. Four levels of features are computed by SAID. The **Particle** level concerns features computed per individual track point while the **Trajectory** level concerns features and statistics computed over all the points in individual tracks. The **Cluster** level concerns features computed over clusters (groups) of tracks. By default all tracks produced by SOS are in one cluster but some particle tracking programs may produce multiple clusters (e.g., they can be manually created in MTrackJ). Finally, the **Overall** level considers all clusters (all tracks) together.

19. For each particle feature selected in the left panel, the selected statistics are computed at the trajectory level (over all the points within the track), at the cluster level (over all the tracks within a cluster), and overall (over all the clusters together). Similarly, for each selected trajectory feature, the selected statistics are computed at the cluster level and overall. And for each selected cluster feature the selected statistics are computed overall.

20. The initially shown values for the sampling time and pixel size are taken from the image metadata and are the same as shown in the Fiji menu **Image > Properties...** If the image metadata does not provide this information the parameters default to 1.

21. Parameter **Angle ALPHA** is needed to compute the McCutcheon index (Table 2).

22. Parameter **Persistence angle** is needed to compute the persistence time (Table 2).

23. In the resulting tables window the user can change the order of the columns and the order (ascending or descending) of the values listed in the columns.

24. A separate file is produced for each of the tabs in the left panel, i.e., for particles (P), trajectories (T), clusters (C), and overall (O). The values in the files are comma-separated so that they can be easily imported in a spreadsheet program such as Microsoft Excel.

25. With this option the background in the visualization result is the original image information shown as a maximum intensity projection over time. It may happen that initially the image information is barely visible. To improve the brightness and contrast of the image, use the Fiji menu item **Image > Adjust > Brightness/Contrast...**

26. Option **Symmetry color** determines whether or not the coloring for the various directional features (such as instant angle, net direction, angular symmetry, turning angle, angular speed) is the same if angles are symmetric (i.e., if they differ by 180°). Option **Histogram equalization** determines whether or not the number of tracks is more or less the same for each color shown. If not selected, the color for each feature value is determined by linear scaling between the minimum and maximum value, and subsequent binning, which may cause very uneven numbers of tracks for the different bins. **Color bins** determines the number of color bins used. The corresponding color legend, from red (maximum value) to blue (minimum value), is shown in the top-left corner of the image window. Interpolated points (originally gaps) and their feature values are shown in gray. **Point size** determines the size (in pixels) with which track points are drawn, while **Point thickness** and **Track thickness** determine the line stroke thickness with which points and tracks are drawn, respectively. Finally, the **Transparency** parameter determines the transparency with which objects (points, tracks, legends) are drawn. All graphical objects are drawn as overlays and can be studied in more detail by zooming in (using the magnifying glass).

Acknowledgments

This work was supported by the Dutch Technology Foundation (STW Grants 10443 and 13391).

References

1. Moser M, Frühwirth M, Kenner T (2008) The symphony of life: importance, interaction, and visualization of biological rhythms. IEEE Eng Med Biol Mag 27:29–37

2. Akhmanova A, Steinmetz MO (2015) Control of microtubule organization and dynamics: two ends in the limelight. Nat Rev Mol Cell Biol 16:711–726

3. Spanjaard E, Smal I, Angelopoulos N, Verlaan I, Matov A, Meijering E, Wessels L, Bos H, de Rooij J (2015) Quantitative imaging of focal adhesion dynamics and their regulation by HGF and Rap1 signaling. Exp Cell Res 330:382–397

4. Reuter M, Zelensky A, Smal I, Meijering E, van Cappellen WA, de Gruiter HM, van Belle GJ, van Royen ME, Houtsmuller AB, Essers J, Kanaar R, Wyman C (2014) BRCA2 diffuses as oligomeric clusters with RAD51 and changes mobility after DNA damage in live cells. J Cell Biol 207:599–613

5. Lichtman JW, Conchello JA (2005) Fluorescence microscopy. Nat Methods 2(12):910–919

6. Shaner NC, Steinbach PA, Tsien RY (2005) A guide to choosing fluorescent proteins. Nat Methods 2:905–909

7. Stephens DJ, Allan VJ (2003) Light microscopy techniques for live cell imaging. Science 300:82–86

8. Schermelleh L, Heintzmann R, Leonhardt H (2010) A guide to super-resolution fluorescence microscopy. J Cell Biol 190:165–175

9. Rittscher J (2010) Characterization of biological processes through automated image analysis. Annu Rev Biomed Eng 12:315–344

10. Danuser G (2011) Computer vision in cell biology. Cell 147:973–978

11. Eliceiri KW, Berthold MR, Goldberg IG, Ibáñez L, Manjunath BS, Martone ME, Murphy RF, Peng H, Plant AL, Roysam B, Stuurman N, Swedlow JR, Tomancak P, Carpenter AE (2012) Biological imaging software tools. Nat Methods 9(7):697–710

12. Meijering E, Dzyubachyk O, Smal I (2012) Methods for cell and particle tracking. Methods Enzymol 504:183–200

13. Cheezum MK, Walker WF, Guilford WH (2001) Quantitative comparison of algorithms for tracking single fluorescent particles. Biophys J 81:2378–2388

14. Smal I, Loog M, Niessen W, Meijering E (2010) Quantitative comparison of spot detection methods in fluorescence microscopy. IEEE Trans Med Imaging 29:282–301

15. Ruusuvuori P, Aijö T, Chowdhury S, Garmendia-Torres C, Selinummi J, Birbaumer M, Dudley AM, Pelkmans L, Yli-Harja O (2010) Evaluation of methods for detection of fluorescence labeled subcellular objects in microscope images. BMC Bioinform 11:248

16. Stěpka K, Matula P, Matula P, Wörz S, Rohr K, Kozubek M (2015) Performance and sensitivity evaluation of 3D spot detection methods in confocal microscopy. Cytometry A 87:759–772

17. Sage D, Kirshner H, Pengo T, Stuurman N, Min J, Manley S, Unser M (2015) Quantitative evaluation of software packages for single-molecule localization microscopy. Nat Methods 12:717–724

18. Smal I, Meijering E (2015) Quantitative comparison of multiframe data association techniques for particle tracking in time-lapse fluorescence microscopy. Med Image Anal 24:163–189

19. Chenouard N, Smal I, de Chaumont F, Maška M, Sbalzarini IF, Gong Y, Cardinale J, Carthel C, Coraluppi S, Winter M, Cohen AR, Godinez WJ, Rohr K, Kalaidzidis Y, Liang L, Duncan J, Shen H, Xu Y, Magnusson KEG, Jaldén J, Blau HM, Paul-Gilloteaux P, Roudot P, Kervrann C, Waharte F, Tinevez JY, Shorte SL, Willemse J, Celler K, van Wezel GP, Dan HW, Tsai YS, de Solórzano CO, Olivo-Marin JC, Meijering E (2014) Objective comparison of particle tracking methods. Nat Methods 11:281–289

20. Gal N, Lechtman-Goldstein D, Weihs D (2013) Particle tracking in living cells: a review of the mean square displacement method and beyond. Rheol Acta 52:425–443

21. Abràmoff MD, Magalhães PJ, Ram SJ (2004) Image processing with ImageJ. Biophotonics Int 11:36–42

22. Collins TJ (2007) ImageJ for microscopy. Biotechniques 43:25–30

23. Schneider CA, Rasband WS, Eliceiri KW (2012) NIH Image to ImageJ: 25 years of image analysis. Nat Methods 9:671–675

24. Schindelin J, Rueden CT, Hiner MC, Eliceiri KW (2015) The ImageJ ecosystem: an open platform for biomedical image analysis. Mol Reprod Dev 82:518–529

25. Schindelin J, Arganda-Carreras I, Frise E, Kaynig V, Longair M, Pietzsch T, Preibisch S, Rueden C, Saalfeld S, Schmid B, Tinevez JY, White DJ, Hartenstein V, Eliceiri K, Tomancak P, Cardona A (2012) Fiji: an open-source platform for biological-image analysis. Nat Methods 9:676–682

26. Linkert M, Rueden CT, Allan C, Burel JM, Moore W, Patterson A, Loranger B, Moore J, Neves C, Macdonald D, Tarkowska A, Sticco

C, Hill E, Rossner M, Eliceiri KW, Swedlow JR (2010) Metadata matters: access to image data in the real world. J Cell Biol 189:777–782

27. Thompson RE, Larson DR, Webb WW (2002) Precise nanometer localization analysis for individual fluorescent probes. Biophys J 82:2775–2783

28. Zhang B, Zerubia J, Olivo-Marin JC (2007) Gaussian approximations of fluorescence microscope point-spread function models. Appl Optics 46:1819–1829

29. Olivo-Marin JC (2002) Extraction of spots in biological images using multiscale products. Pattern Recognit 35:1989–1996

30. de Chaumont F, Dallongeville S, Chenouard N, Hervé N, Pop S, Provoost T, Meas-Yedid V, Pankajakshan P, Lecomte T, Montagner YL, Lagache T, Dufour A, Olivo-Marin JC (2012) Icy: an open bioimage informatics platform for extended reproducible research. Nat Methods 9:690–696

Chapter 15

Quantitative Image Analysis of Single-Molecule mRNA Dynamics in Living Cells

José Rino, Ana C. de Jesus, and Maria Carmo-Fonseca

Abstract

Single mRNA molecules can be imaged in living cells by a method that consists in genetically inserting binding sites for a bacteriophage protein in the gene of interest. The resulting reporter transgene is then integrated in the genome of cells that express the phage protein fused to a fluorescent tag. Upon transcription, binding of the fluorescent protein to its target sequence makes the RNA visible. With this approach it is possible to track, in real time, the life cycle of a precursor mRNA at the site of transcription in the nucleus and transport of mature mRNA to the cytoplasm. In order to measure the fluorescence associated with individual RNA molecules over time, we developed a semi-automated quantitative image analysis tool termed STaQTool. We describe in detail the implementation and application of the STaQTool software package, which is a generic tool able to process large 4D datasets allowing quantitative studies of different steps in gene expression.

Key words Live-cell imaging, Single-molecule, Fluorescence microscopy, Fluorescence quantification, RNA splicing

1 Introduction

Accuracy in all steps of gene expression is vital for cellular and organismal integrity. Yet a surprising revelation of RNA imaging studies was the occurrence of random fluctuations in transcription of individual genes [1–3]. Stochastic fluctuations are likely important for biological plasticity and many studies link stochastic gene expression with cell-fate decisions during development of higher eukaryotes. There is also evidence that aging is correlated with increased noise in gene expression. An outstanding question is how cells control and tolerate noise in each step of gene expression, from transcription to pre-mRNA processing and translation. Recent developments in imaging

Electronic supplementary material: The online version of this chapter (doi: 10.1007/978-1-4939-6810-7_15) contains supplementary material, which is available to authorized users.

Yolanda Markaki and Hartmann Harz (eds.), *Light Microscopy: Methods and Protocols*, Methods in Molecular Biology, vol. 1563, DOI 10.1007/978-1-4939-6810-7_15, © Springer Science+Business Media LLC 2017

strategies capable of monitoring in real time the dynamic behavior of single molecules in living cells [4–6] are likely to pave the way for future discoveries on this topic.

RNAs were first visualized in living cells by genetic insertion of the binding sites for the MS2 bacteriophage coat protein in a reporter gene; the resulting RNAs became visible upon binding of the MS2 coat protein fused to a fluorescent tag such as GFP [7]. Insertion of the MS2 binding sites in the terminal exon of reporter genes revealed kinetic properties of the entire mRNA life cycle, from transcription to transport in the nucleus and export to the cytoplasm [8, 9], while insertion of binding sites for phage coat proteins in introns has been used to visualize splicing in real time [10, 11]. These studies analyzed an ensemble population of pre-mRNAs synthesized from a gene cluster comprising multiple copies of the reporter gene. Thus, multiple nascent RNAs were simultaneously detected, necessitating a modelling approach to infer kinetic information. To circumvent these significant limitations and potential problems in data interpretation, we developed a strategy that permits direct tracking of single pre-mRNA molecules in live cells [12].

Briefly, our protocol starts with construction of a reporter gene that is integrated as a single copy in the genome of human cells. Cells are then transiently transfected to express fluorescent fusion proteins and maintained live in a spinning disk confocal microscope stage for time-lapse imaging. Nascent transcripts emanating from the reporter gene are imaged in 4D and the fluorescence intensity at the transcription site is measured as a function of time [13]. Using a spinning disk confocal microscope, stacks of optical sections centered on the transcription site are recorded at 5 s intervals and the total fluorescence intensity (TFI) is calculated for each time point by performing a 2D Gaussian fit on the volume of interest at the Z plane corresponding to the highest intensity value. The multiple processing steps required for image analysis are integrated in the STaQTool software package tool that includes an open-source user-friendly graphical user interface [14]. In this chapter we describe in detail the implementation and application of this tool to quantify the dynamics at the site of transcription of individual precursor mRNA molecules containing a fluorescently labelled intron. Although we focus on intron dynamics, STaQTool is a generic tool able to process large 4D datasets, allowing quantitative studies of different steps in gene expression.

2   Materials

2.1   Software List

1. MATLAB (The Mathworks, Inc.) Compiler Runtime (MCR) version 9.0.1 (2016a) for Windows 64-bit, which can be downloaded   from   http://www.mathworks.com/supportfiles/

downloads/R2016a/deployment_files/R2016a/installers/win64/MCR_R2016a_win64_installer.exe or installed automatically when running STaQTool setup (*see* **Note 1**).

2. STaQTool for Windows 64-bit, which can be downloaded from https://imm.medicina.ulisboa.pt/en/servicos-e-recursos/technical-facilities/bioimaging/ (*see* **Note 2**).

3. ImageJ (https://imagej.nih.gov/ij/) and ImageJ Plugin MetroloJ (http://imagejdocu.tudor.lu/doku.php?id=plugin:analysis:metroloj:start) for PSF FWHM calculation.

4. Microsoft Excel, which is required by STaQTool to create results files.

2.2 Installation

1. Install the MATLAB Compiler Runtime.

2. Uncompress the STaQTool_setup.zip file in a temporary folder in your hard drive.

3. Run STaQTool_setup.exe. This will create a new folder (Instituto de Medicina Molecular) in "Program Files" containing all the files required to run STaQTool. If you have not installed the MATLAB Compiler Runtime yet, setup will install it automatically. The software is compatible with 64 bits versions of Windows 7, 8, and 10. You can add a desktop shortcut to the program during setup for easier access.

3 Methods

3.1 Single Spot Tracking

1. The main STaQTool graphical user interface is divided in different modules (Fig. 1). A video tutorial on how to use each one is available (Video S1).

2. Open a time-lapse sequence using "Select LOG file" in the "Single File Processing" section (light blue). STaQTool reads LOG and TIF files generated by the Slidebook 6 software from 3i (https://www.intelligentimaging.com/slidebook.php). The parameter boxes "Timepoints," "Z Planes," "Pixel Size," and "Channels" are automatically updated with the information stored in the log file. The file name is displayed in bold next to "Channels" and the complete file path is shown below. In case you have two channels in different TIF files, the complete file path for both is shown. If you are not using Slidebook, you can create a LOG file with the necessary data acquisition parameters for STaQTool using "Create LOG file" (*see* **Note 3**).

3. StaQTool will automatically select "Single Spot 3D" or "Single Spot 2D" modes based on the number of Z planes. You cannot perform single spot tracking if you have only one time point in your TIF file. A warning message will be displayed if this is the case and "Multiple Spots 3D" or "Multiple Spots 2D" modes

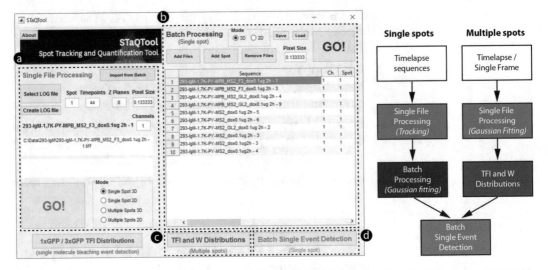

Fig. 1 Screenshot of the main STaQTool graphical user interface (*left*) and workflow for data processing (*right*). The software is divided in different modules: "Single File Processing" (**a**), "Batch Processing" (**b**), "TFI and W Distributions" (**c**), and "Batch Single Event Detection" (**d**) which exchange data and results via Excel files. In this example, a time-lapse sequence from the "Batch Processing" list has been imported to the "Single File Processing" module and is ready to be analyzed in the "Single Spot 3D" mode

will be selected instead. If you do not want to track a single Spot but rather determine the TFI values for multiple spots in each time-lapse frame, select the corresponding "Multiple Spots" mode (2D or 3D) for your analysis. Make sure the appropriate Mode is selected.

4. Set the value for the "Spot" parameter. This variable corresponds to the index of the spot being analyzed. It is set to 1 by default but if your time-lapse contains more than one cell with a spot, you can specify different index values for each spot and analyze each one independently.

5. Click on "GO!" (light blue). STaQTool will open the Timelapse Viewer, where tracking and TFI calculation can be performed for a single time-lapse (consisting of one or two channels) and which consists of a main window with a maximum intensity projection image (3D) or single frame (2D) and additional smaller windows: Z (zoom), FIT (Gaussian fit), Z plot over time (3D only), W plot over time and TFI plot over time (Fig. 2). Start by adjusting the image contrast in the bottom left vertical slider (labelled "MAX"). You can navigate to different time points by using the "Timepoint" slider. If you have two channels, the "<<" and ">>" buttons will allow you to jump to the first time point of the previous or subsequent channel, respectively.

6. Specify which spot will be tracked and analyzed by clicking on its location on the image in the main window. It is not necessary

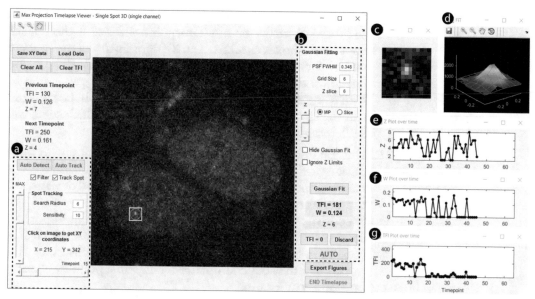

Fig. 2 Screenshot of the Timelapse Viewer graphical user interface (GUI) layout for the "Single File Processing" module in "Single Spot 3D" mode. The main window shows a zoomed in maximum intensity projection image of a cell nucleus with a detected spot (*white* square with *green* circle). Interactive controls allow for adjustment of spot tracking (**a**) and Gaussian fitting (**b**) parameters. Buttons with green text correspond to automated functions. The right side windows show a zoomed in image of the spot (**c**), a 3D surface plot of the 2D Gaussian fit (**d**) and plots of Z slice position (**e**), W (**f**), and TFI (**g**) over time

to click on the spot with pixel precision. A white square with a green circle with radius specified in the "Search Radius" parameter will be drawn around the pixel corresponding to the brightest intensity in the area you clicked and its XY coordinates are displayed below the "Click on image to get XY parameters" text. For 2D time-lapse data, the area corresponding to the white square with the spot at its center will be shown in the Zoom window on the top right corner. For 3D time-lapse data, the "Z" window will display the squared area in the Z plane corresponding to the highest intensity. STaQTool can show all spots detected in nuclei present in the image with the "Auto Detect" function, highlighting their position with green circles. If a spot is not detected within the specified "Search Radius," a white square with a red circle indicating absence of a spot will be displayed instead.

7. If you are analyzing a 3D time-lapse sequence, you can switch the image in the main window from maximum intensity projection (MIP) to single slice by selecting "Slice" on the right and adjusting the Z slider to select individual Z-stack planes. You can click on the image to redefine the spot coordinates either in MIP or Slice modes. Use the zoom and pan controls on the top left corner to adjust the image zoom and spot screen size if needed.

8. Spot tracking is automatically performed when you click on the forward arrow of the Timepoint slider and the "Track Spot" checkbox is checked. The XY coordinates of the spot are update for each time point. In the "Spot Tracking" box, you can adjust the "Search Radius" and "Sensitivity" parameters to specify the size of the search area where a spot will be detected and the signal-to-noise ratio threshold above which spots will be detected (*see* **Note 4**).

9. You can also click on "Auto Track" to automatically perform tracking of the selected spot for the entire time-lapse. If the ratio between the mean intensity and the standard deviation of the intensity values inside the search area is lower than the "Sensitivity" parameter, the spot coordinates are not updated. This ensures that whenever a spot is not present the search area remains in the location where the spot was last observed. You can correct the spot coordinates for any time point by clicking on a different location.

10. After you finish tracking the spot for all time points, press "Save XY data." This will save the spot coordinates in an Excel file which is associated with the TIF file you are analyzing (*see* **Note 5**).

11. If you are working with two channels and have just defined the XY coordinates for the first channel, you can select the first time point of the second channel by pressing ">>" and use the "Load XY Other Channel" button to load the spot coordinates which correspond to the first channel and apply them to the second channel as well. This function is only available in two-channel time-lapses. Press "Save XY data" to save the spot coordinates for the second channel as well.

12. If you do not want to perform Gaussian fitting at this time, you can exit the Timelapse Viewer and go back to the main user interface by selecting the "End Timelapse" checkbox. You can later start the Timelapse Viewer for a particular time lapse and use the "Load Data" button to load the XY coordinates you have exported previously. Alternatively, you can use the Batch Processing mode to perform Gaussian fitting on several time-lapse sequences.

3.2 Single Spot Gaussian Fitting

1. Set the Gaussian Fitting parameters. The "PSF FWHM" is the full-width at half-maximum of the Point Spread Function which can be determined for your particular system by imaging sub-diffraction beads (e.g., 170 nm in diameter) and using MetroloJ (http://imagejdocu.tudor.lu/doku.php?id=plugin:analysis:metroloj:start), a plugin for ImageJ that analyzes the acquired Point Spread Functions to determine the resolution in x, y, z. MetroloJ outputs a pdf report file with a table where you can check the FWHM value for the objective you used. STaQTool

automatically sets the grid size to twice the value of the PSF FWHM, taking into account the pixel size (*see* **Note 6**).

2. If you are analyzing a 3D time-lapse sequence, the "Z Slice" parameter will be present and corresponds to the Z slice where the spot is brightest. You can use the Z slider and change the Z slice where Gaussian fitting is performed (*see* **Note 7**).

3. By default, Gaussian fitting will not be performed if a spot has not been detected (indicated by a red circle in the search area) or if the brightest spot is in the first or last slice of a Z-stack (for 3D time-lapse sequences). To override these rules, uncheck the "Filter" checkbox and check the "Ignore Z limits," respectively (*see* **Note 8**).

4. Click "Gaussian Fit" to perform a Gaussian fitting on the selected spot for the current time point. The TFI, Gaussian Width (W), and Z plane ("Single Spot 3D" mode only) corresponding to the brightest intensity value will be displayed below the "Gaussian Fit" button. The Gaussian fit will be displayed in top right window. The Z plane, W and TFI values will also be plotted in graphs on the right Plot windows, with the current time point shown as black spot with a red outline. The TFI, W, and Z parameters for the previous and subsequent time points are shown on the left of the MIP image, for comparison (*see* **Note 9**).

5. To manually set the TFI value to zero click the "TFI = 0" button. The TFI is automatically set to 0 if the Gaussian peak value is not higher than the intensity standard deviation in the border of the fitting area (defined by the "Grid Size" parameter). To discard a TFI value from the time-lapse data click the "Discard" button.

6. Gaussian fitting can be performed one time point at a time. Alternatively, you can click the "AUTO" button to automatically perform the Gaussian fitting on every time point for which XY coordinates have been defined. Click on "Export Figures" to create images for Z, W, and TFI plots as well as the zoomed in spot and the Gaussian fit for each time point, which will be exported as TIF files.

7. To load previous fitting data for any time-lapse sequence click on the "Load Data" button, which imports the XY coordinates, TFI and W values, Z plane ("Single Spot 3D" mode only), fitting parameters, and other data from the results file. You can delete all data in this results file by pressing the "Clear All" button or just the TFI values (keeping the XY coordinates) by pressing the "Clear TFI" button.

8. Once you have finished calculating the TFI values for each time point, press the "END Timelapse" button to exit the Timelapse Viewer and go back to the main STaQTool user interface.

3.3 Batch Processing Single Spot Time-Lapses

1. In the main STaQTool window, click on "Add Files" to add individual or multiple files to the file list for batch processing. If a specific file has more than one spot to be analyzed, select it in the file list and press "Add Spot" to add another row that corresponds to the sequence you selected but with the spot index increased by 1. You can remove files from the list with the "Remove Files" button.

2. STaQTool will automatically select 2D or 3D Mode depending on the data added to the file list. It is not possible to process both 2D and 3D simultaneously in Batch Processing mode, the software will display a warning message in case you try to do so.

3. Press "Save" to save the file list to an Excel file. You can load it later using the "Load" button (*see* **Note 10**).

4. Check the pixel size for the data in the file list, which is shown in the "Pixel Size" textbox. It is not possible to analyze time-lapse sequences acquired with different pixel sizes, the software will display a warning message in case you try to do so.

5. Press "GO!" (dark blue). This launches the Timelapse Viewer window for Batch Processing where tracking and TFI calculation can be performed for a list of time-lapse sequences (each of them consisting of one or two channels).

6. If you have already performed tracking for the time-lapse sequences specified in the batch mode file list, press "LOAD ALL" to load the tracking coordinates. Check the value of "PSF FWHM" in the Gaussian Fitting parameters and press "AUTO" to perform Gaussian fitting for all time points where tracking has already been performed. To speed up the analysis, check the "Hide Gaussian Fit" option which prevents STaQTool from plotting the Gaussian fit for each time point in a separate window.

7. After Gaussian fitting has been performed, you can review the TFI, W, and Z plots for each time-lapse sequence using ">>" and "<<" to navigate between the different files. You can use the batch mode Timelapse Viewer to perform all the functions available in the Single File Processing mode.

8. To redo Gaussian fitting for all time points in a fully automated mode, press "AUTO REDO". STaQTool will clear the TFI values for all time points where XY coordinates are available (i.e., where tracking has been performed) and repeat the automated Gaussian fitting. Press "END Timelapse" when finished.

9. To review only a particular time-lapse sequence in the batch list, you can also select it and press "Import from Batch" in STaQTool main window to import all the necessary informa-

tion for that sequence from the Batch Processing mode to the Single File Processing Mode, which allows you to open that sequence only and not all the data in the batch mode file list.

3.4 Multiple Spots Gaussian Fitting

1. To perform Gaussian fitting for multiple spots in a single image or a sequence of time-lapse images (2D or 3D), select "Multiple Spots 2D" or "Multiple Spots 3D" in the main STaQTool window after loading information from a LOG file in Single File Processing mode.

2. Press "GO!" (light blue). In Multiple Spots mode, the Timelapse Viewer has no tracking option (Fig. 3). You can specify the coordinates for multiple spots in each time point (by clicking on them) and the software will perform the Gaussian fitting algorithm for each particle while keeping count of the total amount of quantified spots. The results for each time-lapse sequence are automatically saved to an Excel file (*see* **Note 11**).

3. To perform automatic spot detection and Gaussian fitting for a single time-point, press "Auto Fit." To perform automatic spot detection and Gaussian fitting for the complete time-lapse sequence, press "AUTO FIT ALL."

4. You can use the "<" and ">" buttons to review all analyzed spots. To redo the Gaussian fitting for a particular spot, make sure the spot number next to the "Gaussian Fit" button matches the spot you want to redo and press "Gaussian Fit." Press "END Timelapse" when finished.

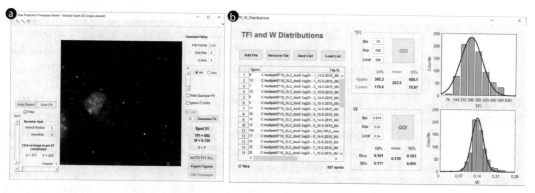

Fig. 3 Screenshots of the Timelapse Viewer GUI for the "Single File Processing" module in "Multiple Spots 3D" mode (**a**) and the "TFI and W Distributions" module (**b**). In this example, all the spots in a single time point of a time-lapse sequence are being automatically detected and Gaussian fitted using the "Auto Fit" function. Spots that were already fitted are indicated by a white circle, whereas spots that have not been fitted yet are surrounded by a *green circle*. The histogram distributions of TFI and W were plotted from a total of 927 spots from 37 results files. Gaussian fitting allows for the calculation of mean TFI and W values, as well as the upper and lower values for 1 standard deviation (68%) and 2 standard deviations (95%) range (Reproduced from [14] with permission from Elsevier)

3.5 Multiple Spots TFI and W Distributions

1. Press "TFI and W Distributions" in STaQTool main window. This brings up a new window where you can specify which files containing multiple spots results data are going to be used to determine the TFI and W distributions and the range of values to be used in the "Single Event Detection" module.

2. Press the "Add File" button to add Excel files from the Multiple Spots Gaussian Fitting to the file list.

3. You can remove files from the file list using the "Remove File" button. The file list can also be saved with the "Save List" button and loaded with the "Load List" button at any time.

4. Set the histogram and Gaussian distribution fitting parameters for TFI and W. "Bin" is the histogram bin value. "Max" is the maximum value for histogram plotting. "Limit" is the upper limit that will be considered for Gaussian fitting: values higher than "Limit" will be discarded from the fitting procedure (*see* **Note 12**).

5. Press "GO!" (light brown) on the TFI box to plot the TFI histogram distribution and perform Gaussian fitting. The mean TFI value and the lower and upper limits corresponding to 68% (one standard deviation) and 95% (two standard deviations) of the population are displayed in the TFI box. Write down these values as they will be used in the "Batch Single Event Detection" module. The histogram and the Gaussian fitting curve will also be displayed.

6. Press "GO!" (dark red) on the W box to plot the W histogram distribution and perform Gaussian fitting. The mean W value and the lower and upper limits corresponding to 68% (one standard deviation) and 95% (two standard deviations) of the population are displayed in the W box. Write down these values as they will be used in the "Batch Single Event Detection" module. The histogram and the Gaussian fitting curve will also be displayed.

3.6 Batch Single Event Detection

1. Press "Batch Single Event Detection" in STaQTool main window. This brings up a new window where you can specify the parameters which will be used to search for cycles of fluorescence gain and loss that correspond to a defined pattern for all the time-lapse sequences in the Batch Processing file list (Fig. 4).

2. Define the number of time points above background levels that constitute the event itself in the "Event Timepoints" box. Specify the number of time points at background level ("ZERO timepoints") that must occur before and after the event. Set the time interval between each time point in the text box "T(s)."

3. Define the "TFI Range" and "W Range" for the event time points. These correspond to the values determined in the "TFI and W Distributions" module for 68% (one standard deviation) or 95% (two standard deviations) distribution values.

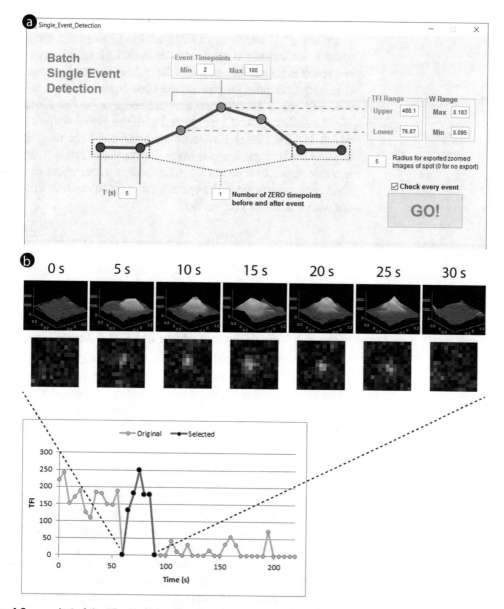

Fig. 4 Screenshot of the "Batch Single Event Detection" GUI (**a**), in which the parameters for the fluorescence patterns that correspond to single events (cycles of fluorescence gain and loss) to be searched in the "Batch Processing" file list can be defined (Reproduced from [14] with permission from Elsevier). STaQTool will generate Excel files with plots of TFI values highlighting identified cycles (**b**). If specified, the software will also export images of the zoomed in spot and the Gaussian fit (*top rows*). In this example, a fluorescence cycle corresponding to a single transcript splicing event with a duration of 30 s is shown

4. Specify the "Radius for exported zoomed images of spot". If set to 0, no images will be exported. Otherwise, zoomed-in images of the spot will be exported for the detected events as squared regions with a radius defined by this parameter.

5. Press "GO!" to start the event detection algorithm. If "Check every event" is checked, you can review all detected events and exclude or include them in the analysis individually. For every sequence in the file list, an Excel file will be created if an event was detected, containing a plot of the time lapse sequence with the detected events highlighted in a different color (*see* **Note 13**). Finally, an Excel file will be created with the global analysis results which include histogram distributions of the Time of Synthesis, defined as the time elapsed since fluorescence intensity starts to increase above background until it reaches a maximum level and the Lifetime, defined as the cycle duration. You can save this Excel file with a name of your choice.

4   Notes

1. The MATLAB Compiler Runtime is required to run compiled MATLAB applications without installing MATLAB. It is available free of charge and allows users to run MATLAB code without the need of purchasing a MATLAB license.

2. If you have MATLAB, you can also download STaQTool MATLAB code as a zip file, expand it to a location of your choice and run it from MATLAB (be sure to change MATLAB starting path to STaQTool folder). Please note that the code might not run properly on MATLAB versions earlier than 2015a.

3. STaQTool works with single-file TIF datasets corresponding to 2D or 3D time-lapse sequences. If you have multiple TIF files (single frame or z-stacks), one for each time point, you need to create a single-file TIF using ImageJ (https://imagej.nih.gov/ij/) or any other image processing software. To create a LOG file associated with a given TIF in STaQTool, fill in the number of time points in "Timepoints," the number of Z slices in "Z Planes" (write 1 for 2D datasets), the number of channels in "Channels" (the maximum number of channels is two) and the pixel size in "Pixel Size." Then click on "Create LOG file" and specify the TIF file (or two TIF files in case you specified two channels) which should be associated with the LOG file. STaQTool will create a LOG file with the same name as the TIF file. You should open this LOG file in "Select LOG file" to proceed with the analysis.

4. Increase the "Sensitivity" parameter if STaQTool is not detecting spots you see in the image. Decrease the "Sensitivity" parameter if the software is detecting spots which correspond to noise.

5. If your TIF is named *filename.tif* and you are analyzing Spot 1 then the Excel file will be named *filename_spot_1_results.xls* and will later also contain the TFI values, fitting parameters and other relevant data.

6. If the software is unable to perform the Gaussian fitting for a very dim spot, decrease the Grid Size and try again.

7. It is advisable to change the image view in the main window from "MIP" to "Slice" when manually changing the Z slice where Gaussian fitting will be performed. Make sure you select the Z slice that corresponds to the brightest spot.

8. Spot detection is performed only inside nuclei. If there are nuclei with different average intensity values, the automatically determined intensity threshold for nuclei detection might be too high for the dimmer ones and spot detection will fail inside of these. If there is a very bright nucleus in your image and spot detection is failing inside your nucleus of interest, uncheck the "Filter" checkbox and manually set the coordinates for the spot.

9. Gaussian fitting can fail if a spot is too dim or very close to a brighter structure such as a nucleolus. In case a spot is not detected, a red circle is displayed in the image. Try do decrease the "Grid Size" and check the "Z" position in the "Slice" viewing mode to avoid neighboring brighter objects. Uncheck the "Filter" checkbox to perform Gaussian fitting even if a spot is not detected by the software.

10. The file list includes the path to the files that will be processed. If you change the location of the LOG, TIF and results files, you need to redo the file list to update the files locations.

11. If your TIF is named *filename.tif* then the Excel file will be named *filename_MULTIPLE_results.xls* and will contain the TFI values, fitting parameters and other relevant data which can be analyzed with the "TFI and W Distributions" module.

12. The "Limit" parameter allows you to truncate the TFI and W data by discarding values higher than a given threshold. This should only be applied if your data distribution has higher intensity values that do not correspond to single mRNAs but to transcription sites or aggregates in time-lapses that have been analyzed automatically.

13. If a TIF file in the file list is named *filename.tif* and corresponds to Spot 1, then the Excel file will be named *filename_spot_1_events.xls*

Acknowledgments

We gratefully acknowledge Tomas Kirchhausen and members of the Kirchhausen lab for advice and insightful discussion. This work was supported by Fundação para a Ciência e Tecnologia, Portugal (PTDC/SAU-GMG/118180/2010; FCT-ANR/BIM-ONC/0009/2013), and the Harvard Medical School-Portugal Program in Translational Research and Information.

References

1. Munsky B, Neuert G, van Oudenaarden A (2012) Using gene expression noise to understand gene regulation. Science 336(6078):183–187. doi:10.1126/science.1216379

2. Sanchez A, Golding I (2013) Genetic determinants and cellular constraints in noisy gene expression. Science 342(6163):1188–1193. doi:10.1126/science.1242975

3. Sanchez A, Choubey S, Kondev J (2013) Regulation of noise in gene expression. Annu Rev Biophys 42:469–491. doi:10.1146/annurev-biophys-083012-130401

4. Knight SC, Xie L, Deng W, Guglielmi B, Witkowsky LB, Bosanac L, Zhang ET, El Beheiry M, Masson JB, Dahan M, Liu Z, Doudna JA, Tjian R (2015) Dynamics of CRISPR-Cas9 genome interrogation in living cells. Science 350(6262):823–826. doi:10.1126/science.aac6572

5. Morisaki T, Lyon K, DeLuca KF, DeLuca JG, English BP, Zhang Z, Lavis LD, Grimm JB, Viswanathan S, Looger LL, Lionnet T, Stasevich TJ (2016) Real-time quantification of single RNA translation dynamics in living cells. Science. doi:10.1126/science.aaf0899

6. Wu B, Eliscovich C, Yoon YJ, Singer RH (2016) Translation dynamics of single mRNAs in live cells and neurons. Science. doi:10.1126/science.aaf1084

7. Bertrand E, Chartrand P, Schaefer M, Shenoy SM, Singer RH, Long RM (1998) Localization of ASH1 mRNA particles in living yeast. Mol Cell 2(4):437–445

8. Janicki SM, Tsukamoto T, Salghetti SE, Tansey WP, Sachidanandam R, Prasanth KV, Ried T, Shav-Tal Y, Bertrand E, Singer RH, Spector DL (2004) From silencing to gene expression: real-time analysis in single cells. Cell 116(5):683–698

9. Shav-Tal Y, Darzacq X, Shenoy SM, Fusco D, Janicki SM, Spector DL, Singer RH (2004) Dynamics of single mRNPs in nuclei of living cells. Science 304(5678):1797–1800. doi:10.1126/science.1099754

10. Schmidt U, Basyuk E, Robert MC, Yoshida M, Villemin JP, Auboeuf D, Aitken S, Bertrand E (2011) Real-time imaging of cotranscriptional splicing reveals a kinetic model that reduces noise: implications for alternative splicing regulation. J Cell Biol 193(5):819–829. doi:10.1083/jcb.201009012

11. Coulon A, Ferguson ML, de Turris V, Palangat M, Chow CC, Larson DR (2014) Kinetic competition during the transcription cycle results in stochastic RNA processing. Elife 3. doi:10.7554/eLife.03939

12. Martin RM, Rino J, Carvalho C, Kirchhausen T, Carmo-Fonseca M (2013) Live-cell visualization of pre-mRNA splicing with single-molecule sensitivity. Cell Rep 4(6):1144–1155. doi:10.1016/j.celrep.2013.08.013

13. Rino J, Martin RM, Carvalho C, de Jesus AC, Carmo-Fonseca M (2015) Single-molecule imaging of RNA splicing in live cells. Methods Enzymol 558:571–585. doi:10.1016/bs.mie.2015.01.013

14. Rino J, de Jesus AC, Carmo-Fonseca M (2016) STaQTool: Spot tracking and quantification tool for monitoring splicing of single pre-mRNA molecules in living cells. Methods 98:143–149. doi:10.1016/j.ymeth.2016.02.005

Chapter 16

Analysis of Protein Kinetics Using Fluorescence Recovery After Photobleaching (FRAP)

Nickolaos Nikiforos Giakoumakis*, Maria Anna Rapsomaniki*, and Zoi Lygerou

Abstract

Fluorescence recovery after photobleaching (FRAP) is a cutting-edge live-cell functional imaging technique that enables the exploration of protein dynamics in individual cells and thus permits the elucidation of protein mobility, function, and interactions at a single-cell level. During a typical FRAP experiment, fluorescent molecules in a defined region of interest within the cell are bleached by a short and powerful laser pulse, while the recovery of the fluorescence in the region is monitored over time by time-lapse microscopy. FRAP experimental setup and image acquisition involve a number of steps that need to be carefully executed to avoid technical artifacts. Equally important is the subsequent computational analysis of FRAP raw data, to derive quantitative information on protein diffusion and binding parameters. Here we present an integrated in vivo and in silico protocol for the analysis of protein kinetics using FRAP. We focus on the most commonly encountered challenges and technical or computational pitfalls and their troubleshooting so that valid and robust insight into protein dynamics within living cells is gained.

Key words Live-cell imaging, Fluorescence recovery after photobleaching, Protein kinetics, Parameter inference, Stochastic hybrid models, Artificial neural networks, easyFRAP

1 Introduction

Advancements in modern microscopy systems and computational methods, coupled with the increasing availability of fluorescent protein variants, have made it possible to visualize, track, and quantify a number of proteins within living cells. Functional imaging techniques such as fluorescence recovery after photobleaching (FRAP) are gaining popularity amongst biology laboratories and are widely used to elucidate the dynamic properties of proteins, such as their expression, interactions, and mobility, in vivo [1, 2]. FRAP is based on the physicochemical principle of photobleaching, the irreversible loss of fluorescence that occurs as a result of

---

*These authors contributed equally to this work.

Yolanda Markaki and Hartmann Harz (eds.), *Light Microscopy: Methods and Protocols*, Methods in Molecular Biology, vol. 1563, DOI 10.1007/978-1-4939-6810-7_16, © Springer Science+Business Media LLC 2017

illuminating a fluorescent protein with a high intensity light. The most commonly used fluorescent protein for photobleaching assays is the enhanced green fluorescent protein (eGFP), due to its brightness, photostability, and non-toxicity, properties which permit its use for monitoring protein activity over large time-frames [3].

During a typical FRAP experiment, a strong laser pulse is applied on a selected area within the cell, resulting in the irreversible loss of fluorescence of the molecules that are found within this region (photobleaching). Standard time-lapse microscopy is used to quantify the intensity of the fluorescence in the region as a function of time before (pre-bleach period) and after (post-bleach period) the bleaching step. The resulting fluorescence measurements, referred to as FRAP recovery curves, reflect the rate at which fluorescence is restored after this perturbation (Fig. 1). If the protein under study is mobile and all protein particles are free to diffuse, all bleached particles will diffuse away from the region and will be substituted by fluorescent particles diffusing back into the region, evident by complete recovery of the fluorescence in the area in a short time-scale. At the other extreme, if all protein

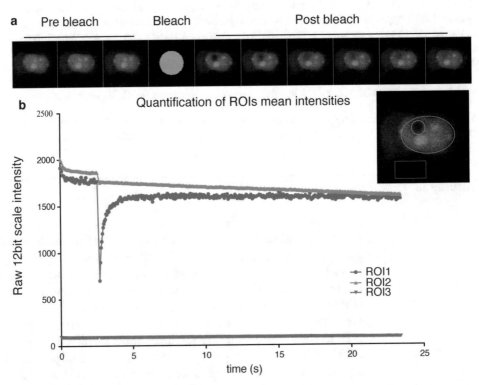

Fig. 1 Example of FRAP experimental images and raw mean intensity curves of the three standard regions of interest. (**a**) During FRAP image acquisition, a number of images are collected before, during and after photobleaching of a defined area. (**b**) Quantification of the mean fluorescence in the regions of interest. ROI1 (*green*) represents the bleaching area, ROI2 (*cyan*) represents the total area of fluorescence and ROI3 (*red*) a random nonfluorescent background area

particles within the bleached region are immobile, no recovery of fluorescence will be observed. Different shapes of the recovery curve reflect the percentage of molecules that are free to diffuse or bind at any given time, as well as their diffusion properties and their binding kinetics within the region of interest. Analysis of FRAP recovery curves can thus allow inference of the kinetic properties of the protein under study such as the rate of diffusion, the fraction of mobile and immobile molecules and the duration of immobilization (residence time) [4].

FRAP is considered a photoperturbation technique; the steady-state distribution of the fluorescence in the region of interest before the bleach is intentionally perturbed by the bleaching step and, by examining the rate at which fluorescence gradually regains equilibrium after the bleaching, conclusions on the mobility of the studied proteins can be reached [5, 6]. For biologically relevant conclusions, ensuring that the experimental setup does not affect cell physiology is pivotal. In addition, the validity of conclusions drawn is heavily influenced by the quality of the raw data, the type of preprocessing steps and the methods and models employed during the kinetic parameter identification process. During the experimental process and before data analysis, raw images and FRAP curves must be carefully inspected and problematic curves, due for example to cell movement, loss of focus, or excessive recording photobleaching, must be removed. Two additional parameters, commonly computed at this stage of the analysis, are bleaching depth and gap ratio; their values reflect bleaching efficiency and total loss of fluorescence respectively and can be used for quality control and assessment of the experiment [7].

Following quality assessment of raw data, raw recovery curves must be preprocessed to remove noise, systematic bias and minor artifacts and produce clean and comparable data. Background subtraction is initially performed and eliminates noise, autofluorescence, and reflected light that contribute to the total detected intensity. Then, normalization of the curves aims to rescale the curves to a reference axis of arbitrary units, typically between zero and one. Common normalization methods include single, double and full scale normalization and correct for technical variations, such as differences in the absolute pre-bleach fluorescence intensities among different cells or differences in bleaching efficiencies [8, 9]. The effect of normalization in the final recovery curves is paramount; once it is properly carried out, technical sources of variation are eliminated and experimental curves can be compared based on their underlying biological variations only.

Quantitative analysis of the data aims to estimate parameters related to the shape of the recovery curve, such as the fraction of immobile molecules (associated with the plateau of the curve) and the time of half-maximal recovery (associated with the speed of recovery). This step is typically performed using standard curve-fitting techniques and provides a first, rough indication of the recovery dynamics, especially useful for differential analysis [7]. However, to characterize explicitly the underlying kinetics of the protein of interest, such as association and dissociation rates and protein diffusion speed, model-based analysis is necessary [8]. Modeling approaches traditionally involve fitting the recovery curves to analytical expressions of fluorescence recovery, containing diffusion, binding and photobleaching parameters [10–14]. In recent years, the ever-increasing power of computational resources has made it feasible to develop and simulate models of diffusion, binding and bleaching at a particle level and within realistic environments [15–19]. Parameter inference can then be performed either via repeated simulations for varying combinations of the kinetic parameters, or through the use of more sophisticated machine learning systems [20].

In this chapter, we present an integrative FRAP protocol from the cell culture to the model-based analysis. After a presentation of the FRAP experimental process, with focus on how to avoid experimental artifacts and problematic data, we present data analysis and kinetic parameter inference steps, emphasizing their interpretability for robust and reproducible biological insight.

2   Materials

2.1   Chemicals and Cell Culture Disposables

Powdered Eagle's Minimum Essential Medium [MEM] (Sigma M3024).

Sodium bicarbonate ($NaHCO_3$).

L-glutamine.

Fetal bovine serum (FBS).

HEPES.

Hydrochloric acid (HCl).

Sodium hydroxide (NaOH).

Phosphate buffered saline 1× (PBS 1×).

Ibidi μ-Dish 35 mm, high glass bottom dish (Cat No 81158).

2.2   Imaging Medium Preparation

We commonly use Eagle's Minimum Essential Medium [MEM] without phenol red for imaging cells grown in monolayers (*see* **Note 1**). Live-cell imaging MEM is prepared as follows:

1. Measure 90 % of the final required volume of water. Water temperature should be 15–20 °C. Use double distilled H_2O, milli-Q grade H_2O or water for injection (WFI).

2. While stirring the water, add the appropriate mass of powdered medium according to the manufacturer's instructions. Stir until dissolved and without heat. The bottle is covered by foil as the medium is light-sensitive.

3. Add 1.1 g $NaHCO_3$ or 14.65 ml of $NaHCO_3$ solution (7.5 % w/v) for 500 ml final volume of medium prepared. Stir until dissolved.

4. Since the pH of the medium may rise during filtration, adjust it while stirring to 0.1–0.3 pH units below the desired pH level, with 1 N HCl or 1 N NaOH.

5. Add extra water to bring the solution to the final volume.

6. Sterilize immediately by filtration with a 0.22 μm porosity membrane.

7. Store at 2–8 °C in the dark.

8. Prior to use, add L-glutamine 2 mM final concentration, HEPES to 25 mM final and FBS as required (*see* **Note 1**).

2.3 Cell Growth and Preparation

Cultured cells should be grown to approximately 80–90 % confluency in glass bottom dishes and incubated in optimal CO_2 and temperature conditions with full medium with the required serum. Before image acquisition:

1. Remove the medium from the cells.

2. Wash well with prewarmed PBS 1× in order to remove any residuals of the full medium that contains phenol-red.

3. Add 2 ml of prewarmed live-cell imaging medium. If other types of glass bottom dishes are used, add the required volume of imaging medium according to the manufacturer.

2.4 Microscope and Imaging Instrumentation

Different microscope setups can be used for photoperturbation experiments. FRAP experiments can be performed using single point scan confocal units, with the disadvantage of lower time resolution. This can be surpassed with the use of resonant scanners available from different microscope companies. Widefield microscopes equipped with a light source capable of photoperturbing fluorescent proteins and coupled with a highly sensitive and fast camera (emCCD or sCMOS) can be used for FRAP experiments. When high acquisition rates, spatial resolution, and low phototoxicity are needed, spinning-disk microscopes may also be used as an appropriate instrumentation setup. Other specialized microscope setups are also possible [5, 21–23]. Since FRAP is a live-cell imaging technique, the microscope setup must include an incubation chamber or a small incubation box on the stage to ensure controlled CO_2 flow, humidity, and temperature.

This protocol is optimized for a Leica TCS SP5 microscope, equipped with an incubation chamber with controlled CO_2 flow, humidity, and temperature, with an Argon laser, 63 × 1.4 numerical aperture (NA) oil objective and equipped with FRAP booster.

3 Methods

This protocol can be applied for FRAP analysis of fluorescent proteins, either transiently transfected or stably expressed in cultured mammalian cells [24–27]. Fluorescent proteins should ideally be expressed to levels lower than the endogenous proteins. High protein expression levels can affect protein kinetics and mask the immobile fraction, due to saturation of binding sites. It should be noted that transient expression levels are often several fold higher than endogenous levels, and care should be taken to ensure that data reflect the behavior of the endogenous protein. Similarly, addition of the fluorescent moiety must be shown not to affect the functionality of the protein under study, for example by showing that the fluorescent protein behaves like the endogenous protein and can replace it. The three fluorescent proteins most commonly used are eGFP, YFP, and mCherry. GFP or YFP can be photobleached with a ~488 nm laser, whereas for mCherry photobleaching can be carried out with a ~561 nm laser. In the following examples, experiments were conducted with the use of eGFP nuclear proteins.

3.1 Microscope Preparation and Experimental Parameter Setup

Proper live-cell conditions (temperature, pH, and CO_2 concentration) should be met during a FRAP experiment. Failing to keep optimal environmental conditions may result in inducing stress responses, altering cellular processes and eventually protein kinetics [34].

3.1.1 Hardware Setup

1. Preheat the incubation chamber of the microscope to 37 °C. Evaporation of the medium should be minimized in order to avoid osmolarity changes and therefore a humidifier of the sample's atmosphere is strongly suggested. This can be easily achieved with the use of a humidity and CO_2 microscope stage box.

2. A 63× immersive lens with higher than 1 NA is optimal for FRAP experiments. If there is a temperature correction ring this should be properly set up. Water, oil, and silica or glycerol immersive lenses are available. The refractive index of the lens and immersive medium should be as close as possible to the refractive indices of the sample (*see* **Note 2**).

3.1.2 Software Setup

1. Set the image bit depth to at least 12 bit.

2. Open fully the pinhole of the confocal.

3. Set the scanning speed according to the total time frame of the experiment (*see* **Notes 2** and **3**).

3.2 Image Acquisition Per Cell

Since phototoxicity can trigger stress responses, it is important to keep recording photobleaching and free radical production as low as possible. For this reason, image acquisition should be carefully executed so that the duration and intensity of illumination are minimized. The total number of images acquired during the time frame of the experiment should be sufficient for an adequate observation of the biological phenomena under study, while avoiding excess acquisition photobleaching and phototoxic events. The experimental setup should be carefully designed so that problematic experimental curves, such as the ones shown in Fig. 2, are avoided.

1. Select nuclei with moderate fluorescent protein expression level at low zoom. Cells with very low fluorescence intensity will produce noisy curves due to a suboptimal signal-to-noise ratio, whereas high expression levels might be difficult to bleach and could affect fluorescence recovery rates due to saturation of binding sites.

2. Zoom in on one selected nucleus and keep the zoom constant through the experiment as it affects the resolution in a confocal laser-scanning microscope. In this example, a 10× digital

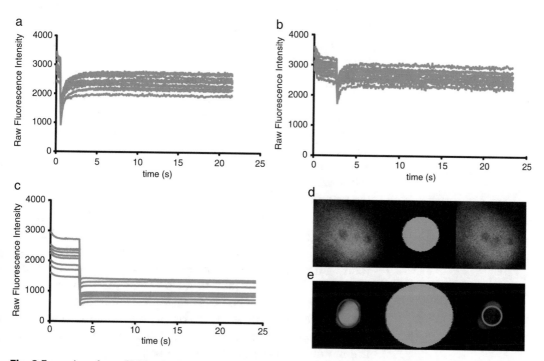

Fig. 2 Examples of raw FRAP experimental curves that should be excluded due to a suboptimal experimental setup. (**a**) Insufficient number of pre-bleach images. (**b**) and (**d**) Unsatisfactory values of bleaching depth as shown in the raw recovery curves (**b**) and the fluorescence levels of ROI1 (*red circle*) in the first post-bleach acquired images (**d**). (**c**) and (**e**) Unsatisfactory values of gap ratio can be recognized by observing the mean fluorescence intensity of ROI2 ((**e**), *green circle*) which indicates that the total fluorescence in the cell is reduced to less than half after the photobleaching step

zoom with a 63×1.4 NA Oil lens and a resolution of 128×128 pixels and full scanning speed at 1400 Hz were used (*see* **Note 3**). Averaging of the image frame should be avoided since it reduces the signal and significantly increases the time interval between image acquisitions (*see* **Note 4**).

3. Find the single middle plain of the nucleus on the Z-axis. The offset of the detector should be set so that background pixels have a mean intensity slightly greater than zero. The gain of the detector should be set up so that the amount of saturated pixels per nucleus is minimized.

4. Draw a circular bleaching region (ROI1) with a diameter of 4 μm, located away from the fluorescent protein expression boundaries, as shown in Fig. 1 (*see* **Note 5**).

5. Select the laser lines, the intensity at which the bleaching will be conducted and the number of bleaching pulses at full scanning speed. To increase the bleaching effectiveness and decrease the time needed to bleach a region, it is recommended to use the zoom-in option at confocal systems during bleaching, and FRAP booster if available. Laser lines selected for bleaching should be chosen according to the transmission spectra of the fluorescent protein under study. In this example, for effective bleaching of eGFP on an SP5 Leica system, 488 nm and 514 nm at 100 % intensity with a single pulse of 60 % of Argon laser was used (*see* **Note 6**).

6. A minimum of 50 pre-bleach images are captured (*see* **Note 7**), followed by a single bleach pulse and a number of post-bleach images until the recovery of the fluorescence reaches a plateau without leading to high acquisition bleaching (Fig. 2, *see* **Note 8**). For pre- and post-bleach image acquisition, laser intensity is set as low as possible (ideally 3–5 % of the lines), in order to avoid recording bleaching and extended phototoxicity during the experiment.

7. Select the experimental time frame and minimal intermediate time step between image acquisitions (*see* **Note 8**). We routinely record 400 postbleach images. For fast recovering proteins, intervals between images are kept to a minimum (0.066 s). It is important to keep the acquisition frequency during an experiment constant; changing the frequency during the experiment will lead to observing intensity variations attributed to photophysical changes and not to differences in the mobility of the proteins (*see* **Note 9**).

8. For normalization purposes, select and quantify in addition to the bleaching region (ROI1), the total area of fluorescence (ROI2) as well as a random background nonfluorescent region (ROI3), as shown in Fig. 1.

9. Save raw quantifications for further analysis in .txt or .csv format and raw images for reference or reanalysis (*see* **Note 10**).

10. Repeat **steps 1–9** to analyze a sufficient number of cells for each experimental time-point. We routinely analyze 50 cells per condition (*see* **Note 11**).

4   Analysis of FRAP Curves

Once the raw experimental data have been exported, analysis of FRAP recovery curves can elucidate the mobility of the proteins under study. For unbiased conclusions on the underlying biology to be made, FRAP data analysis must be carefully executed ensuring the quality of the data and the robustness and accuracy of the computational methods at every step of the analysis. A typical FRAP analysis pipeline consists of the following steps [28]:

1. **Preprocessing** of the raw curves, which aims to eliminate noise, experimental artifacts, and bias so that data from different experiments can be compared.

2. First-level **quantitative analysis**, where a number of parameters related to the shape of the recovery curves are computed in order to provide a first indication of the protein's mobility.

3. **Model-based inference**, where analytical or numerical FRAP models are used to derive estimates of the kinetic parameters, namely diffusion coefficient and association/dissociation rates.

Steps 1 and **2** are typically executed either manually of with the use of dedicated software [29, 30]. Here, we show how this process can be automated using the software easyFRAP (Fig. 3), a standalone application that simplifies data preprocessing and normalization and additionally extracts quantitative parameters associated with protein dynamics from the recovery curves [7]. Modifications of EasyFRAP have been developed which allow estimation of additional quantitative parameters depending on experimental requirements [31].

4.1   Preprocessing and Quantitative Analysis

1. **Installation:** Download and install easyFRAP following the instructions on the website: http://ccl.med.upatras.gr/easy-frap.html. Documentation, source files, and sample data sets are also available.

2. **Data upload:** Once you run the software, upload the raw data in Panel 1 by (optionally) naming the experiment, selecting the data format and selecting the folder containing the files. A large number of single-cell curves under a given experimental condition can be processed simultaneously. EasyFRAP is compatible with .csv, .txt and .xls data formats (different microscopes support different

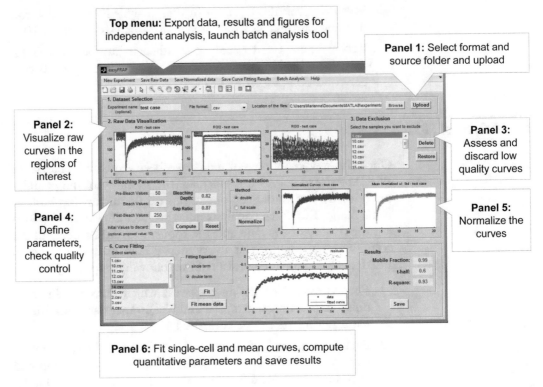

Fig. 3 Main Graphical User Interface of easyFRAP. Different functionalities such as plotting, normalization and fitting, are organized in different Panels

formats), as long as the data files contain measurements from the three regions of interest (Bleaching region—ROI1, total area of fluorescence—ROI2 and background region—ROI3) and a time vector, containing the exact time points of the quantification. Upon clicking the Upload button, easyFRAP checks the data for consistency (e.g., if all data files contain four columns), and plots the raw FRAP curves from the 3 ROIs in Panel 2.

3. **Quality check:** Inspect the plots of Panel 2 for quality; by clicking on them, plots are exported from the main GUI for better evaluation. Curves with intensity fluctuations due to cell movement, high acquisition photobleaching or high background intensity should be excluded (*see* examples in Fig. 4). To discard any problematic curves, select them from the list box in Panel 3 and click Delete (*see* **Note 12**).

4. **Initial values:** Insert the number of images taken before (pre-bleach values), during (bleach values) and after the bleach (post-bleach values) in Panel 4. EasyFRAP checks again the data files for consistency and returns error messages in case of incompatibility. For the reasons explained in **Note 7**, a number of initial values must be deleted from the measurements. Indicate the number of initial pre-bleach measurements to be deleted and press Compute.

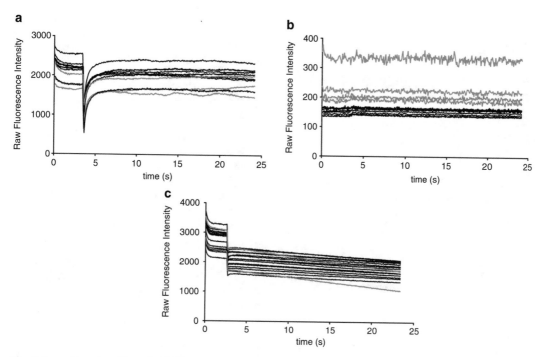

Fig. 4 Examples of problematic FRAP curves that should be excluded, marked in *red*. (**a**) ROI1 (region of interest): Raw recovery curves with fluctuations due to cell movement. (**b**) ROI3 (*background*): Fields of view that have high background noise or very low signal-to-noise ratio should be avoided. Curves indicated with pink should be further evaluated by assessing the corresponding image files for background biases or problematic image acquisition. (**c**) ROI2 (total fluorescence) Experimental curves with high acquisition photobleaching

5. **Bleaching depth–Gap ratio:** After subtraction of the background intensity that aims to eliminate noise, autofluorescence, and reflected light, easyFRAP computes the values of bleaching depth and gap ratio, two parameters associated with the quality of the experimental process. As shown in Fig. 5, bleaching depth reflects the loss of fluorescence in the bleaching region and thus indicates the efficiency of the bleaching; values of 1 indicate absolute bleaching whereas values equal to 0 indicate that no bleaching occurred. Gap ratio reflects the total fluorescence remaining after the bleaching; values of 1 indicate no loss of fluorescence whereas values of 0 indicate total loss of fluorescence (details and formulas in the Appendix). Evaluate bleaching depth as sufficient when approximately 80 % of the fluorescence in ROI1 is bleached. A small value of bleaching depth (smaller than 0.6) indicates insufficient bleaching of the region of interest. Similarly, evaluate gap ratio as acceptable when its value is around 0.8; a small value of gap ratio (smaller than 0.6) indicates excessive bleaching; a large portion of the total fluorescence was

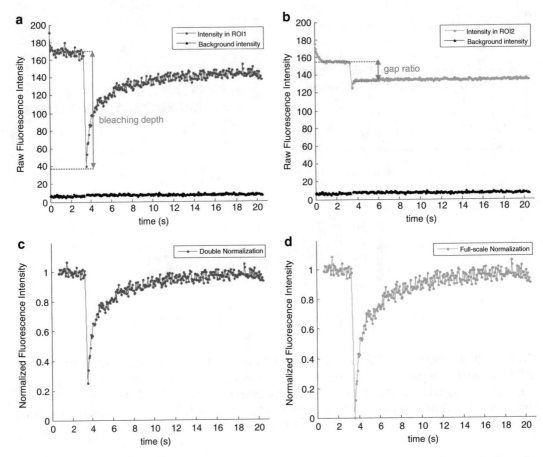

Fig. 5 *Top*: Bleaching depth (**a**) and gap ratio (**b**). Bottom: Results of different normalization methods on the same raw curve, (**c**): double, (**d**): full-scale normalization

eliminated and recovery will appear partial because of lack of available diffusive fluorescent particles (*see* also **Note 13**).

6. **Normalization:** Single cells exhibit variability in their fluorescence levels (e.g., fluorescence intensity of the bleaching region and the total area of fluorescence) as well as the experimental process (e.g., efficiency of the bleaching step). Normalization aims to rescale the data to a reference axis of 0 to 1, removing these effects and enabling the comparison of curves across different cells or different experiments. Double normalization accounts for differences in the starting intensity of the bleaching region and the total fluorescence, attributed for example to recording photobleaching, and full scale normalization additionally corrects for the differences in bleaching efficiencies by subtracting the first post-bleach measurement (see formulas in the Appendix). Proceed to normalize the data by selecting either double or full-scale normalization and pressing the Normalize button in Panel 5. Since full-scale normalization forces all curves to start from zero values, it tends to distort the

shape of the curves, an effect more pronounced for the cases of small bleaching depth. For this reason, we suggest using the double normalization method (*see* **Note 14**).

7. **Quantitative analysis:** Once the curves have been normalized, quantitative parameters can be estimated through standard curve fitting techniques. EasyFRAP computes the mobile fraction, defined as the fraction of bleached particles that are mobile (free to diffuse or transiently binding) and therefore the respective fluorescence recovers during the time-course of the experiment, and the half maximal recovery time (t-half), defined as the time at which the recovery of the fluorescence was equal to half of the maximal recovery (and therefore the time required for 50 % of the mobile molecules to recover, *see* Fig. 6 and the Appendix for formulas). The mobile fraction is associated with the number of molecules which bind or are free to diffuse; a value of mobile fraction close to 1 indicates that the protein exhibits full recovery and thus all the molecules are free to diffuse or bind only transiently, whereas a value smaller than 1 indicates partial recovery attributed to the fact that a fraction of the molecules are bound and are not replaced during the time-course of the experiment. T-half is associated with the speed of recovery; a small value of t-half indicates that the protein reaches its plateau fast because of a high diffusion coefficient and/or small residence times when bound. To compute these parameters, select a single cell from the list in Panel 6 and a fitting equation (single-term or double-term, more information on the Appendix) and press Fit. EasyFRAP proceeds to fit the experimental curve to a parametric equation with one or two exponential terms respectively, plot the fitted curve and residuals and compute the values of mobile fraction and t-half. For each fit, the value of the coefficient of determination (R-square) is also computed (*see* the Appendix). To evaluate the fit, observe the plot of the fitted residuals and the value of R-square; the residuals should be uniformly distributed around 0 with no apparent trend (*see* Fig. 6) and R-square should be close to 1 (*see* **Note 15**). By clicking the Fit mean button, the same process is repeated on the mean of all single-cell curves, providing an indication of the average protein dynamics (*see* **Note 16**). By pressing the Save button and choosing the single cells of interest, easyFRAP repeats the fitting process and saves the results in a separate file for future use (e.g., statistical analysis and plotting).

8. **Top menu:** Use the top menu if you want to start a new experiment, save the raw, normalized data and figures as well as the results of the fitting process in separate files for further use or perform batch analysis of multiple experiments (*see* **Note 17**).

Once the analysis is complete, the values of the estimated parameters can be used as a first-level indication of the underlying protein kinetics. For example, as seen in Fig. 7, proteins with fast

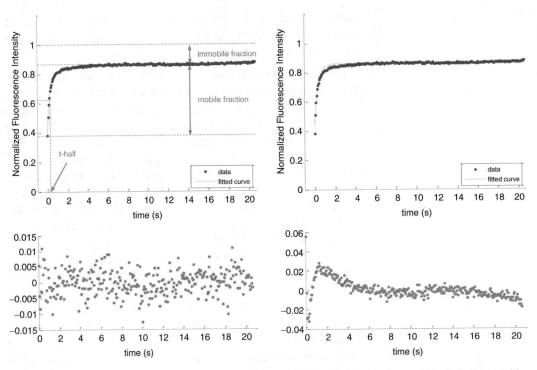

Fig. 6 *Left*: Curve fitting results and plots (*top*: fitted curve, mobile-immobile fraction and t-half, *bottom*: residuals of the fit). *Right*: When the fitting is poor (*top*), the residuals are not uniformly distributed and exhibit a clear trend, such as here for the first post-bleach time points

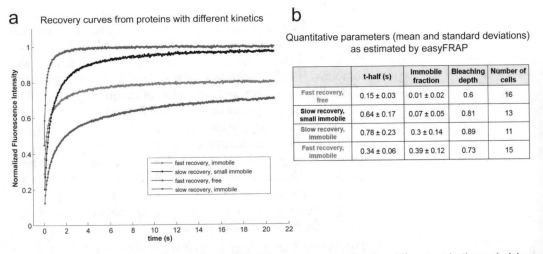

Fig. 7 (**a**) Hypothetical FRAP normalized curves of different shapes, indicating differences in the underlying kinetic parameters. (**b**) Quantitative parameters of the respective hypothetical curves, as derived from the analysis with easyFRAP

recovery are expected to have small values of t-half while proteins with slow recovery will have relatively larger values. Similarly, fully mobile proteins will have a mobile fraction approximately equal to 1, whereas if a percentage of the protein molecules is bound, mobile fraction will be smaller than 1. Although useful in a context of differential analysis, both parameters are dependent on the experimental setup and more specifically on the time frame of the observation [5] (*see* **Note 8**). To overcome this limitation, model-based analysis can identify the physical parameters associated with protein kinetics, such as the diffusion coefficient and the pool of bound and unbound molecules.

4.2 Model-Based Kinetic Parameter Inference

In FRAP literature, traditional model-based approaches involve developing parametric expressions of the physical processes that govern the underlying kinetics, namely diffusion, binding, and photobleaching. For simplification reasons, in each modeling approach a number of assumptions regarding the underlying processes were made, focusing occasionally only on the dominant processes and ignoring the rest (e.g., diffusion vs. reaction models [9, 11, 32, 33]). At the same time, in most models additional simplifications concerning the cell geometry, the properties of diffusion or the number and distribution of binding sites needed to be made. Inference of the kinetic parameters is possible by fitting these parametric expressions to the experimental data; however the robustness of this approach has been disputed since multiple studies fail to agree on the reported estimates, possibly due to the variability in the underlying assumptions [10].

Here, we briefly discuss an alternative approach for parameter estimation from FRAP data, based on the work presented in [20]. Our method is based on numerical simulations of a stochastic model of FRAP recovery [17], coupled to a machine learning step that maps simulated curves to kinetic parameters. As shown in Fig. 8, it consists of two main parts: an in silico training process, where simulated curves with their corresponding input parameters are used to learn the desired mapping, and an estimation process, executed once per experimental curve to derive kinetic parameter estimates with the aid of the abovementioned mapping.

In our stochastic model of FRAP experiments, diffusion, binding and photobleaching are modeled at a particle level in a realistic spatial environment representing the nucleus. Diffusion is modeled by a continuous state representing the spatial coordinates of each particle; its evolution is governed by stochastic dynamics through a stochastic differential equation. The bound state of each molecule is represented by a discrete state that takes a value of 1 if the protein is bound and zero if it is free to diffuse; to capture the stochastic nature of binding events, bind and release propensities are used. Last, the FRAP process is modeled by associating each

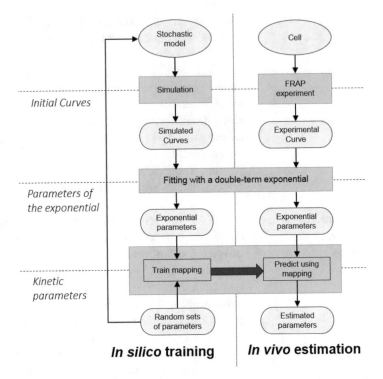

Fig. 8 Simplified representation of the parameter inference method. *Left:* In silico training process to generate the desired mapping. *Right:* In vivo estimation executed once per experimental curve in order to infer kinetic parameters

particle with an additional discrete state representing its fluorescence and assuming that the molecules that enter the bleaching region during the bleaching time interval will get bleached with a probability proportional to the time spent there (more details on the stochastic hybrid model of FRAP experiments can be found in [17, 20]).

Simulations of the model for various combinations of the physical parameters (diffusion coefficient, bound fraction, residence time) give rise to a set of simulated curves corresponding to different kinetics. Then, the simulated curves are fitted to a parametric equation with two exponential terms. This serves as a representation of the curves in a space of reduced dimensions, while at the same time preserving the information of their shape. Last, the parameters of the exponential together with the corresponding sets of physical parameters are used to train an Artificial Neural Network (ANN), which learns the relationships and correspondence between these two sets of parameters. At the same time, a bootstrap process is used to assess the sensitivity of the exponential parameters to the fitting and derive confidence intervals of the mapping. The second part of the method deals with the inference of physical parameter estimates from actual experimental curves. This is achieved by simply fitting the experimental curves to the double-term exponential using the same process as above and subsequently feeding the parameters of the exponential to the already trained ANN. In this sense, the ANN functions as a predictor, applying the knowledge acquired through simulated data to actual experimental data. The same bootstrap process as before is used to derive confidence intervals of the estimates and study local identifiability of the physical parameters.

An illustration of the resulting estimates is shown in Fig. 9, where the inference process was applied to the hypothetical recovery curves of Fig. 7 resulting in clusters of estimates (different clusters correspond to different hypothetical curves, colors same as in Fig. 7). As we can see, estimates from the green protein are located in an area of the space characterized by high diffusion coefficient, small bound fraction and zero residence time, indicating a purely diffusive behavior. On the contrary, estimates of the red and blue proteins are characterized by high residence times, indicating permanent interactions, varying bound fraction (higher for the blue protein, as also indicated by their differences in plateau) and varying diffusion coefficient (the red protein appear faster than the blue). Last, the black protein appears to recover with a slower rate, indicated by small values of diffusion coefficient, and participate in shorter-lived interactions. These observations are in accordance with not only the shape of the curves but also the corresponding estimates from easyFRAP. Moreover, the shape and the spread of the clusters, derived through the bootstrap process described in [20], indicate the confidence intervals and the identifiability of the parameters.

5 Notes

1. Different types of media can be used depending on cell type. For live-cell imaging, media without phenol-red must be used. Live imaging media can be supplemented with 25 mM HEPES to avoid fast occurring toxic effects on cells due to pH changes and fluctuations in CO_2 in the live-imaging chamber [34]. If background fluorescence is a problem, consider reducing FBS.

2. The higher the numerical aperture of the objective and the deeper the structures of interest inside the sample, the more important it is to match the refractive indices of the sample and the immersion medium. Different refractive indices may lead to various spherical aberrations and geometrical distortions of the structures, leading to loss of contrast and definition as well as structural compression or stretch.

3. The scanning speed of the laser scanner in the confocal microscope (also referred to as pixel dwell time) depends on the resolution parameters, namely scan size in pixels and scan area (lens magnification and zoom). High speed and therefore low

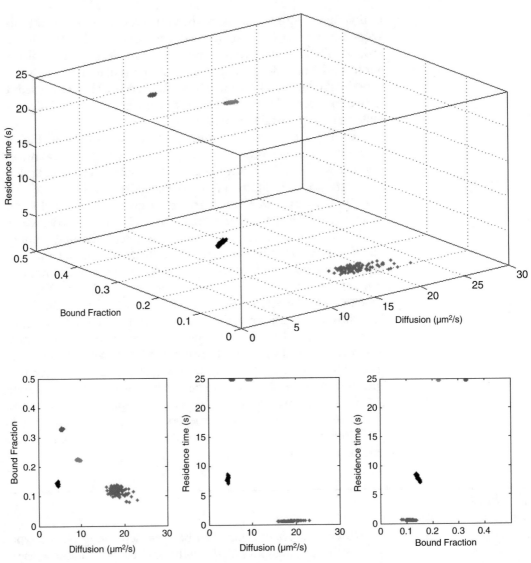

Fig. 9 Kinetic parameter estimates for the hypothetical curves of Fig. 7. *Top*: estimates shown in the three-dimensional space of kinetic parameters (diffusion coefficient, bound fraction, and residence time). *Bottom*: pairwise plots of all respective two-dimensional projections. Different *colors* correspond to confidence regions for the estimates of the different curves

resolution is essential when studying fast processes (time scale of milliseconds to seconds), whereas lower scanning speed and higher image resolution formats can be used when studying processes occurring over larger time scales (time scale of seconds to minutes).

4. In confocal microscopes bidirectional scanning should be active with the proper X axis-phase correction. Bidirectional scanning doubles the speed of the scanning laser, decreasing significantly image acquisition time and thus enabling the observation of

fast-occurring processes. Incorrect phase correction can result in fuzzy images due to misaligned image rows.

5. The size, shape and relative position of the bleaching region (ROI1) can affect both the bleaching effectiveness and the observed recovery. For example, if a very small ROI is used to bleach a free-to-diffuse protein, fast recovery during the bleaching step will result in inefficient bleaching. On the contrary, a large ROI will result in bleaching a significant fraction of the total fluorescence (*see* also **Note 13**). Both will affect the shape of the resulting recovery curve. For a thorough investigation of the effects of different geometries to the recovery curves see [20]. Therefore, size, shape and relative location of ROI1 should ideally be kept constant for all cells to be compared. If however cells with very different sizes need to be compared, one should consider keeping the ratio of bleaching region to total area of fluorescence (ROI1/ROI2) constant among different cells. Such concerns become less crucial when recovery curves are not compared directly but modeling is used to derive underlying kinetic parameters (*see* Subheading 4.2).

6. Additional bleaching pulses can be used, to ensure efficient bleaching. However, increasing the duration of the bleaching steps will lead to fluorescence recovery during the bleaching, and selective loss of fluorescence of the free-to-diffuse fraction from the unbleached region, affecting recovery kinetics. This is utilized in a related photoperturbation technique—fluorescence loss in photobleaching (FLIP).

7. Due to the physicochemical properties of fluorescent proteins, the initial pre-bleach values, corresponding to the first images taken at the beginning of the time lapse, exhibit non-intentional loss of fluorescence in the form of exponential decay. This phenomenon is especially pronounced in the case of high acquisition rates and can interfere with the quality of the identified parameters. For this reason the number of pre-bleach images should be sufficiently large (i.e., **50**) so that fluorescence intensity reaches steady state before the bleach. Then, the first pre-bleach measurements can be deleted during the data analysis steps.

8. The number of post-bleach images recorded and the interval of image acquisition depends on the kinetics of the protein under study. To capture initial fluorescence recovery, which is governed by diffusion and fast on-off binding behavior, images should be recorded as fast as possible, over a few seconds (typically 25 s). To analyze long-lived interactions, fluorescence recovery should be monitored over longer time-frames (over minutes and sometimes over hours). To reduce phototoxicity during long FRAP experiments, the total number of images recorded must be kept low and therefore intervals between images must be increased. Preserving cell physiology is crucial

during a long FRAP experiment. Cell movement is another important consideration in long FRAP experiments—cell type will affect the amount of cell movement while tracking can be used for correct assignment of ROIs. If both initial and long-term behavior needs to be analyzed, separate FRAP experiments must be set up (*see* **Note 9**). The shape of the recovery curve, and therefore curve derived parameters such as immobile fraction and t-half (*see* Subheading 4.1) will inevitably depend to the time-frame of observation. A protein appearing to have an immobile fraction over a short time interval for example, may have recovered fully (no immobile fraction) over a longer period of time, with a concomitant increase in the t-half of the recovery. Model-based protein kinetic inference can be used to derive underlining protein behavior, irrespective of experimental setup (*see* Subheading 4.2)

9. All fluorescent proteins fluctuate between a dark state and a fluorescent state [35]. Due to the illumination, during image acquisition a fraction of the fluorescent proteins are driven to a dark state. Changes in the image acquisition step and consequently on the illumination frequency result in alterations of the equilibrium between the dark and fluorescence state of the proteins and therefore to a change in fluorescence intensity, observed as a discrete step coinciding with the change in the image acquisition parameters.

10. ROI selection and quantification can be carried out at the time of the experiment using microscope software, or raw images can be saved and analyzed with image analysis software (such as FIJI). This is particularly important in long FRAP experiments, when ROI tracking may be necessary due to cell movement. In any case, saving the raw images is essential for quality control later in the analysis.

11. Cell-to-cell heterogeneity in FRAP kinetics is observed even in apparently homogeneous populations of cells, therefore analyzing many cells per condition is pivotal for robust conclusions. Cell-to-cell heterogeneity due to technical reasons (levels of protein expression, cell size, size, shape and location of ROI, differences in bleaching depth, etc.) must be kept to a minimum, to allow insight into the underlying biological heterogeneity. Note that comparison to control cases analyzed in parallel is essential for robust biological conclusions. During a typical FRAP experimental therefore, hundreds of individual cells are analyzed. When modeling is employed to estimate underlying kinetic parameters (see Subheading 4.2), variations due to technical heterogeneity can be minimized, permitting comparisons between experiments and assessment of biological variations at the single-cell level.

12. Low quality curves due to technical artifacts (such as cell movement, excessive photobleaching, low signal to noise ratios, out of focus data-points etc.) need to be removed from the dataset prior to analysis. However care must be taken to ensure that curves are excluded for technical reasons which are apparent in the raw data, not because they differ from the majority of curves (as this would constitute cherry-picking of results).

13. The value of bleaching depth depends also on the recovery kinetics; proteins with high recovery rates (e.g., fast-diffusing proteins) will tend to have smaller bleaching depth than proteins with slower recovery (e.g., bound proteins), as they diffuse back into the bleaching region during the bleaching step. Although a bleaching depth of 0.9 is unrealistic for fast-diffusing proteins such as GFPnls, it must be ensured that a bleaching depth of at least 0.6 is reached. At the same time, the values of gap ratio are affected by the duration and intensity of the bleaching pulse as well as the relative size of the bleaching region with respect to the total region. Bleaching a relatively large area with respect to the total nucleus results in small values of gap ratio, affecting the observed recovery (*see* also **Notes 5** and **6** and Fig. 2).

14. If comparing across different datasets, the choices of normalization method and fitting equation must be kept constant across the analysis to avoid introducing bias to the resulting estimates.

15. To evaluate the fit, the values of R-square must be taken into consideration together with the residual plot. Values of R-square close to 1 suggest that a high degree of the variability in the data is captured, however the fitted equation might still miss a local part of the curve, most usually the first post-bleach points. When comparing between different fits, choose the one that has the higher value of R-square while at the same time no trend is apparent in the residual plot.

16. The Fit Mean functionality must be used with caution and only as a rough indication of the "mean cell" behavior. It must be stressed out that, since the average curve is artificial and not a real measurement, its use can in many cases be misleading (e.g., when two distinct populations of single cells exist) and has no physical meaning. At the same time, we note that computing quantitative estimates by fitting the mean curve does not coincide with fitting all single-cell curves and averaging the resulting estimates. Since FRAP is a single-cell method, we strongly suggest to use it for analyzing cell-to-cell heterogeneity of protein kinetics by closely studying not only the average values but also the variance and distribution of all singe-cell derived parameters.

17. The Batch analysis module of easyFRAP allows the simultaneous analysis of a number of FRAP experiments, organized in multiple folders. It has limited visualization capabilities but can be used for speed, if the analysis steps have already been visually inspected through the main easyFRAP GUI. Before analyzing your data with the Batch analysis tool, make sure that all experiments were performed under the same setup (e.g., time step, number of images before and after bleaching).

Acknowledgments

We thank the Advanced Light Microscopy Facility of the University of Patras for assistance with live-cell imaging experiments and all members of the Cell Cycle and Stem Cell labs, Medical School, University of Patras for helpful discussions.

Work in our lab is supported by a grant from the European Research Council (DYNACOM, 281851).

Appendix

Let $y(t)_{ROI1}$, $y(t)_{ROI2}$, and $y(t)_{ROI3}$ represent the fluorescence intensity in the bleaching region, the total area of fluorescence, and a random background area. Background correction is performed by simply subtracting the background measurements from the rest:

$$y(t)_{ROI1*} = y(t)_{ROI1} - y(t)_{ROI3}$$
$$y(t)_{ROI2*} = y(t)_{ROI2} - y(t)_{ROI3}$$

Let y_{ROI1}^{pre} denote the average intensity in the bleaching region during the pre-bleach interval and $t_{bleach+1}$ denote the first time point after the bleach. Bleaching depth (bd) is computed as follows:

$$bd = \frac{y_{ROI1}^{pre} - y(t_{bleach+1})_{ROI1*}}{y_{ROI1}^{pre}} \tag{1}$$

Similarly, let $y_{ROI2}^{pre}, y_{ROI2}^{post}$ denote the average intensities in the total area of fluorescence during the pre- and post-bleach interval respectively. Gap ratio (gr) is computed as follows:

$$gr = \frac{y_{ROI2}^{post}}{y_{ROI2}^{pre}} \tag{2}$$

Double normalization is computed as follows:

$$y(t)_{double} = \frac{y(t)_{ROI1*}}{y_{ROI1}^{pre}} \times \frac{y_{ROI2}^{pre}}{y(t)_{ROI2*}} \tag{3}$$

Similarly, full-scale normalization is computed as follows:

$$y(t)_{\text{fullscale}} = \frac{y(t)_{\text{double}} - y(t_{\text{bleach}+1})_{\text{double}}}{1 - y(t_{\text{bleach}+1})_{\text{double}}} \tag{4}$$

To compute quantitative parameters such as t-half ($t_{1/2}$) and mobile fraction (*Fmob*), only the post-bleach part of the curve is necessary. Dropping normalization index for simplicity, let $y(t_{\text{end}})$ denote the normalized intensity (double or full-scale) when the curve has reached its plateau and $y(t_{\text{bleach}+1})$ denote the first post-bleach measurement. To remove the pre-bleach part of the curve from the measurements, we simply subtract $t_{\text{bleach}+1}$ from the rest of the time points, leading to $y(t_{\text{bleach}+1}) = y(t=0)$. It is:

$$F_{mob} = \frac{y(t_{end}) - y(t=0)}{1 - y(t=0)} \tag{5}$$

Immobile fraction (F_{imm}) is defined as the fraction of bleached molecules that were bound and do not diffuse away from the bleaching area by the end of the experiment. It is:

$$F_{imm} = \frac{1 - y(t_{end})}{1 - y(t=0)} \tag{6}$$

Naturally, $F_{\text{mob}} + F_{\text{imm}} = 1$. It is clear that for curves that exhibit full recovery, $y(t_{\text{end}}) = 1$, leading to $F_{\text{imm}} = 0$ and $F_{\text{imm}} = 1$.

The value of $t_{1/2}$ is computed as follows:

$$y(t_{1/2}) = \frac{y(t_{end}) + y(t=0)}{2} \tag{7}$$

To estimate the values of these parameters, the experimental data are fitted to one of the following exponential equations:

$$y(t)_{\text{single}} = y_0 - \alpha e^{-\beta t} \tag{8}$$

$$y(t)_{\text{double}} = y_0 - \alpha e^{-\beta t} - \gamma e^{-\delta t} \tag{9}$$

If full-scale normalization was used, then it is: $y(t=0) = 0$ and from Eq. (5) it is $F_{\text{mob}} = y(t_{\text{end}}) = y_0$, since for both Eqs. (8) and (9) as $t \to \infty$, $y(t_{\text{end}}) = y_0$. For double normalization, we have:

1. Using single exponential fitting (Eq. (8)) it is $y(t=0)_{\text{single}} = y_0 - a$, and from Eq. (5) it is:

$$F_{mob} = \frac{y_0 - y_0 + a}{1 - y_0 + a} = \frac{a}{1 - y_0 + a}$$

2. Using double exponential fitting (Eq. (9)) it is $y(t=0)_{\text{double}} = y_0 - a - \gamma$, and again from Eq. (5) it is:

$$F_{mob} = \frac{y_0 - y_0 + a + \gamma}{1 - y_0 + a + \gamma} = \frac{a + \gamma}{1 - y_0 + a + \gamma}$$

The value of $t_{1/2}$ is estimated from Eq. (7) as follows:

1. Using single exponential fitting and since similarly as above $y(t=0)_{single} = y_0 - a$

$$\frac{y_0 + y_0 - a}{2} = y_0 - \alpha e^{-\beta t_{1/2}}$$

$$e^{-\beta t_{1/2}} = \frac{1}{2}$$

$$t_{1/2} = \frac{\ln 2}{\beta}$$

2. Using a double exponential fitting equation, the value of $t_{1/2}$ is estimated numerically, since there is no closed form solution.

References

1. Lippincott-Schwartz J, Patterson GH (2003) Development and use of fluorescent protein markers in living cells. Science 300(5616): 87–91

2. Reits EAJ, Neefjes JJ (2001) From fixed to FRAP: measuring protein mobility and activity in living cells. Nat Cell Biol 3(6):145–145

3. White J, Stelzer E (1999) Photobleaching GFP reveals protein dynamics inside live cells. Trends Cell Biol 9(2):61–65

4. Phair RD, Misteli T (2001) Kinetic modelling approaches to in vivo imaging. Nat Rev Mol Cell Biol 2(12):898–907

5. Bancaud A, Huet S, Rabut G et al (2010) Fluorescence perturbation techniques to study mobility and molecular dynamics of proteins in live cells: FRAP, photoactivation, photoconversion, and FLIP. Cold Spring Harb Protoc 2010(12):pdb.top90

6. Beaudouin J, Mommer MS, Bock HG et al (2013) Experiment setups and parameter estimation in fluorescence recovery after photobleaching experiments: a review of current practice. In: Bock H G, Carraro T, Jäger W et al (eds) Model based parameter estimation. Springer, Berlin Heidelberg

7. Rapsomaniki MA, Kotsantis P, Symeonidou IE et al (2012) easyFRAP: an interactive, easy-to-use tool for qualitative and quantitative analysis of FRAP data. Bioinformatics 28(13):1800–1801

8. Phair RD, Gorski SA, Misteli T (2003) Measurement of dynamic protein binding to chromatin in vivo, using photobleaching microscopy. Methods Enzymol 37:393–414

9. Ellenberg J (1997) Nuclear membrane dynamics and reassembly in living cells: targeting of an inner nuclear membrane protein in interphase and mitosis. J Cell Biol 138(6):1193–1206

10. Mueller F, Mazza D, Stasevich TJ et al (2010) FRAP and kinetic modeling in the analysis of nuclear protein dynamics: what do we really know? Curr Opin Cell Biol 22(3):403–411

11. Sprague BL, McNally JG (2005) FRAP analysis of binding: proper and fitting. Trends Cell Biol 15(2):84–91

12. Carrero G, McDonald D, Crawford E et al (2003) Using FRAP and mathematical modeling to determine the in vivo kinetics of nuclear proteins. Methods 29(1):14–28

13. Beaudouin J, Mora-Bermúdez F, Klee T et al (2006) Dissecting the contribution of diffusion and interactions to the mobility of nuclear proteins. Biophys J 90(6):1878–1894

14. Sprague BL, Pego RL, Stavreva DA et al (2004) Analysis of binding reactions by fluorescence recovery after photobleaching. Biophys J 86(6):3473–3495

15. Royen ME, Farla P, Mattern KA et al (2012) Fluorescence recovery after photobleaching (FRAP) to study nuclear protein dynamics in living cells. In: Hancock R (ed) The nucleus: chromatin, transcription, envelope, proteins, dynamics, and imaging, vol 2. Humana Press, New York, pp 2363–2385

16. Schaff JC, Cowan AE, Loew LM, Moraru II (2009) Virtual FRAP - an experiment-oriented simulation tool. Biophys J 96(3 Supplement 1):30

17. Cinquemani E, Roukos V, Lygerou Z, and Lygeros J (2008) Numerical analysis of FRAP experiments for DNA replication and repair. Proceedings of the 47th IEEE conference on decision and control. Cancun, Mexico pp. 155–160

18. Farla P, Hersmus R, Geverts B, Mari PO, Nigg AL, Dubbink HJ, Trapman J, Houtsmuller AB

(2004) The androgen receptor ligand-binding domain stabilizes DNA binding in living cells. J Struct Biol 147(1):50–61

19. Geverts B, van Royen ME, Houtsmuller AB (2015) Analysis of biomolecular dynamics by FRAP and Computer Simulation. In: PJ V (ed) Advanced Fluorescence Microscopy, vol 1251. Springer, New York, pp 109–133

20. Rapsomaniki MA, Cinquemani E, Giakoumakis NN et al (2015) Inference of protein kinetics by stochastic modeling and simulation of fluorescence recovery after photobleaching experiments. Bioinformatics 31(3):355–362

21. Mazza D, Abernathy A, Golob N et al (2012) A benchmark for chromatin binding measurements in live cells. Nucleic Acids Res 40(15):e119 p. gks70

22. Cole R (2014) Live-cell imaging: The cell's perspective. Cell Adh Migr 8(5):452–459

23. Hagen GM, Caarls W, Lidke KA et al (2009) FRAP and photoconversion in multiple arbitrary regions of interest using a programmable array microscope (PAM). Microsc Res Tech 72(6):431

24. Xouri G, Squire A, Dimaki M et al (2007) Cdt1 associates dynamically with chromatin throughout G1 and recruits geminin onto chromatin. EMBO J 26(5):1303–1314

25. Roukos V, Kinkhabwala A, Colombelli J et al (2011) Dynamic recruitment of licensing factor Cdt1 to sites of DNA damage. J Cell Sci 124(3):422–434

26. Symeonidou IE, Kotsantis P, Roukos V et al (2013) Multi-step loading of human minichromosome maintenance proteins in live human cells. J Biol Chem 288(50):35852–35867

27. Kourti M, Ikonomou G, Giakoumakis NN et al (2015) CK1δ restrains lipin-1 induction, lipid droplet formation and cell proliferation under hypoxia by reducing HIF-1α/ARNT complex formation. Cell Signal 27(6):129–1140

28. Rapsomaniki MA (2014) Applications of stochastic hybrid models in biological systems. University of Patras, Doctoral dissertation

29. Halavatyi A (2008) Mathematical model and software FRAPAnalyser for analysis of actin-cytoskeleton dynamics with FRAP experiments, in Proceedings of FEBS/ECF workshop. Potsdam, Germany

30. Kota M (2011) Analysis of FRAP curves, online available via EMBL: http://cmci.embl.de/documents/frapmanu. Accessed 05 May 2011

31. Vakaloglou KM, Chrysanthis G, Rapsomaniki MA et al (2016) IPP complex reinforces adhesion by relaying tension-dependent signals to inhibit integrin turnover. Cell Rep 14(11):2668–2682

32. Soumpasis DM (1983) Theoretical analysis of fluorescence photobleaching recovery experiments. Biophys J 41(1):95–97

33. Axelrod D, Koppel DE, Schlessinger J et al (1976) Mobility measurement by analysis of fluorescence photobleaching recovery kinetics. Biophys J 16(9):1055–1069

34. Frigault MM, Lacoste J, Swift JL, Brown CM (2009) Live-cell microscopy–tips and tools. J Cell Sci 122(6):753–767

35. Dickson RM, Cubitt AB et al (1997) On/off blinking and switching behaviour of single molecules of green fluorescent protein. Nature 388(6640):355–358

Chapter 17

Fluorescence-Based High-Throughput and Targeted Image Acquisition and Analysis for Phenotypic Screening

Manuel Gunkel, Jan Philipp Eberle, and Holger Erfle

Abstract

Applying the right acquisition method in a fluorescence imaging-based screening context is of great importance to obtain an appropriate readout and to select the right scale of the screen. In order to save imaging time and data, we have developed routines for multiscale targeted imaging, providing both a broad overview of a sample and additional in-depth information for targets of interest identified within the screen. These objects can be identified and acquired on-the-fly by an interconnection of image acquisition and image analysis.

Key words High-throughput screening, High content screening, Targeted imaging, Automated imaging, KNIME

1 Introduction

Microscopic image acquisition is a crucial step in high-throughput or high content screening experiments [1, 2]. In most cases, a compromise has to be found between duration of the screen and quality and quantity of the data, especially if the scope of the screen comprises thousands of conditions or multiple cell lines or specimen to be tested. In some cases, it is sufficient to get a broad and fast overview for each condition to quantify the desired readout (Fig. 1). In other cases in-depth insight for instance in structural conformations or colocalization information is needed. For both cases appropriate image acquisition routines are presented here.

In-depth information can only be obtained by increasing the sample rate in one or more of the five classical image dimensions (X, Y, Z, time, color), leading in the same extent to prolonged acquisition durations. Preferably, this higher sampling is only performed at regions of interest to save acquisition time, to avoid acquisition of unusable data, and to preserve the microscopic equipment (light sources, mechanical components) as long as possible.

We have developed imaging routines that enable the fast scanning of a specimen or cell plate with a low sampling rate and switch

Yolanda Markaki and Hartmann Harz (eds.), *Light Microscopy: Methods and Protocols*, Methods in Molecular Biology, vol. 1563, DOI 10.1007/978-1-4939-6810-7_17, © Springer Science+Business Media LLC 2017

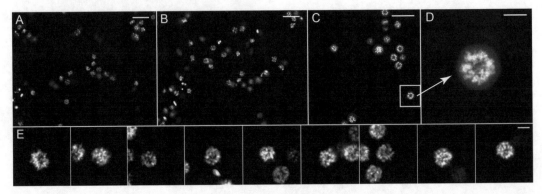

Fig. 1 Comparison of different acquisition modi. Phenotypic HeLa cell nuclei arrested in prometaphase upon siRNA induced knockdown of KIF11 acquired with wide field (**a**), spinning disc confocal (**b**), and point scanning confocal microscopy (**c**). Scale bars are 50 μm each. Based on the image in **c**, 3D acquisition of phenotypic nuclei is triggered (as marked by the *white* selection). A maximum-projection of this is shown in (**d**), the scale bar represents 10 μm. In (**e**), further examples of identified and acquired phenotypic cells are shown. The scalabar represents 10 μm

to a higher sampling rate if needed. The decision can be made by an experimenter or by image processing after a first screen and identified spots can be relocalized and acquired with appropriate parameters in a secondary screen [3, 4].

Alternatively, a decision-making progress based on direct analysis of the gathered images can also be integrated directly into the acquisition routine by automatic image processing [5] and feedback to the microscope [6, 7].

Here, these routines were implemented using the open source data analytics and integration platform KNIME (www.knime.org) that enables a modular implementation of processes and workflows. Existing image processing plugins (KNIME image processing, KNIP) were used as well as specially developed nodes for microscope control (*see* Fig. 2) to generate these workflows.

By using these software tools it is possible to obtain a broad overview of the experiment on the one hand and in-depth information of specific objects of interest on the other. Since the image processing can be adapted to the need of the experiment, this technique can be used for a broad set of applications in a screening context. Possible use cases are the switch from low to high resolution, acquisition of additional colors or z-planes upon detection of rare phenotypes or in case of sparse sample distribution to prevent unnecessary data acquisition. In live-cell experiments higher temporal sampling upon detection of an interesting event can be triggered or selective photoactivation performed.

We have implemented these tools to identify nuclei for colocalization studies similar to [8] and image them at higher resolution (Fig. 3). The switch from low to high resolution hereby happened

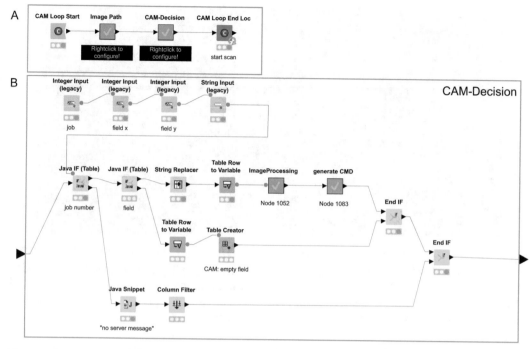

Fig. 2 KNIME workflow for targeted imaging. Image processing and decision making is embedded into a loop structure providing feedback to the microscope (**a**). The decision whether to trigger a CAM event or not is split into an image processing part and a generation of the actual CAM command (**b**)

on-the-fly, as soon as one low-resolution image was recorded, it was analyzed for potential targets by image processing. The coordinates of these targets were fed back to the microscope and high-resolution imaging restricted to these regions of interest (ROIs) was started. We were able to speed up the acquisition time tenfold compared to screening the same area at high resolution and afterward picking the targets by image processing.

2   Materials

2.1   Samples

Various different sample plates and formats exist suitable for screening experiments and accordingly preconfigured layout files for different microscope systems are readily available. Most screening microscopes are additionally configurable to define and use individual plate schemes. As widespread screening plates, microtiter or micro-well plates carrying usually 6, 24, 96, 384, or 1536 individual cavities have been established and standardized by the Society for Biomolecular Sciences (SBS). Alternatively, cell arrays consisting of a single cavity comprising multiple locally different conditions are used for screening experiments. An exemplary protocol for the preparation of siRNA plates is given in [9, 10].

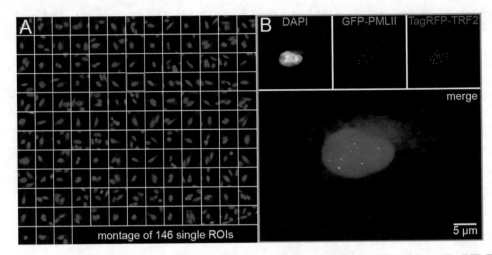

Fig. 3 Example for targeted imaging. 146 individualHeLa cells stained with DAPI, GFP-PMLII, and TagRFP-TRF2 which have been identified in a pre-screen are addressed and imaged at higher resolution in a secondary screen on a Leica SP5 confocal microscope implementing feedback to image processing routines via the CAM interface (**a**). One individual cell of this secondary screen is presented in (**b**), in top row the individual color channels are presented in grayscale values, a color merge is shown below

2.2 Microscopes

Multiple microscope systems are capable of performing screening experiments. A minimum prerequisite is a full automation of excitation settings, sample movement, and image acquisition in combination with suitable autofocusing routines. A comparison of images acquired with different microscope systems is shown in Fig. 1. In the following, a short and non-excluding listing of different types of microscopes suitable for screening experiments is given.

2.2.1 Wide-Field Screening Microscope

Olympus IX81 ScanR screening microscope, 10×, 20× and 40× magnification air and 40× and 60× oil immersion objectives, mercury arc lamp illumination, DAPI, CFP, GFP, YFP, Cy3, Cy5 and triple DAPI, FITC and TexasRed filter sets (triple set with additional excitation filters in the lamp), stage insert for object slides or SBS plates, two-step gradient-based software autofocusing routine.

2.2.2 Spinning Disc Screening Microscope

Perkin Elmer Opera LX spinning disc microscope, 20× and 60× magnification water immersion objectives, 488 nm, 561 nm and 647 nm laser illumination with appropriate filters, additional wide-field UV illumination and separate detection, reflection-based hardware autofocusing.

2.2.3 Point Scanning Confocal Microscope

Leica TCS SP5 point scanning confocal microscope with additional MatrixScreener software, 20× and 40× magnification air and 40× and 63× oil immersion objectives, 405, 458, 476, 488, 496, 514, 561, 594, and 633 nm laser wavelengths, stage insert for object slides and SBS plates, software-based generation of an interpolated focus lookup table prior to screening.

2.3 Image Analysis and Microscope Feedback

For image and metadata processing the open source platform KNIME (www.knime.org) is used, additionally the KNIME image processing plugins (KNIP) and microscope feedback nodes (own development) are installed. Within this software, data and image processing steps like background subtraction, thresholding, connected component analysis, and feature extraction can be performed to identify phenotypic cells by interconnecting appropriate data processing and data handling nodes to complete workflows (Fig. 2). These individual steps are represented as single nodes within the workflow. They can be configured individually and interconnected to be executed subsequently on the images to build whole analysis pipelines. Interactive microscope feedback is provided by the Leica CAM loop nodes that connect to the MatrixScreener and are able to communicate in both ways, and thus query the state of the microscope, retrieve acquired images, and send commands back to the microscope to interfere with the ongoing screen.

3 Methods

Depending on scope of the screen and microscope accessibility, different systems for image acquisition can be chosen, adjusted to the desired readout. Microscopic systems vary in terms of possible lateral and axial resolution, available color channels, sensitivity, live-sell capability, imaging speed, or interactivity. Image acquisition is described here for three different scanning systems, an automated wide-field system (Olympus ScanR), a spinning disc confocal high content screening system (Perkin Elmer Opera), and a point scanning confocal system with direct image processing feedback (Leica TCS SP5 with MatrixScreener). Analysis of the images for quantification as well as for microscope feedback is performed using KNIME.

3.1 Wide-Field Microscopy Image Acquisition

Wide-field imaging allows for high imaging speeds and thus can provide a broad overview over a large set of samples. It is the method of choice for cellular monolayers or thin samples where no additional axial resolution or high lateral resolution is needed. Live cell experiments also with large sample sizes are possible due to the fast acquisition process.

1. Initialize the system.
2. Select the appropriate plate type (*see* **Note 1**).
3. Put the plate in the stage insert, the A1 well at the top left position.
4. Calibrate the position of A1 by marking two opposite corners of the well. If no fluorescence stain is present in A1, use the transmission light configuration of the microscope.

5. Select the 20× objective and the filters matching the staining and adjust the acquisition time and the excitation intensity (*see* **Note 2**). Check whether your settings are appropriate for multiple wells, especially for control wells where possibly high or low fluorescence intensities are expected.

6. Set the software autofocus routine. Specify a coarse range matching the expected well-to-well differences of the plate. 100 μm range with 7 mm step size is sufficient for many types of available screening plates. The fine range should cover roughly two steps of the coarse autofocus scan, a step size of 0.8 μm is appropriate for the 20× objective used. Binning of the camera can be set to 4×4, thus acquisition time per image can be decreased (*see* **Note 3**).

7. Specify the wells of the plate which are to be imaged and the number and arrangement of acquisitions within each well. Nine images arranged in a 3×3 matrix spread over the well provide a good balance between the duration of the acquisition and the images needed for the analysis.

8. Specify the path where the images are to be stored and the name of the plate.

9. Start the screen.

3.2 Spinning Disc Microscope Image Acquisition

Spinning disc microscopy also allows fast imaging speeds and provides similar advantages as wide-field imaging. It can be considered intermediate between wide-field and point-scanning confocal.

1. Initialize the system.

2. Select (if not available: specify) the appropriate plate type.

3. Select the 20× water immersion objective.

4. Put the plate in the holder, A1 at the top left position.

5. For the plate layout, specify which wells should be imaged (*see* **Note4**).

6. Define the sub-layout, which positions in each well should be acquired. If needed, an overlap between adjacent fields can be specified in percent.

7. Set the exposure parameters. For each color channel, a different exposure and binning can be chosen. It is recommended to keep the camera binning consistent to the same value for all channels. In spinning-disc microscopy, only exposure times of a multiple of the disc revolution time, in this case 40 ms, can be chosen. Within the exposure settings, also an offset from the upper plate bottom can be chosen. This offset represents also the reference plane if an image stack should be acquired. (*see* **Note 5**).

8. Define an image stack. Based on the height of the sample and the axial sampling rate, the number of image planes acquired below and above the reference plane can be specified.

9. Compose plate layout, sub-layout, stack, and exposure definitions with an existing reference file into an experiment.

10. Name the plate according to your experiment.

11. Start the screen.

3.3   Point Scanning Confocal Microscope (Targeted) Image Acquisition

Point scanning microscopy offers a great degree of freedom in image acquisition, since also parameters like pixel size, scan speed, field of view, etc. can be configured and adapted to the job at hand. Usually, it is slower, but offers high lateral and axial resolution. The CAM interface integrated into the MatrixScreener of the Leica SP5 confocal used here offers additional possibilities to interfere with the screen. In these cases, the necessary steps are labeled as CAM-only.

1. Initialize the system.

2. Turn on the lasers needed.

3. Start the MatrixScreener module.

4. Specify the path where the images will be saved.

5. Define the plate layout (*see* **Notes 1** and **4**). Start coordinates and distances can also be taught within the software by moving the plate to appropriate positions and click "learn".

6. Create a new confocal imaging job and define it as autofocus job for the color channel the focusing should be performed (*see* **Note 6**).

7. Define a job for confocal screening. In order to identify phenotypic cells, an image size of 2048 × 2048 pixel at 120 nm pixel size, covering a field of view of 245 × 245 μm [2] can be chosen (*see* Fig. 1c). See also **Note 7**.

8. CAM-only: If targeted imaging applying the CAM-interface is performed, define a job for target acquisition. Identified phenotypic cells as shown in Fig. 1are imaged in 3D with 49 planes at 0.5 μm spacing and 512 × 512 pixel at 96 nm pixel size.

9. CAM-only: Create a pattern comprising the prescreen job and a subsequent wait command to synchronize image acquisition and analysis.

10. Specify the wells you want to acquire by assigning the specified jobs or patterns to them.

11. CAM-only: Activate the CAM interface.

12. Define the autofocus pattern. Depending on the flatness of the used plates, a dense or wide pattern can be chosen. Z-positions of fields not part of the autofocus pattern are interpolated (*see* **Note 8**).

13. Create the focus map.

14. non-CAM: start the screen.

15. CAM-only: Open the microscope feedback workflow within KNIME.

16. CAM-only: In the Cam-loop Start node, specify the same path as in **step 4**.

17. CAM-only: Specify the job with which identified objects should be acquired (job of **step 8**) (*see* **Note 9**).

18. CAM-only: Run the workflow, which starts and controls the screen automatically.

3.4 *Image Analysis*

Image processing is performed to identify individual objects and to classify them based on morphological (like size or shape) and textural (like intensity or intensity distribution) features of these objects. All necessary steps are available as nodes in KNIME by the KNIP image processing repository. Depending on the task at hand, alternative or additional steps might be applied.

Image processing usually consists of several steps performed subsequently and based on one another:

Preprocessing of the images:

In order to prepare the images for further analysis, it is often necessary to process them to retrieve a good (reliably detectable) contrast between objects of interest and background of the images. Gradients in background intensities can be leveled by background subtraction. Noisy images can be smoothed by Gaussian filtering or other filters like variance or median filters can be applied to enhance or suppress specific regions of the images.

Separating signal from background:

In order to identify objects from background, global or local thresholding methods based on the distribution of the grayscale values can be applied to transform the images to binary images. This can also be achieved by watersheding of the images.

Identifying individual objects:

By determining connected areas within these binary images, individual objects can be identified and given unique IDs, in most cases consecutive numbers starting with 1 for each image. Usually, the type of connection can be specified, in 2D images 8 adjacent pixels for each pixel or 4 adjacent pixels (top, bottom, left, and right).

Adapting the objects:

By morphological operations like opening, closing, eroding, or dilating, holes in the segmentation can be closed, the regions extended or shrinked and small objects consisting of one or few pixels excluded. By Voronoy segmentation, the resulting image space can be divided evenly between the identified objects to get an estimate for the area of influence for each object.

Feature extraction:

Within each obtained segment of the image, features like Tamura features (granularity, contrast, kurtosis of directionality, standard deviation of directionality, maximal directionality, skewness), segment geometry (size, perimeter, centroid, circularity, convexity, diameter,…), first-order statistics (min, max, mean, geometric mean, sum, square of sums, standard deviation, variance, skewness, kurtosis, quantil25, quantil50, quantil75, user defined quantil, and histogram) and Haralik features (statistical features based on gray-level co-occurrence matrix) can be retrieved to further determine and classify each object.

The image processing workflow depicted here is implemented to identify phenotypic cells in the images and should be adapted for each analysis.

1. Load the images. The folder containing the image data is specified as well as the data format of the images.

2. Perform background subtraction.

3. Smooth the images by Gaussian convolution.

4. Threshold the images locally.

5. Segment individual objects by connected component analysis.

6. Calculate the features for each object.

7. Apply filters based on the retrieved features.

8. Match the data with appropriate metadata (plate, well number, treatment etc.).

3.5 Microscope Feedback

In order to select only structures of interest for targeted microscopy with improved resolution and additional 3D information, the workflow for identification of phenotypic cells from Subheading 3.4 can be embedded in a microscope feedback structure (Fig. 2a). By this, structures of interest are directly identified during the screen, their positions are given back to the microscope and images with higher content are acquired directly.

1. The CAM Loop Start and CAM Loop end nodes provide a feedback loop between microscopic image acquisition and image processing. The output of the CAM server, which provides information about the status of the screen and locations of the recently acquired images, is constantly checked. If commands for the imaging procedure—typically locations of structures of interest—are generated during image processing, these are transferred back to the CAM server (*see* **Note 10**).

2. Image processing should be set up according to Subheading 3.4 to process all images of one well once the whole well is completely imaged (field filter in Fig. 2b) (*see* **Note 11**). Only images

with the job-number of the acquisition job are considered for image processing (job filter in Fig. 2b), additionally stored images from autofocus jobs or drift-correction jobs are filtered out and not considered for image processing. Thus, structures of interest are identified automatically and their coordinates determined within the image and—together with the image metadata providing stage position information—on the microscope.

3. These coordinates are fed back to the microscope as a string embedded in a CAM syntax. These structures are then imaged subsequently with the specified imaging job (*see* Subheading3.3, **step 8**).

4. The next well is acquired as specified within the MatrixScreener.

5. Once all wells are imaged, the CAM-loop also ends.

4   Notes

1. If your plate type is not available, please check the data sheet and information of the manufacturer. Well-to-well distance in x- and y direction, shape, and dimensions of the wells as well as thickness of the plate bottom need to be specified.

2. Fluorescence signals should be well above background but not higher than 75 % of the maximum count rate of the camera. For the camera used the brightest signals should not exceed 3000 counts.

3. Since the autofocusing routine is based on the gradient of the images, please make sure that the signals are well above background noise level, but also not oversaturated compared to **Note 2**.

4. Different groups of wells can be imaged using different sublayouts and exposure settings. If applied, these need to be specified separately.

5. Focusing is performed by a laser-based hardware autofocus, 0 μm represents the surface of the wellplate.

6. This job does not need to have the resolution and speed of the later imaging jobs, it can be set more coarse and faster, but the observed objects should still give a good contrast.

7. Imaging of one well took 39 s on the Olympus wide-field microscope with software autofocusing, 12 s on the Perkin-Elmer spinning disk system with hardware autofocusing, and 15 min on the Leica point scanning microscope, including 3D imaging of 10 phenotypic cells at high resolution.
   Acquisition of one 3D stack took 84 s.

8. If z-drift due to long or repetitive imaging is expected, additional points for drift-correction can be specified. After each drift-correction, all reference points are shifted accordingly.

9. Take care to provide the number of the job, not the name.

10. In order to keep image acquisition and image processing synchronized, a "Wait for Cam" job is inserted in the acquisition routine. This can be omitted, but might lead to unwanted sample movement, since the image acquisition then runs on a "first-come, first-served" basis switching between primary and secondary screen.

11. The image processing workflow should be tested with a set of data containing potential targets acquired similar to Subheading 3.3, **step 7**.

Acknowledgment

The authors wish to thank Michael Berthold and the KNIME/KNIP developers for their help with the development of the KNIME nodes and workflows. This work was funded within the project CancerTelSys (grant number 01ZX1302) in the e:Med program, the project HD-HuB (grant number 031A537C) in the de.NBI program and within the project RNA-Code (grant number 031A298) in the e:Bio program, all of the German Federal Ministry of Education and Research (BMBF). The ViroQuant-CellNetworks RNAi Screening Facility was also supported by the CellNetworks-Cluster of Excellence (grant number EXC81).

References

1. Neumann B, Held M, Liebel U, Erfle H, Rogers P, Pepperkok R, Ellenberg J (2006) High-throughput RNAi screening by time-lapse imaging of live human cells. Nat Methods 3(5):385–390. doi:10.1038/nmeth876

2. Neumann B, Walter T, Hériché J-K, Bulkescher J, Erfle H, Conrad C, Rogers P, Poser I, Held M, Liebel U, Cetin C, Sieckmann F, Pau G, Kabbe R, Wünsche A, Satagopam V, Schmitz MHA, Chapuis C, Gerlich DW, Schneider R, Eils R, Huber W, Peters J-M, Hyman AA, Durbin R, Pepperkok R, Ellenberg J (2010) Phenotypic profiling of the human genome by time-lapse microscopy reveals cell division genes. Nature 464(7289):721–727. doi:10.1038/nature08869

3. Gunkel M, Flottmann B, Heilemann M, Reymann J, Erfle H (2014) Integrated and correlative high-throughput and super-resolution microscopy. Histochem Cell Biol 141(6):597–603. doi:10.1007/s00418-014-1209-y

4. Flottmann B, Gunkel M, Lisauskas T, Heilemann M, Starkuviene V, Reymann J, Erfle H (2013) Correlative light microscopy for high-content screening. Biotechniques 55(5):243–252. doi:10.2144/000114099

5. Eliceiri KW, Berthold MR, Goldberg IG, Ibanez L, Manjunath BS, Martone ME, Murphy RF, Peng H, Plant AL, Roysam B, Stuurman N, Swedlow JR, Tomancak P, Carpenter AE (2012) Biological imaging software tools. Nat Methods 9(7):697–710. doi:10.1038/nmeth.2084

6. Conrad C, Wünsche A, Tan TH, Bulkescher J, Sieckmann F, Verissimo F, Edelstein A, Walter T, Liebel U, Pepperkok R, Ellenberg J (2011) Micropilot: automation of fluorescence microscopy-based imaging for systems biology. Nat Methods 8(3):246–249. doi:10.1038/nmeth.1558

7. Tischer C, Hilsenstein V, Hanson K, Pepperkok R (2014) Adaptive fluorescence microscopy by online feedback image analysis. Methods Cell Biol 123:489–503. doi:10.1016/B978-0-12-420138-5.00026-4

8. Osterwald S, Wörz S, Reymann J, Sieckmann F, Rohr K, Erfle H, Rippe K (2011) A three-dimensional colocalization RNA interference screening platform to elucidate the alternative lengthening of telomeres pathway. Biotechnol J. doi:10.1002/biot.201000474

9. Gunkel M, Beil N, Beneke J, Reymann J, Erfle H (2015) Fluorescence microscopy-based RNA interference screening. Methods Mol Biol 1251:59–66. doi:10.1007/978-1-4939-2080-8_4

10. Erfle H, Neumann B, Liebel U, Rogers P, Held M, Walter T, Ellenberg J, Pepperkok R (2007) Reverse transfection on cell arrays for high content screening microscopy. Nat Protoc 2(2):392–399. doi:10.1038/nprot.2006.483

Index

A

Acceptor 12, 53, 54, 85–89
Action potentials (APs) 74
Aging..20, 229
Alzheimer...173
Amyloid plaque 43–45, 173
Anesthetize..43, 59, 60, 62, 63, 147
Antibody
    monoclonal 94
    primary 42, 103, 146, 148
    secondary.....................................94, 98, 99, 103, 144–146, 148
Artificial neural network (ANN)....................................258
Ascospores...19
Autofluorescence 81, 82, 253
Autofocus 159, 274, 275, 278
Autophagosome..24, 25, 27, 29, 30

B

Background 3, 4, 7, 78, 82, 97, 131, 140, 155, 156, 158, 161–163, 187, 193, 195, 197–199, 205, 212, 221, 223, 224, 226, 238, 240, 244, 245, 250, 252, 253, 259, 264, 273, 276–278
Batch processing....................................... 232, 234, 236–239
Biosensor.. 13, 53, 54, 85–88
Bleedthrough..87–89
Blocking buffer.. 146, 148
Brain slice... 83, 144–145, 149
Brain stem 37, 41

C

Calcium 54
    indicator
        Fluo-3..54
Calcofluor...94, 97–99
Camera
    CCD..139
    emCCD..154, 247
    sCMOS 75, 77, 247
Cell-cell interactions 51, 54
Cell chamber 87, 88
Cell culture 20, 96, 118, 152–154, 156–157, 246

Cell cycle reporter
    Fucci 52
    Histone 2B 52
Cells
    endocrine 151–163
    HeLa 119, 120, 272
    INS-1 ....155, 156, 158, 160, 162
    leukocytes 52
    neuronal..10, 13, 73, 74, 81
    PC12 156
    tumor..52, 53
Cell wall 91–104
Chromatic correction..117
Clearing method
    3DISCO 35, 36, 42
    BABB 35
    CLARITY..35
    CUBIC..35
    Scale 144
Collagen
    type I 52
Colocalization
    intensity correlation 191
    overlap 191
Contrast
    DIC 2, 139
    Laplacian filter...198
    phase contrast 2
    unsharp masking operator 198
Counting objects 189
Coverslip chamber.. 154, 157, 159, 160, 162, 163
Coverslip preparation 155, 156
    etch protocol...155
    plasma cleaning 140
    surface additives
        poly-D-lysine 155, 156
        poly-L-lysine 155, 156
CRISPR/Cas9..11
Cryosectioning 147
Cytoskeletal elements
    actin 108
    microtubules 108

Yolanda Markaki and Hartmann Harz (eds.), *Light Microscopy: Methods and Protocols*, Methods in Molecular Biology, vol. 1563,
DOI 10.1007/978-1-4939-6810-7, © Springer Science+Business Media LLC 2017

D

Danio 20
DAPI...140, 272
Deconvolution...3, 198
Dehydration 35, 40, 42, 46, 66, 67
Descriptors 8, 187, 189, 190
Diffraction......................... 1, 3–6, 11, 109, 129, 131,
143, 158, 160, 161, 169, 234
Diffusion 40–42, 157, 197, 245, 246,
251, 255, 257, 259–261
DNA breaks 108
Donor 12, 53, 54, 85–89
3D printing..22, 27, 28
3D reconstruction...............................33, 43–45
Drosophila..........................8, 41, 43, 108, 143–149
Dynamic range 20, 27, 159, 160, 202

E

Electrode 73, 76, 77, 81
Electrophysiology......................................73, 76, 81
Embryos
Drosophila.. 8, 108, 109
zebrafish 20, 109, 120, 121
Environmental chambers.....................................10
Evanescent field..152
Exocytosis..163
Explant 10, 55, 57, 59–60
Ex vivo intravital imaging..55

F

Feature
extraction..273, 277
tabulation...215, 220
visualization..215–222
Fiji....................... 23, 27, 29, 187, 204, 211, 212,
215, 222, 226, 262
Fixation 9, 35, 36, 39–42, 46, 48, 59,
92, 131, 146, 147, 149
Fluorescent beads 137, 157, 198
Fluorescent protein
Butterfly 75, 77, 79, 82
CFP.. 53, 86, 272
Dendra2.................................... 52, 130, 132, 136
Dronpa 135
eGFP 244, 248, 250
GFP.................................2, 11, 20, 23, 28, 35, 36, 40, 46,
119, 120, 154, 157, 230, 248, 272
Kaede...52
mCherry 154, 157, 248
mEOS3.2 132
mNeonGreen..................................... 132, 133, 135, 136
Padron 135
PAGFP...135
PAmCherry.. 132, 134–136, 139

photoconvertible 13, 52
PS-CFP2...136
PSmOrange2...136
TdTomato 144–145, 149
YFP 86, 248, 272
Fluorophore..131
blinking rate..131
live time 5, 10, 11
quantum yield
ratio 131
Fungi
filamentous 19–28

G

Gaussian fit
2D 230, 233, 237
3D 232, 233, 235, 237
single spot..234–236
Geodesic reconstruction 200
GRIN lenses..74

H

Hemicelluloses...91
High-throughput.....................................8, 269–279
Huygens's principle...1

I

Image analysis
colocalization...191
counting objects..189
Gaussian fit...239, 241
intensities.. 190, 195
particle tracking.......................................8, 210
quantitative.................. 103, 193, 200, 210, 245, 251–257
ratio 234
segmentation 7, 8, 191–194, 203
shapes 189–190, 195, 197
ImageJ 23, 86, 90, 161, 204, 211, 222, 231, 234, 240
Image processing 195, 197, 199
filter
morphological...195
noise.. 197, 199
localisation...130
normalization...254
Imaging chamber
cleaning 137, 139
Imaging window.............................53, 55, 58, 61, 63–65, 67
Immunolabeling
live-cell 96–99
Incubation chamber.. 76, 247, 248
In vivo intravital imaging
skin 55
Ionomycin... 154, 159

K

Kinetic 73, 161, 230, 264
KNIME 270, 271, 273, 276

L

Laser 115–118
   ablation 108, 119, 121, 122
   femtosecond pulses 114
   infrared 109
   pulsed 107, 109, 114, 117
   sanner
      calibration 115–118
   UV-A 111
LC3 .... 20, 23
Lectin 36, 38, 42–43
Lineage tracing 52, 53
Live-cell imaging 4–6, 9–11, 246, 247, 259
Living animal 51, 54
Localization 5, 12, 29, 30, 52,
      140, 144, 210
Low fluorescence medium 136
Low-melting point agarose 21, 24

M

MATLAB 75–77, 161, 230, 231, 240
Measuring positions
   center-of-mass 190
   centroid 190
   Euclidean distances 190
   radial analysis 190
Metamorph 161
Micropuncture 108, 121, 122
Microscope feedback 273, 276–278
Microscopy techniques 3, 12, 19, 51–67, 74,
      95, 109–112, 114, 121, 122, 130, 136, 138, 140,
      152–154, 157, 159, 160, 270, 272–276
   confocal
      point scanning 270, 272–276
      spinning disc 270, 273
   differential interference contrast (DIC) 2, 139
   electron microscopy
      variable pressure scanning 95
   fluorescence lifetime imaging (FLIM) 54
   fluorescence recovery after photobleaching
      (FRAP) 13, 111, 264
   Förster resonance energy transfer (FRET) 12, 13,
      53, 54, 77, 82, 85–90
   I^5 M microscopy 4
   intravital microscopy (IVM) 51, 54, 55
   lattice light sheet 6
   light sheet-based fluorescence microscopy
      (LSFM) 19
   multi-photon imaging 51–52, 54–56, 66
      second harmonic generation (SHG) 52, 53
      two-photon intravital microscopy
         (2P-IVM) 52, 54–56, 66
   phase contrast 2
   4Pi microscopy 4
   polarized light microscopy 2
   super-resolution imaging 4–7, 13, 110,
      114, 129–140, 144, 149
      FPALM 5
      multi-colour 136
      PALM 5, 7, 110, 114,
         129–140, 144
      STED 5, 6, 13, 149
      STORM 5, 7, 130, 144
      SIM 4, 5
   time-lapse 120, 210, 212, 244
   total internally reflected fluorescence
      (TIRF) 3, 12, 130, 136, 138, 140,
      152–154, 157, 159, 160
   ultramicroscopy 33–48
Micro-well plates 271
Migration 20, 51–53, 209
Modeling 7, 210, 246, 257, 261, 262
Morphological filters
   dilation 195, 198–200, 205
   erosion 195, 198, 205
   filling holes 195
   opening 195, 199, 200, 276
   skeletonization 197
Mouse
   brain 6, 33, 35, 37, 40, 41, 46,
      48, 75, 144, 173
   embryo 36, 38, 42
mRNA 51, 229
Mycelium 19, 20, 24, 25, 27

N

Nail polish 23, 147–149
Nanoscopy 5
Nanosurgery
   laser 110–115, 120
Nearest Neighbor 212, 214, 224
Neurons 2, 73, 74, 108,
      144–145, 149, 196
Noise 197, 276
   filter
      adaptive 197
      Gaussian 197
      linear 197
      median 276
      sigma 197
Normalization 190, 245, 250–252,
      254, 263–265
Nyquist-Shannon criterion 202

O

Objective lens 4, 5, 9, 21, 23, 25–27, 111, 114–117, 163, 169

Organic fluorescent dye 73

P

PaATG8 ....20, 23

Particle
    linking 210, 212, 214–215, 224
    tracking 210–215, 225

Patch clamp 73, 76

Pectin 91, 97, 101–103

Perfusion
    chamber 57, 59, 65

Photobleaching.............................. 10, 12, 20, 21, 52, 54, 89, 110, 119, 121, 157, 160, 202, 243–264

Phototoxicity 6, 9, 10, 21, 52, 60, 247, 249, 250, 261

Pixel...................................6–8, 74, 75, 83, 87, 121, 130, 161, 161, 162, 168, 174, 187, 189–198, 200, 202–205, 212–216, 220, 223, 225, 226, 231, 233, 235, 236, 240, 250, 259, 275, 276

Plant
    Green alga 91
    Penium margaritaceum 104

Plasma cleaning..140

Podospora anserina 19, 20, 28, 29

Point spread function (PSF) 129, 132–134, 171, 198, 201, 212, 213, 223, 231, 234, 236

Polymer 104

Polysaccharides..91

Proliferation...51–53

Protein-protein interaction...............................86

Q

Quantifying 189, 190, 201
    intensities...............................190
    shapes
        circularity...............................190
        ellipsis 189
        Fourier descriptors 190
        Shape Factor 190
        solidity 190, 201

Quantitative
    analysis........................ 193, 245, 251–257
    measurement................................ 99, 187, 201

R

Rab GTPases..151

Ratio..............................3, 4, 7, 27, 75, 81, 86–89, 132, 162, 202, 204, 207, 217–219, 224, 234, 245, 249, 253, 254, 261, 263, 264

Resolution
    Abbe's law..............................3, 5

Rayleigh criterion 129

Reversible switchable optical linear fluorescence transition (RESOLFT) 5, 6

RNA imaging...229

S

Sample holder.............................. 22–25, 147

Screening
    high content...............................269, 273
    high throughput 8, 279

Segmentation
    binarization...............................191–193
    edge detection...............................192, 193
    pixel classifcation 192–194
    watershed transform 193–194

Signal-to-noise ratio (SNR) 13, 224

Single-molecule..................... 12, 130, 132, 229

siRNA 270, 271

Skin...............................55, 58, 60–64, 66, 167, 174, 175

SNARE proteins
    SNAP-25...............................151
    Syntaxin1a 151
    VAMP 151, 156, 163

Snell's law 1

Software
    Fiji 23, 27, 29, 186, 187, 204, 211, 212, 215, 222, 226, 262
    ImageJ 23, 86, 90, 161, 204, 211, 222, 231, 234, 240
    KNIME................ 270, 271, 273, 276
    MATLAB 75–77, 161, 230, 231, 240
    STaQTool................... 230–233, 235–240

Spatial statistics
    clusters...............................191
    point pattern analysis.......................191
    random 191
    regular...............................191

Spot tracking 231–234

STaQTool...............................230–233, 235–240

Statistics 185, 191, 215, 225, 277

Stochastic 5, 130, 143, 197, 229, 257

Surface............... 4, 12, 25, 26, 43, 44, 74, 80, 92, 97, 99–103, 116, 118, 121, 140, 152, 155, 192–194, 233, 278

Surgery 55, 62–64, 67, 76, 107, 115, 122

Surgical exposure 55, 58, 61–63

T

Tagged image file format (TIFF) 160, 161, 222

TDE Mounting Medium................................ 146, 148, 149

Texture descriptors 187

Time-lapse 4, 8, 9, 20, 27, 99, 110, 119, 120, 210, 212, 230–238, 240, 241, 244, 261

Top-hat transform 198, 199
Tracking 8, 10, 191, 210, 212, 215, 221,
            225, 230–234, 236, 237, 262
Trajectory analysis 210, 212, 215–222
Transfection..11, 86, 87, 89, 156–157

V

Vesicle...151, 156–158, 160, 162, 163
    cargo marker
        chromogranin 156
        NPY-GFP 156–158, 160, 162
        phogrin 156

Rab 151, 156
    tissue plasminogen activator 156
    VAMP 151, 156, 163
dense-core.. 156, 158, 162
fusion 161, 162
Voltage indicator...73–83
Voxel.. 187, 189,
        195, 205

W

Whole-mount 36, 38, 42,
        144–145

Printed in the United States
By Bookmasters